# Medication-Related Osteonecrosis of the Jaws

Sven Otto

**Editor**

# Medication-Related Osteonecrosis of the Jaws

## Bisphosphonates, Denosumab, and New Agents

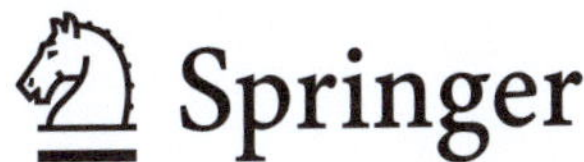 Springer

*Editor*
Sven Otto, MD, DMD, FEBOMFS
Department of Oral and
Maxillofacial Surgery
Ludwig-Maximilians-University
of Munich
Munich
Germany

ISBN 978-3-662-52433-6          ISBN 978-3-662-43733-9   (eBook)
DOI 10.1007/978-3-662-43733-9
Springer Heidelberg New York Dordrecht London



Printed on acid-free paper

Springer is part of Springer Science+Business Media (www.springer.com)

# Foreword

What began as a link between intravenous bisphosphonates in cancer patients and osteonecrosis of the jaw has greatly expanded to a definitive causation from two intravenous bisphosphonates as well as several oral bisphosphonates for osteoporosis patients and a RANK ligand inhibitor for either cancer patients or osteoporosis patients. Furthermore, the route of administration for the RANK ligand inhibitors is subcutaneous rather than intravenous or oral. Adding to the complexity of jaw osteonecrosis are more rare reports from drugs which inhibit the vascular endothelial growth factor and others which inhibit certain tyrosine kinase receptors as their main mechanism of action.

The textbook *Medication-Related Osteonecrosis of the Jaws: Bisphosphonates, Denosumab, and New Agents* by Sven Otto explores the science, pharmacodynamics, diagnosis, and treatment options in a complete and comprehensive manner. Each chapter contains extensive evidence-based as well as experience-based data designed to help the reader fully understand the nuances of this complex and interesting disease as well as how it can be managed and many times resolved.

Sven Otto himself has been one of the pioneers and leaders internationally that brought to clinicians a clearer understanding of this complex pathophysiology. Together with the experience and expertise of each chapter author, this text becomes a required read and one that serves as a reference that helps everyone in the treatment of osteonecrosis of the jaw.

As a recognized disease entity in the published literature, osteonecrosis of the jaw was unheard of prior to 2003. In just a few years, it has become a condition seen in nearly every dental office throughout the world. While this book thoroughly prepares the reader related to the current drugs causing osteonecrosis of the jaw, new targeted drugs are coming to the marketplace with similar and profound effects on normal cellular functions. Only the naïve would think we have seen the last of jaw osteonecrosis.

FL, USA                                                                     Robert E. Marx, DDS

# Contents

# Pharmacological Aspects of Antiresorptive Drugs: Bisphosphonates and Denosumab

**1**

Reiner Bartl and Emmo von Tresckow


**Abstract**

Bisphosphonates and denosumab are the most widely used classes of antiresorptive osteotrop drugs worldwide. They are used to treat a variety of bone disorders including osteoporosis, metastatic bone disease and hypercalcemia of malignancy. Bisphosphonates are administered either orally or intravenously, while denosumab is injected subcutaneously. While bisphosphonates are not metabolized and have a strong affinity to the bone and a very long half-life in the bone (months–years), denosumab is an antibody which is metabolized, not specifically stored, in the bone and has a short half-life (weeks). Both substance classes have strong inhibitory effects towards bone resorption and are therefore used for the treatment of osteoporosis and metastatic bone disease as well as other bone disorders with great success. Generally, bisphosphonates and denosumab are well tolerated and have few side effects. However, both substance classes of osteotrop antiresorptives have one side effect in common, namely, osteonecrosis of the jaw.


## Introduction

Bone fulfils two mechanical tasks: weight bearing and flexibility at the lowest possible weight. This is accomplished by the combination of an elastic matrix for flexibility hardened by the deposition of calcium and phosphate which gives bone its rigidity, while the highly developed architecture contributes to both. The macroscopic skeleton consists of two major components: compact or cortical bone and the cancellous or spongy bone [1] (Fig. 1.1).

Modeling is continuous during skeletal development, then it is greatly reduced and ceases completely after skeletal maturity, while remodeling takes place throughout life. Modeling results in changes in the shape and size of the bone, while remodeling maintains but usually does not change size and shape. It is carried out by two major bone cells: the osteoclasts which resorb the bone and the osteoblasts which form the bone [1]. Characteristic of active osteoclasts are their "ruffled borders" which lie directly on the surface of the bone. Howship's lacunae are formed as the osteoclasts carve out the bone [1].


R. Bartl
Ehrenfelsstrasse 5, 81375 Munich, Germany
e-mail: Reiner.Bartl@osteologie-online.de

E. von Tresckow (✉)
Rosenstrasse 2, 82319 Starnberg, Germany
e-mail: emmo.von_tresckow@bendalis.com



S. Otto (ed.), *Medication-Related Osteonecrosis of the Jaws: Bisphosphonates, Denosumab, and New Agents*,
DOI 10.1007/978-3-662-43733-9_1, © Springer-Verlag Berlin Heidelberg 2015

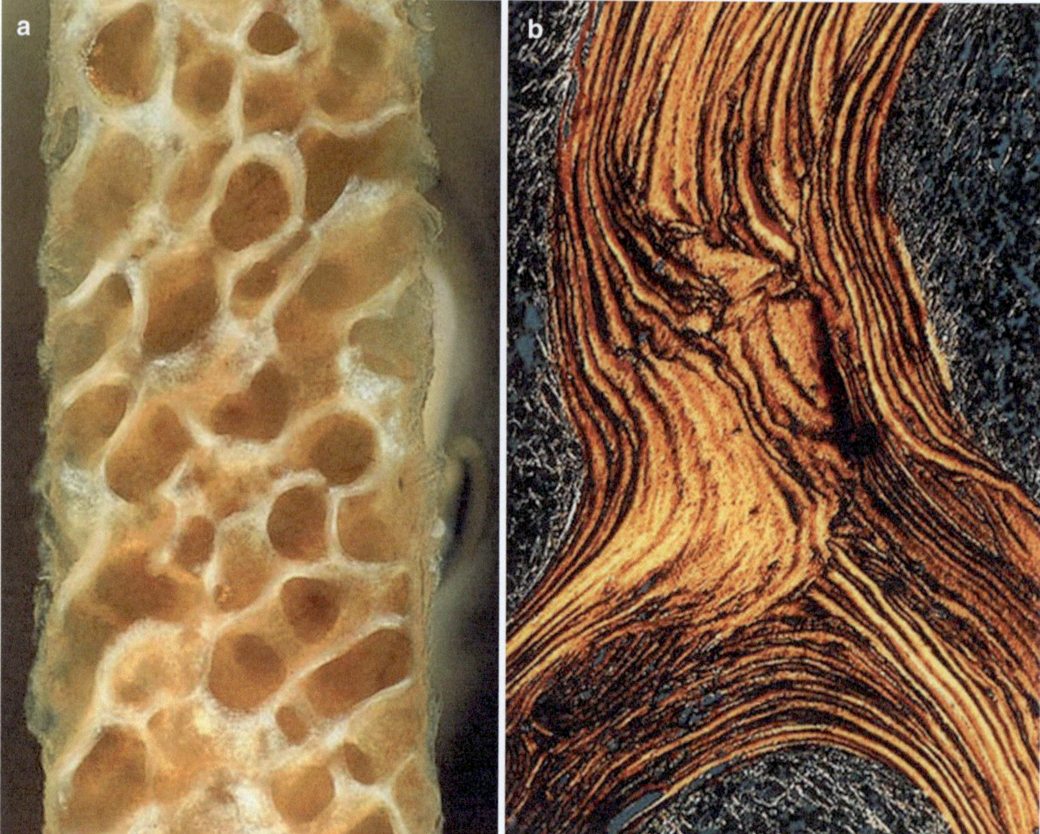

**Fig. 1.1** (**a**, **b**) Normal trabecular bone. (**a**) Cut surface of a bone biopsy showing trabecular network and intertrabecular spaces. Note the honeycomb-like arrangement of the interconnected horizontal and vertical trabeculae and the nodes connecting them. The density of these "nodes" ensures mechanical strength. (**b**) Trabecula consisting of parallel layers of collagen fibrils. These lamellae ensure flexibility of bone (Reprinted with kind permission of Springer Business and Media from [1])

Osteoblasts form an epithelial-like lining at the surface of the bone and are connected by gap junctions. They synthesize osteoid and the organic bone matrix and are responsible for its mineralization. When osteoblasts are embedded in the bone matrix, they become osteocytes. Osteocytes are essential for survival of the bone; if deficient osteocytes are not replaced, the involved bone cannot be maintained and a sequestrum is formed, rejected, and removed [1].

Hyperactive, abnormally activated osteoclasts are characterized by a higher resorptive capacity and therefore a high destructive potential, so that numerous osteoblasts need months to repair an osteolytic lesion accomplished by a few osteoclasts in a week [1]. Deregulation of osteoclasts is the main cause of nearly all osteopathies such as osteoporosis (systemic) or osteolysis (local), potentially accompanied by spontaneous fractures and hypercalcemia. Therefore, antiresorptive drugs such as bisphosphonates and denosumab which effectively reduce osteoclastic activity are of major clinical importance in the treatment of a variety of bone disorders especially osteoporosis and metastatic bone disease [1].

## Bisphosphonates

### Historical Review

The bisphosphonates constitute a group of pharmacological agents first synthesized in the 1880s but developed over the past 40 years for diagnosis and treatment of disorders of the bone and anomalies of calcium metabolism. The fundamental research carried out by H. Fleisch in the 1960s laid the ground work for the rapid development of the bisphosphonates in medicine [1–3].

*The starting point was provided by the natural pyrophosphates which have a central P-O-P binding.* Pyrophosphate was widely employed in industry due to its ability to dissolve calcium carbonate. Consequently, pyrophosphates were used in washing powders and other soapy solutions to inhibit scale formation. Interestingly, today they are also used worldwide in toothpaste to prevent and to reduce plaque formation. Due to its strong affinity for calcium phosphate and therefore for bone, pyrophosphate can be bound to 99mTc and utilized for scintigraphy of the skeleton (bone scans) [1].

Moreover, in vivo studies demonstrated an inhibitory effect of pyrophosphates on calcification. Various forms of ectopic calcification could be effectively avoided by parental, but not by oral, administration. However, there was no influence on osteoclastic resorption due to enzymatic splitting of pyrophosphate when taken orally (half-life of only 16 min) [1].

The bisphosphonates were then discovered during the search for analogues of pyrophosphate. They have similar physical and chemical effects but are resistant to enzymatic splitting and to metabolic breakdown. *This is because, in contrast to the P-O-P binding of pyrophosphate, the P-C-P binding of the bisphosphonates is stable and above all cannot be broken down enzymatically so that their activity is retained. This switch of the binding from P-O-P to P-C-P represented a genuine breakthrough which enabled the development of the potent bisphosphonates which are now in use for therapy of disorders of bone all over the world* [1].

The first medical application of a bisphosphonate was published in the Lancet in 1969. A 16-month-old baby, diagnosed as having progressive myositis ossificans, was successfully treated with oral etidronate to inhibit the extraosseous calcification [2].

Subsequently, H. Fleisch and co-workers demonstrated, by means of animal experiments, that bisphosphonates inhibit osteoclastic bone resorption and thereby achieve a positive calcium balance.

The rapid advances in the diagnosis and therapy of the osteopathies is thus closely bound up with the history of the bisphosphonates [1, 3–5].

During the past 30 years, new, more potent bisphosphonates have been developed. These have now been extensively applied in medicine, particularly in the fields of osteology, orthopedics, surgery, as well as in hematology, and particularly in oncology. *All osteopathies characterized by excess (absolute or relative) of osteoclastic activity are now treated with bisphosphonates and more recently denosumab, and it should be noted that this comprises about 90 % of all disorders of the bone* [1]. Bisphosphonates are now the major drugs used in the treatment of postmenopausal osteoporosis and represent the first-line therapy in the majority of patients. The latest applications of bisphosphonates include their administration for prevention of osseous metastases (administered during adjuvant chemotherapy), for alleviation of bone pain, and for their modulation of the immune and stromal systems in the bone marrow and the bone [1].

## Chemistry

Bisphosphonates are analogues of pyrophosphates which occur physiologically and in which the oxygen atom of the central P-O-P structure has been replaced by carbon, resulting in a P-C-P group (see Fig. 1.2), and this exchange has made them resistant to heat and enzymatic hydrolysis. These bisphosphonates exert strong effects on bone. Further substitutions have enabled synthesis of a series of biologically active bisphosphonates, each of which has its own characteristic potential activity and effect on bone. Therefore, every bisphosphonate has to be evaluated individually [1].

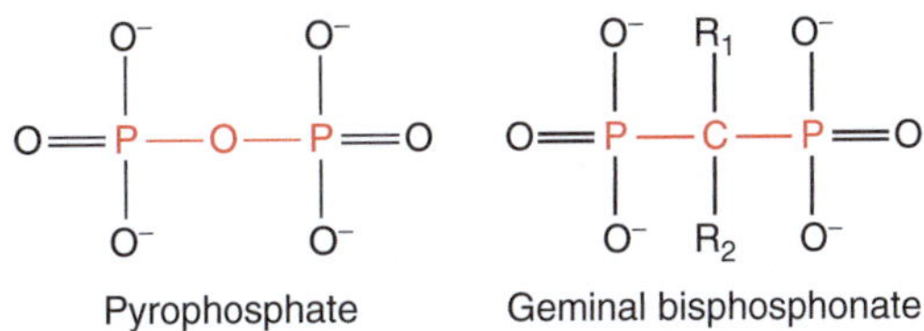


**Fig. 1.2** Chemical structure of pyrophosphate and of bisphosphonates (Reprinted with kind permission of Springer Business and Media from [1])

*For practical purposes, the bisphosphonates are subdivided into chemical groups according to the alphabetic order of the side chains:*
- Bisphosphonates without nitrogen substitution: etidronate and clodronate
- Aminobisphosphonates: pamidronate and alendronate
- Aminobisphosphonates with substitution of the nitrogen atom: ibandronate
- Bisphosphonates with basic heterocycles containing nitrogen: risedronate, pyridine-ring, and zoledronate, imidazole-ring

*The bisphosphonates used to be given in grams, now only milligrams, are given because of their greatly increased potency* [1].

## Pharmacodynamics

The bisphosphonates are poorly absorbed when taken orally, but this is compensated for by their greatly increased potency – *even 1 % of a given dose is effective!* They are distributed in the body via the blood stream, stored in the bones, and excreted unchanged by the kidneys. Interactions with other pharmaceutical agents have not been observed. Four compartments of bisphosphonate distribution are distinguished; these determine their pharmacodynamics (Fig. 1.3): the gastrointestinal tract, blood, bone, and kidneys [1].

## Administration and Absorption

Bisphosphonates may be taken orally as tablets or given intravenously as infusions (Fig. 1.3). The intestinal absorption of modern bisphosphonates is minimal to low. It varies from <1 to 3 %. However, as mentioned above, these doses are effective [1].

Two characteristics of bisphosphonates are responsible for their poor absorption: their low affinity for lipids, which hinders transport through membranes and into the cell, and their polarity, their negative charge, which prevents paracellular transport. Bisphosphonate absorption is further decreased when ingested together with food, especially food rich in calcium, such as milk and milk products because bisphosphonates form insoluble chelates with the calcium in these products [1].

## Distribution Half-Life

Bisphosphonates are bound to albumin in the blood. There are big differences in the strength of the albumin bonds (from 22 % for zoledronate to 87 % for ibandronate) and therefore in the time it takes for the bisphosphonates to be eliminated from the plasma. The half-life of zoledronate in the plasma is only 1–2 h, while that of ibandronate is 10–16 h. But the half-life in the bone is much longer [1].

Bisphosphonates from the plasma are actively bound to the surface of the bones, especially in the resorption lacunae where they are attached to calcium (Fig. 1.4a, b). *The amount of deposition depends on the extent of resorption surface of bone available* [1].

## Affinity to Bone

By binding to hydroxyapatite, bisphosphonates accumulate at sites of bone resorption and are selectively internalized by actively resorbing osteoclasts. *The different bisphosphonates have different affinities for hydroxyapatite crystals.*

*These differences in binding affinities and effects on mineral surface properties are likely to be reflected in the clinical differences among these bisphosphonates: uptake and retention on the skeleton, diffusion of the drug within the bone, release of absorbed drug from the bone, potential recycling of the desorbed drug back onto bone surface, effects on mineral dynamics, and effects on bone cellular function* [1].

## Uptake and Desorption of Bisphosphonates

Few studies have addressed the question of how bisphosphonates actually enter the cell. Since no specific transport mechanisms have yet been

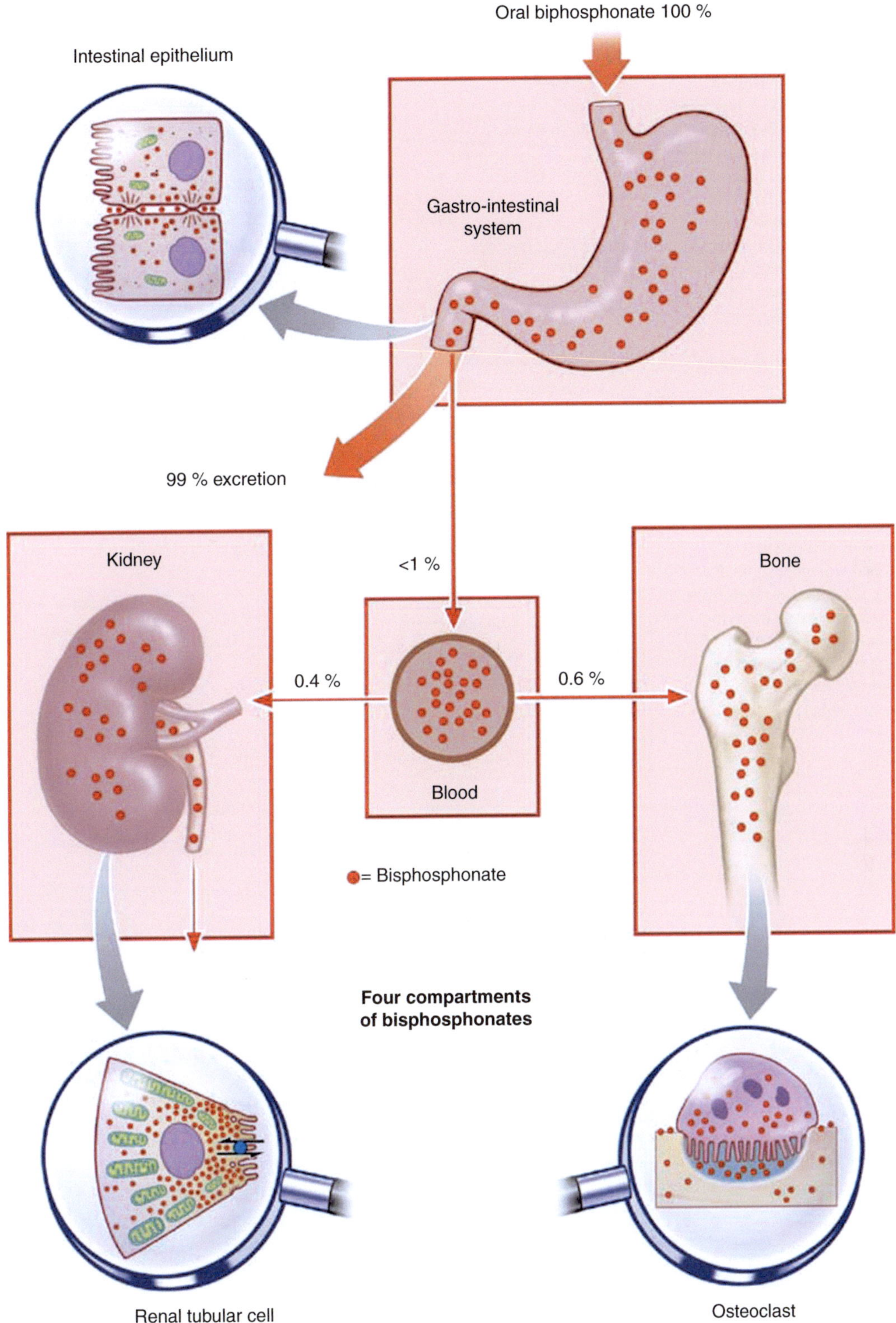



**Fig. 1.3** Diagrammatic representation of the four compartments of bisphosphonate absorption and excretion: the gastrointestinal tract, blood, bone, and kidney (Reprinted with kind permission of Springer Business and Media from [1])

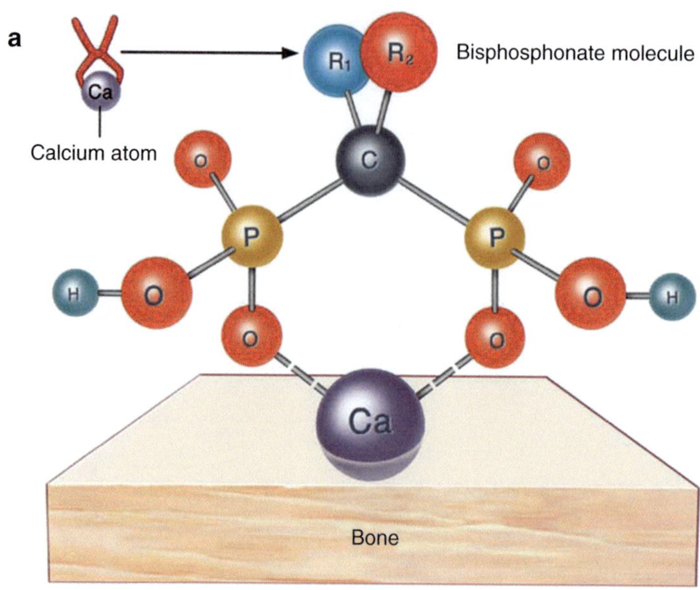



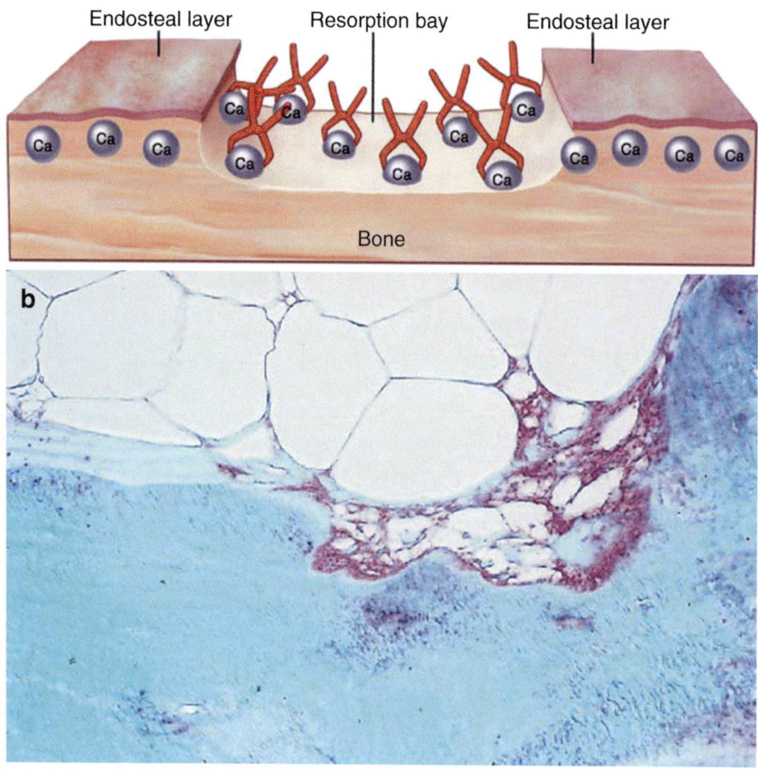



elucidated, the assumption has been made that bisphosphonates are taken up from the surrounding fluid by nonspecific pino- and endocytosis. Bisphosphonates have been demonstrated in the cytoplasm, in mitochondria, and in other organelles within the cytoplasm of the osteoclasts.

Relatively speaking, macrophages, a cell line to which osteoclasts belong, are also active in their uptake. *However, the concentration of bisphosphonates in extraosseous cells is very low, which explains the lack of toxicity and the paucity of side effects in these tissues* [1].

Twenty to fifty percent of the bisphosphonate in the plasma is deposited on the bone and the rest is eliminated by the kidneys into the urine. There are considerable differences between the various bisphosphonates with respect to their elimination. Bisphosphonates exhibit a very strong affinity for hydroxyapatite crystals which are avid bisphosphonate grabbers, and this "binding" process is strictly pH-dependent, so that when, during active resorption, the interface between osteoclasts and bone becomes strongly acidic, the previously bound bisphosphonate is released from its binding to calcium. In contrast to the blood (half-life of 1–15 h), the half-life on the surface of the bone varies from 150 to 200 h; but once inside the bone, and after the resorption cavity has been filled by the osteoblasts, the bisphosphonates remain attached even for years [1, 6].

Skeletal retention varies with the different bisphosphonates and a major factor in retention is the rate of bone turnover and the amount of bone surface available [7]. This retention in bone is similar to that of substances such as tetracyclines, fluoride, and strontium. The prolonged surface attachment of bisphosphonates explains their extended duration of action. The earliest pharmacological effect is manifest 24 h after administration [1].

While some will enter the circulation and will appear in the urine, it is not known whether and to what extent the released bisphosphonate will be active for the suppression of bone resorption. In all studies with alendronate, risedronate, and pamidronate, cessation of bisphosphonate treatment given for 2–7 years was not associated with a rebound increase in bone turnover and rapid bone loss, as it occurs after stopping hormone therapy. *These results support the hypothesis that some of the embedded bisphosphonate that is released later is active again at the bone surface* [1, 8].

## Elimination of Bisphosphonates

Bisphosphonates are eliminated without prior metabolism via the kidneys. This renal clearance of bisphosphonates is accomplished by glomerular filtration as well as active tubular excretion. Bisphosphonates are passively bourne by the blood stream to the kidneys; the quantity depends on the concentration gradient of the bisphosphonate in the blood. Bisphosphonates released from the surface of the bone (T½ 150–200 h) also reach the kidneys by way of the blood stream and are actively eliminated by the proximal tubules [1].

Consequently, excretion of bisphosphonates given by intravenous infusion is multiphasic – a fast biphasic elimination *from the blood stream, followed by a lengthier phase with a final elimination half-life of several days. Even after administration of a number of doses, accumulation in the plasma does not occur* [1].

*About half of the amount of bisphosphonate given at any time is excreted unchanged by the kidneys within 24 h. The half-life time of the bisphosphonates in renal tissue is very variable. It is clear that these differences are responsible for differences in toxicity to the kidney, particularly if and when administration is repeated. Therefore, when dealing with patients with impaired renal function, precautionary measures have to be applied* [1].

## Actions of Bisphosphonates

*Clinically, bisphosphonates act almost exclusively on bone as outlined above. The mechanisms of action of the bisphosphonates* include the following:

*The most important therapeutic action of bisphosphonates is inhibition of bone resorption, which commences within 1–2 days after administration, regardless of the route and frequency of administration. The total amount given determines the overall effect.* The reduction in bone resorption is accompanied by a positive calcium balance (Fig. 1.5). The target cells are osteoclasts and their precursors. At the biochemical level, bisphosphonates interfere with the mevalonate pathway by inhibiting formation of the lipid chains of prenylated proteins and thus also with metabolism of steroids. Bisphosphonates inhibit the formation of lipid chains of prenylated proteins. While statins effect the synthesis of mevalonic acid by inhibition of HMG-CoA-reductase, the bisphosphonates interfere with the earlier phases of prenylation and of steroid synthesis [1] (Fig. 1.5).

The following steps in the process of mevalonic acid synthesis are clinically relevant and are targets of the bisphosphonates:

1. *The first-generation bisphosphonates* (non-nitrogen-containing bisphosphonates) – together with adenosine monophosphate, they form an ATP analogue which cannot be hydrolyzed and thereby withholds the energy required for the synthesis of isopentenyl pyrophosphate.
2. *The second-generation bisphosphonates* (nitrogen-containing) – these prevent the enzymatic switch of Dimethylallyl pyrophosphate to geranyl pyrophosphate.
3. *The third-generation bisphosphonates* (nitrogen-containing) – these additionally block the next step in the enzymatic reaction, i.e., conversion of geranyl pyrophosphate to farnesyl pyrophosphate or to geranylgeranyl pyrophosphate [1].

Consequently, the cells become inactive, lose their membrane-specific properties, and eventually induce programmed cell death, i.e., apoptosis (Fig. 1.6a, b). Initially, this blockage takes place in the osteoclasts, due to their uptake of bisphosphonates from the osseous surface. Within osteoclasts, bisphosphonates cause many changes that affect their ability to resorb bone, such as loss of the ruffled border, disruption of the cytoskeleton, and inability to migrate or bind to bone [9]. Because of the inhibitory effect of nitrogen-containing bisphosphonates, there is an increase in the concentration of IPP, which in turn results

in the formation of *isopentenyl ATP* by means of its reaction with AMP. *This combination triggers the excretion of caspases and thereby programmed cell death, i.e., apoptosis.* It should be stressed that the same process occurs in all cells in which bisphosphonates accumulate and it is responsible for the (desired) effects as well as the (unwanted) side effects of the bisphosphonates. Nowadays, mainly containing bisphosphonates (second and third generation) are widely used in clinical practice. Their activity is strongly dependent on local pH values. In acidic milieus nitrogen-containing bisphosphonates are released and activated and exert their therapeutical effects as well as their side effects (Fig. 1.7) [1].

*In summary, inhibition of osteoclastic resorption is accomplished by means of three different mechanisms corresponding to the three generations of bisphosphonates* (Fig. 1.5) [1].

## Direct Effects on Osteoclasts

- Reduction of osteoclastic activity: As soon as the bisphosphonates have entered the osteoclasts, their cellular activity decreases. Structural alterations of the cytoskeleton can be seen on electron microscopy. Microtubules are depolymerized and the "ruffled membrane" is retracted. The levels of products of bone resorption in the serum such as CTX (C-terminal polypeptide) are reduced, and the serum calcium concentration is lowered [1].
  Bisphosphonates inhibit osteoclast adhesion. The layer of bisphosphonates on the surface of bone prevents attachment of osteoclasts and thereby development of the appropriate acidic environment essential for resorption. Furthermore, there is a decreasing number of osteoclasts because bisphosphonates inhibit the proliferation of macrophages that are recruited and undergo fusion to become osteoclasts. Bisphosphonates induce osteoclast

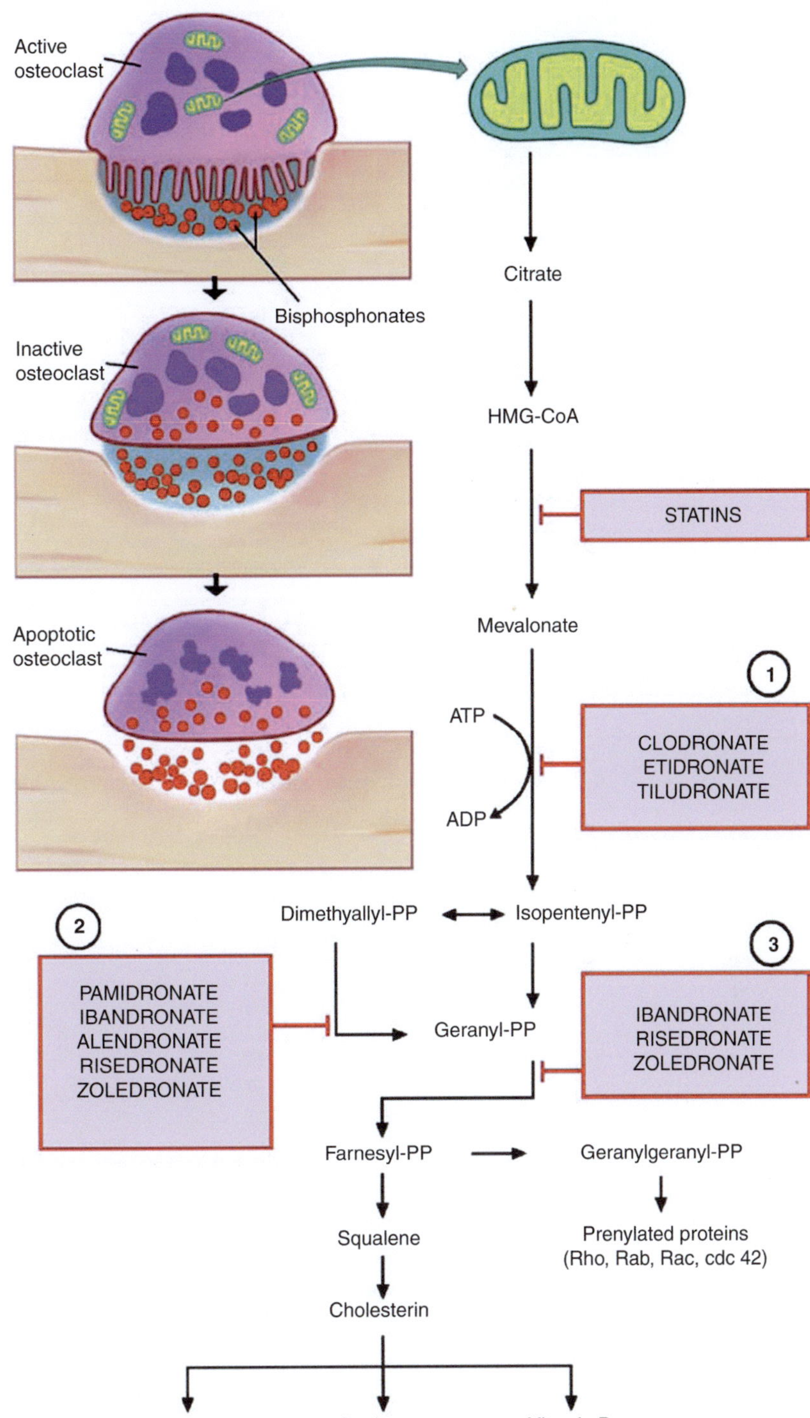



**Fig. 1.5** Cellular and biochemical mechanisms of action of the nitrogen-containing bisphosphonates: *Left*: Layer of bisphosphonate (*red dots*) on bone beneath osteoclasts in resorption lacunae. The bisphosphonates are taken up by the osteoclasts which leads to their inactivation and retraction of the ruffled membrane. Higher doses lead to increased apoptosis of the osteoclasts. *Right*: Biosynthetic pathway for sterols and isoprenoids, which takes place in the cytoplasm of the osteoclasts. Steps of inhibition by statins and bisphosphonates. *HMG Co-A* 3-hdroxy-3-methylglutaryl-Co-A, *PP* pyrophosphate. *1*, *2*, and *3* shows the different generations of bisphosphonates each with its own specific targets. Effects of the 2nd and 3rd generation lead to an accumulation of isopentenyl-PP, which in turn stimulates the acute phase reaction. However, this may be reduced by previous administration of clodronate (Reprinted with kind permission of Springer Business and Media from [1])

**Fig. 1.6** (**a**) The four most important cellular targets for bisphosphonates in the bone-remodeling unit (*BRU*). ORI, osteoclast resorption inhibitor. (**b**) Bisphosphonates inhibit the production of membrane proteins in the osteoclast causing its inactivation and apoptosis (Reprinted with kind permission of Springer Business and Media from [1])

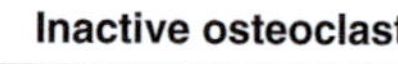
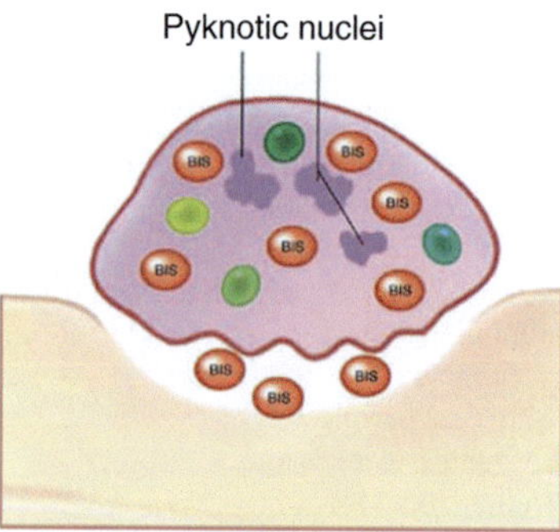
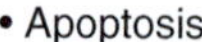

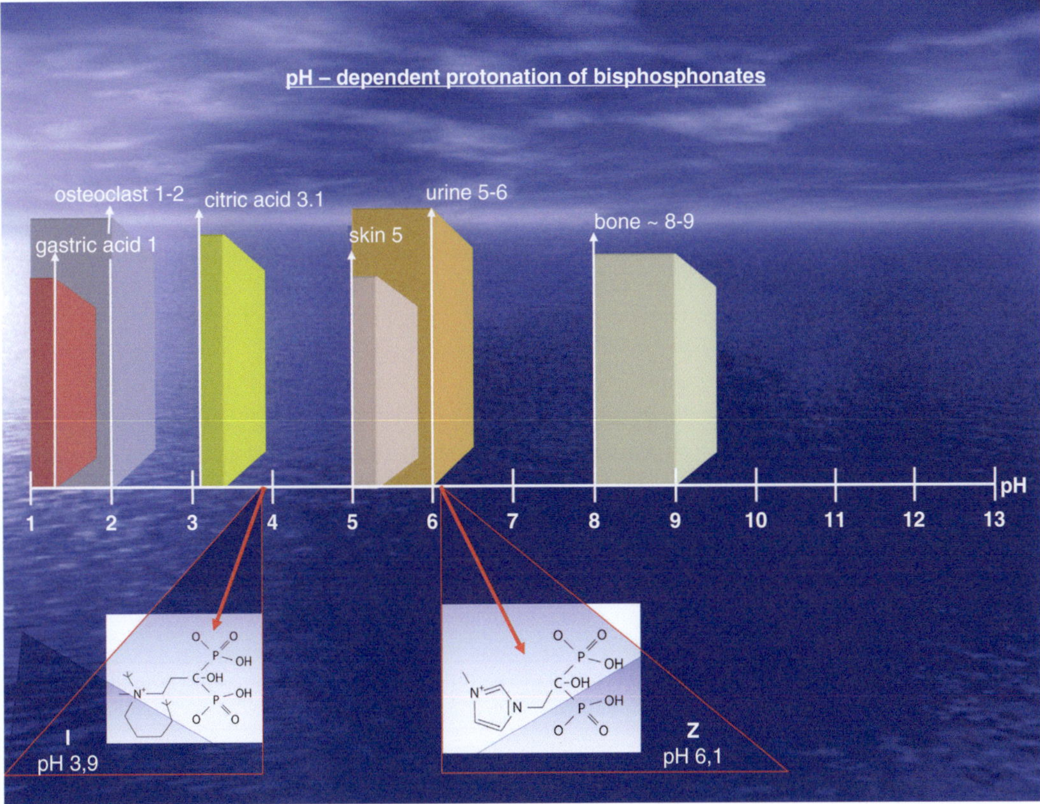



**Fig. 1.7**  pH-dependent protonation of nitrogen-containing bisphosphonates

apoptosis, which is premature cell death. This leads to a reduction in osteoclast numbers [1].

- To summarize: the bisphosphonates inhibit lipopolysaccharide and parathyroid hormone-induced osteoclast differentiation, fusion, attachment, and actin-ring formation and activation, in simple terms, the whole process of resorption of bone [1, 10].

## Effects on Osteoblasts and Osteocytes

*It was recently shown that low concentrations of bisphosphonates stimulate osteoblasts to produce a factor which inhibits osteoclast recruitment and activation (Fig. 1.6a). Bisphosphonates stimulate proliferation and osteogenic differentiation of bone marrow stromal cells and thus promote osteoblastic bone formation* [11] (Fig. 1.6b). Few studies have dealt with the influence of bisphosphonates on osteocytes. However, high concentrations in solutions have inhibitory effects towards osteoblasts and osteocytes [1].

## Effects on Immune System

Some bisphosphonates stimulate cytokine production by macrophages and other immunocompetent cells. There is also a significant decrease in the number of circulating lymphocytes, especially natural killer cells and T lymphocytes both CD4- and CD8-positive. This decrease is probably caused by an increase in acute-phase reactants such as C-reactive protein, IL-6, and TNFα. In contrast, ibandronate stimulates a moderate increase in lymphocytes within 10 h, whereas clodronate has no apparent effect [1].

## Antiangiogenic Effects

Both in vivo and in vitro studies have demonstrated the qualitative and quantitative antiangiogenic actions of bisphosphonates in high concentrations. The mechanism of endothelial cell inhibition presumably includes downregulation of integrins and laminin receptors. Possibly negative actions on vascular endothelial growth factors (VEGFs) are also involved. *Enrichment on the bone surface and combinations with chemotherapeutic agents such as the taxanes increase the antiangiogenic action of bisphosphonates* [1].

## Effects on Tumor Cells

Bisphosphonates appear to slow down the rate of tumor growth by inhibiting intracellular signal transduction, which stimulates apoptosis, i.e., an antiproliferative effect. This apoptotic effect of pamidronate has been demonstrated in human myeloma cells. There are indications that bisphosphonates interfere with the establishment of osseous and probably also visceral metastases [12]. Recent in vitro studies have highlighted the direct toxic effect of the modern bisphosphonates on tumor cells leading to their apoptosis [13]. They also prevent cancer adhesion to bone by their inhibitory effect on protein prenylation [14]. In addition, as shown in these experiments, bisphosphonates together with standard chemotherapeutic agents induced a greater degree of toxicity and apoptosis of tumor cells than that achieved by chemotherapy alone [1].

## Side Effects

*The bisphosphonates are well tolerated. Their side effects are few and dependent on the route of administration.* Mild gastrointestinal side effects may occur when bisphosphonates are taken orally. These include diarrhea, nausea, bloating, gastric pain, and other uncharacteristic abdominal complaints, which had previously been reported in 2–10 % of patients [1].

In case of intravenous administration, mild to moderate acute-phase reactions in 20–40 % of all patients experience fever and lymphocytopenia as well as a rise in C-reactive protein, in IL-6, and in TNFα especially after the first infusion of a nitrogen-containing bisphosphonate. These patients experience flu-like symptoms such as headache, bone and joint pains, and fatigue. Normally, these circumstances are self-limiting. Symptomatic therapy can be given but is rarely required [1].

Furthermore, impairment of renal function can occur after intravenous administration especially after rapid intravenous infusion of nitrogen-containing bisphosphonates. Normally, the impairment of renal function is transitory. However, permanent renal insufficiency has been described in rare cases. Therefore, renal function (creatinine clearance) should be measured prior to intravenous administration of bisphosphonates. Due to the inhibition of osteoclast function, hypocalcemia can occur. Interestingly, especially after long-term treatment with bisphosphonates, atypical fractures of the femur have occurred. The exact etiology is under intensive investigation [1].

Other side effects of bisphosphonate treatment are extremely rare. They include ocular side effects (conjunctivitis, scleritis, episcleritis, and uveitis) [15]. In extremely rare cases, visual, olfactory, and auditory hallucinations have also been reported after therapy with pamidronate [1, 16].

## Osteomyelitis/Osteonecrosis of the Jaw Bones

In 2003, the first scientific publications dealing with a side effect of bisphosphonates in the jaw bone were reported [17–19]. Ever since, this so-called bisphosphonate-related osteonecrosis of the jaw (BRONJ) has become a well-known and severe side effect which predominantly occurs in patients who received intravenous administrations of nitrogen-containing bisphosphonates due to malignant underlying disease [20–22]. The epidemiology, clinical and radiological presentation, and surgical and nonsurgical treatment concepts are discussed in detail in the following chapters.

## Effects of Cessation of Bisphosphonate Therapy

Within 2–4 months of stopping therapy with bisphosphonates, indices of bone turnover begin to increase – a negative bone balance, that is, bone loss, becomes evident 1–2 years later. These considerations might play a role with regard to potential drug holidays prior to dentoalveolar surgery in patients under bisphosphonate treatment. However, there is no valid data available whether or not and how long an appropriate drug holiday should be prior to dentoalveolar surgeries in patients with bisphosphonates [1].

## The RANK/RANKL/Osteoprotegerin System

*The RANK/RANKL/Osteoprotegerin cytokine system plays a key role in the regulation of and in "coupling" within the processes of remodeling.* Osteoprotegerin is an important member of the tumor-necrosis factor-receptor family which is produced by osteoblasts and which blocks the differentiation of osteoclasts from their precursor cells and thus inhibits resorption of bone. RANKL (receptor activator of NF-kb ligand) and its receptors RANK and osteoprotegerin (OPG) are the key components of the regulation of remodeling units. RANKL, a member of the TNF family, is the main stimulus for osteoclast maturation and is essential for osteoclast survival. *The elucidation of the RANK/RANKL/osteoprotegerin system constitutes a breakthrough for understanding the processes of local remodeling* (Fig. 1.8) [1].

Thus, an increase in the expression of RANKL leads directly to increased resorption and loss of bone. RANKL is also produced by osteoblastic cells and by activated T lymphocytes. Its specific receptor RANK is located on the surface membranes of osteoclasts, dendritic cells, smooth muscle cells, and endothelial cells. The production of RANKL by T lymphocytes and the consequent activation of dendritic cells represent a connection between the immune system and bone tissues.

The effect of RANKL is regulated by OPG. This is secreted in various organs, including the bone, skin, liver, stomach, intestine, lungs, kidneys, and placenta, and acts as a soluble endogenous receptor antagonist. Numerous cytokines, hormones, and drugs may stimulate or inhibit the effects of RANKL or of OPG [1].

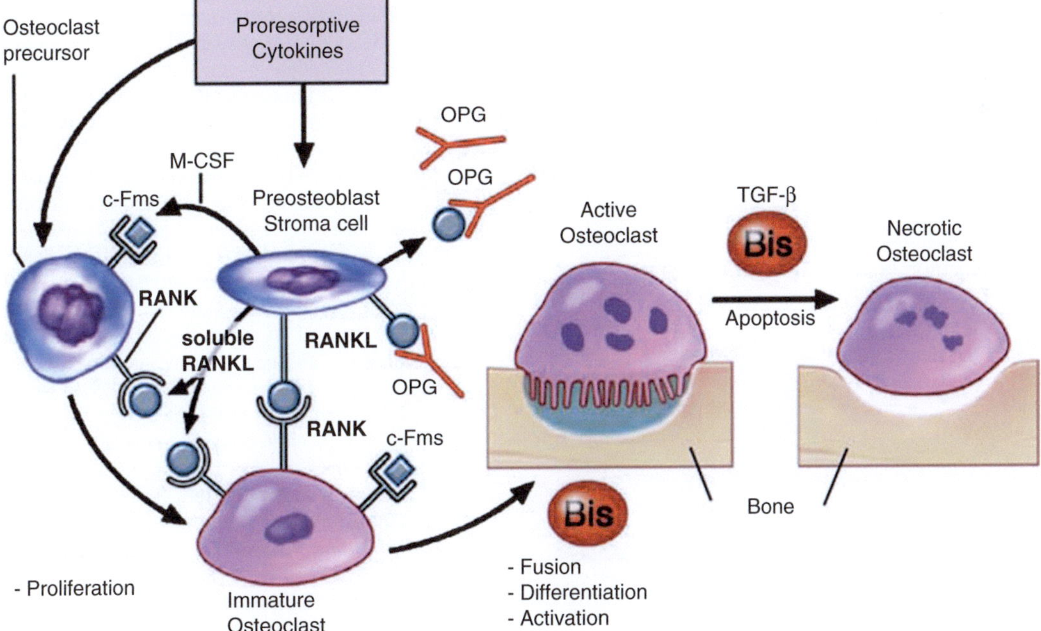


**Fig. 1.8** The OPG/RANK/RANKL system and its control of bone resorption (Reprinted with kind permission of Springer Business and Media from [1])

Denosumab, a human monoclonal antibody to RANKL, was developed to block the binding of RANKL to RANK. By this way, differentiation and activity of osteoclasts are inhibited and bone resorption is decreased [23]. Denosumab is administrated subcutaneously and used for the management of osteoporosis (60 mg every 6 months) as well as metastatic bone disease (120 mg every 4 weeks) [23, 24]. Denosumab is cleared by the reticuloendothelial system (half-life 26d), subsequently not interfering with renal function [25].

The effective inhibition of osteoclastic activity by denosumab needs a careful control of the calcium level as serious hypocalcemia can occur. On the other hand, therapies with high doses should be slowly reduced, as cessation may result in a rebound with hypercalcemia.

The interference of denosumab with the "coupling" between osteoclasts and osteoblasts especially under high dosages may lead to a disbalance in remodeling of the bone. This could explain the similar rates of jaw bone necrosis of patients receiving denosumab or zoledronate [26, 27]. As described above, the RANK/RANKL/OPG system does not only interfere with bone remodeling, but also with the immune system and may therefore cause immunomodulatory effects resulting in atypical infections and which may be involved in tumorigenesis [28].

### Conclusions

Bisphosphonates and denosumab are potent inhibitors of bone resorption which are routinely and successfully used in the treatment of bone disorders especially osteoporosis and metastatic bone disease (Table 1.1).

**Table 1.1** Antiresorptive drugs and respective trade names

| Bisphosphonate | Trade names |
| --- | --- |
| Alendronate | Fosamax®, Fosavance® |
| Clodronate | Ostac®, Bonefos® |
| Ibandronate | Bondronat®, Bon(v)iva® |
| Pamidronate | Aredia® |
| Risedronate | Actonel®, Actonel® plus calcium |
| Zoledronate | Zometa®, Aclasta® |
| Denosumab | Prolia®, XGEVA® |

According to Bartl et al. [1]
(Reprinted with kind permission of Springer Business and Media) [1]

**Ackowledgements:** This chapter contains excerpts of parts of the book „Bisphosphonates in medical practice-actions, side effects, indications and strategies" by ReinerBartl et al. [1], Reprinted with kind permission of Springer Science and Business Media.

## References

1. Bartl R, Frisch B, von Tresckow E, Bartl C. Bisphosphonates in medical practice actions, side effects, indications, strategies. Berlin/New York: Springer; 2007.
2. Bassett CA, Donath A, Macagno F, Preisig R, Fleisch H, Francis MD. Diphosphonates in the treatment of myositis ossificans. Lancet. 1969;2(7625):845. PubMed PMID: 4186297. eng.
3. Fleisch HA, Russell RG, Bisaz S, Mühlbauer RC, Williams DA. The inhibitory effect of phosphonates on the formation of calcium phosphate crystals in vitro and on aortic and kidney calcification in vivo. Eur J Clin Invest. 1970;1(1):12–8. PubMed PMID: 4319371. eng.
4. Fleisch H. Bisphosphonates: mechanisms of action. Endocr Rev. 1998;19(1):80–100. PubMed PMID: 9494781. eng.
5. Fleisch H. Bisphosphonates in bone disease. 4th ed. San Diego: Academic Press; 2000.
6. Sato M, Grasser W, Endo N, Akins R, Simmons H, Thompson DD, et al. Bisphosphonate action. Alendronate localization in rat bone and effects on osteoclast ultrastructure. J Clin Invest. 1991;88(6):2095–105. PubMed PMID: 1661297. eng.
7. Cremers SC, Pillai G, Papapoulos SE. Pharmacokinetics/pharmacodynamics of bisphosphonates: use for optimisation of intermittent therapy for osteoporosis. Clin Pharmacokinet. 2005;44(6):551–70. PubMed PMID: 15932344. eng.
8. Landman JO, Hamdy NA, Pauwels EK, Papapoulos SE. Skeletal metabolism in patients with osteoporosis after discontinuation of long-term treatment with oral pamidronate. J Clin Endocrinol Metab. 1995;80(12):3465–8. PubMed PMID: 8530584. eng.
9. Russell RG, Rogers MJ, Frith JC, Luckman SP, Coxon FP, Benford HL, et al. The pharmacology of bisphosphonates and new insights into their mechanisms of action. J Bone Miner Res. 1999;14 Suppl 2:53–65. PubMed PMID: 10510215. eng.
10. Suzuki K, Takeyama S, Sakai Y, Yamada S, Shinoda H. Current topics in pharmacological research on bone metabolism: inhibitory effects of bisphosphonates on the differentiation and activity of osteoclasts. J Pharmacol Sci. 2006;100(3):189–94. Epub 2006 Mar 4. PubMed PMID: 16518076. eng.
11. Plotkin L, Aquirre J, Kousteni S, et al. Bisphosphonates and estrogens inhibit osteocyte apoptosis via distinct molecular mechanisms downstream of extracellular signal-regulated kinase activation. J Biol Chem. 2005 280:7317–325.

12. Diel IJ, Solomayer EF, Costa SD, Gollan C, Goerner R, Wallwiener D, et al. Reduction in new metastases in breast cancer with adjuvant clodronate treatment. N Engl J Med. 1998;339(6):357–63. PubMed PMID: 9691101. eng.

13. Mönkkönen H, Auriola S, Lehenkari P, Kellinsalmi M, Hassinen IE, Vepsäläinen J, et al. A new endogenous ATP analog (ApppI) inhibits the mitochondrial adenine nucleotide translocase (ANT) and is responsible for the apoptosis induced by nitrogen-containing bisphosphonates. Br J Pharmacol.2006;147(4):437–45. PubMed PMID: 16402039. eng.

14. Roelofs AJ, Thompson K, Gordon S, Rogers MJ. Molecular mechanisms of action of bisphosphonates: current status. Clin Cancer Res. 2006;12(20 Pt 2): 6222s–30. PubMed PMID: 17062705. eng.

15. El Saghir NS, Otrock ZK, Bleik JH. Unilateral anterior uveitis complicating zoledronic acid therapy in breast cancer. BMC Cancer. 2005;5:156. PubMed PMID: 16332258. eng.

16. Coleman CI, Perkerson KA, Lewis A. Alendronate-induced auditory hallucinations and visual disturbances. Pharmacotherapy. 2004;24(6):799–802. PubMed PMID: 15222671. eng.

17. Marx RE. Pamidronate (Aredia) and zoledronate (Zometa) induced avascular necrosis of the jaws: a growing epidemic. J Oral Maxillofac Surg. 2003;61(9): 1115–7. PubMed PMID: 12966493. eng.

18. Migliorati CA. Bisphosphonates and oral cavity avascular bone necrosis. J Clin Oncol. 2003;21(22): 4253–4. PubMed PMID: 14615459. eng.

19. Wang J, Goodger NM, Pogrel MA. Osteonecrosis of the jaws associated with cancer chemotherapy. J Oral Maxillofac Surg. 2003;61(9):1104–7. PubMed PMID: 12966490. eng.

20. Bamias A, Kastritis E, Bamia C, Moulopoulos LA, Melakopoulos I, Bozas G, et al. Osteonecrosis of the jaw in cancer after treatment with bisphosphonates: incidence and risk factors. J Clin Oncol. 2005; 23(34):8580–7. PubMed PMID: 16314620. eng.

21. Abu-Id MH, Warnke PH, Gottschalk J, Springer I, Wiltfang J, Acil Y, et al. "Bis-phossy jaws" – high and low risk factors for bisphosphonate-induced osteonecrosis of the jaw. J Craniomaxillofac Surg. 2008;36(2):95–103. PubMed PMID: 18234504. Epub 2008/01/30. eng.

22. Otto S, Abu-Id MH, Fedele S, Warnke PH, Becker ST, Kolk A, et al. Osteoporosis and bisphosphonates-related osteonecrosis of the jaw: not just a sporadic coincidence–a multi-centre study. J Craniomaxillofac Surg. 2011;39(4):272–7. PubMed PMID: 20580566. Epub 2010/07/02. eng.

23. Cummings SR, San Martin J, McClung MR, Siris ES, Eastell R, Reid IR, et al. Denosumab for prevention of fractures in postmenopausal women with osteoporosis. N Engl J Med. 2009;361(8):756–65. PubMed PMID: 19671655. Epub 2009/08/11. eng.

24. Stopeck AT, Lipton A, Body JJ, Steger GG, Tonkin K, de Boer RH, et al. Denosumab compared with zoledronic acid for the treatment of bone metastases in patients with advanced breast cancer: a randomized, double-blind study. J Clin Oncol. 2010; 28(35):5132–9. PubMed PMID: 21060033. Epub 2010/11/08. eng.

25. Baron R, Ferrari S, Russell RG. Denosumab and bisphosphonates: different mechanisms of action and effects. Bone. 2011;48(4):677–92. PubMed PMID: 21145999. Epub 2010/12/09. eng.

26. Van den Wyngaert T, Claeys T, Huizing MT, Vermorken JB, Fossion E. Initial experience with conservative treatment in cancer patients with osteonecrosis of the jaw (ONJ) and predictors of outcome. Ann Oncol. 2009;20(2):331–6. PubMed PMID: 18953067. Epub 2008/10/26. eng.

27. Henry DH, Costa L, Goldwasser F, Hirsh V, Hungria V, Prausova J, et al. Randomized, double-blind study of denosumab versus zoledronic acid in the treatment of bone metastases in patients with advanced cancer (excluding breast and prostate cancer) or multiple myeloma. J Clin Oncol. 2011;29(9):1125–32. PubMed PMID: 21343556. Epub 2011/02/22. eng.

28. Anastasilakis AD, Toulis KA, Polyzos SA, Anastasilakis CD, Makras P. Long-term treatment of osteoporosis: safety and efficacy appraisal of denosumab. Ther Clin Risk Manag. 2012;8:295–306. PubMed PMID: 22767993. Epub 2012/06/19. eng.

# Bisphosphonate and Denosumab Therapy: Fields of Application

2

Cornelia Then, Emmo von Tresckow, Reiner Bartl, and Fuat S. Oduncu

**Abstract**

Bisphosphonates are highly effective in preserving bone mineral density and have a favorable benefit-risk profile. Thereby, bisphosphonates became the preferred antiresorptive drug for malignant and nonmalignant diseases characterized by various kinds of bone loss. In general, bisphosphonates may be considered as treatment option for preserving bone mineral density in any disease accompanied by increased bone resorption, regardless of the pathogenic mechanisms involved. Typical and frequent indications are postmenopausal osteoporosis, breast cancer, prostate cancer, and multiple myeloma.

Bisphosphonates exert beneficial effects beyond their antiresorptive properties and reduce morbidity and mortality in malignant and nonmalignant diseases. Especially, the antitumor activity described in several malignancies is intriguing. The molecular mechanisms generating these additional beneficial effects are still incompletely understood.

Among bisphosphonates, zoledronic acid is the most potent and most thoroughly studied substance. Of all bisphosphonates, zoledronate displays the most beneficial effects in reducing fracture risk, antitumor activity, and additional effects but also the highest risk of adverse events, including BRONJ/MRONJ.

Denosumab has a similarly high antiresorptive capacity as zoledronic acid. In certain settings, it may be a suitable alternative to bisphosphonate therapy.

C. Then, MD (✉)
Medizinische Klinik IV, Klinikum der
Ludwig-Maximilians-Universität München,
Ziemssenstrasse 1, Munich, Germany
e-mail: cornelia.then@med.uni-muenchen.de

E. von Tresckow
Rosenstrasse 2, 82319 Starnberg, Germany
e-mail: emmo.von_tresckow@bendalis.com

R. Bartl
Ehrenfelsstrasse 5, 81375 Munich, Germany
e-mail: Reiner.Bartl@osteologie-online.de

F.S. Oduncu, MD, PhD
Department of Hematology and Oncology,
Medizinische Klinik und Poliklinik IV,
Klinikum der Universität München,
Ziemssenstrasse 1, Munich, Bavaria
D-80336, Germany
e-mail: fuat.oduncu@med.uni-muenchen.de

S. Otto (ed.), *Medication-Related Osteonecrosis of the Jaws: Bisphosphonates, Denosumab, and New Agents*,
DOI 10.1007/978-3-662-43733-9_2, © Springer-Verlag Berlin Heidelberg 2015

## Introduction

Due to their effective antiresorptive properties, bisphosphonates are the first-choice treatment in many disorders involving an increase or disruption in bone resorption. Bisphosphonates help to ameliorate quality of life and furthermore have the potential to improve survival in malignant and nonmalignant diseases [1, 2]. The overall good tolerability results in a continuous and prolonged use in many patients. Adverse effects are infrequent and primarily constituted by acute-phase reactions with transient influenza-like symptoms, hypocalcemia, impaired renal function, and complications of the upper aerodigestive tract, such as esophageal ulceration [3]. Additionally, rare cases of atypical femoral fractures have been connected with long-term use of bisphosphonates [4, 5], and an association of atrial fibrillation and esophageal cancer with bisphosphonate use has been suggested [6]. The most problematic adverse event, bisphosphonate-related osteonecrosis of the jaw, has emerged as a severe complication of bisphosphonate therapy [7, 8] and has primarily been described in patients with prolonged intravenous bisphosphonate therapy. Of all available bisphosphonates, the intravenous nitrogen-containing bisphosphonate zoledronic acid displays the most distinct beneficial effects both in reducing skeletal-related events and in improving overall survival in malignant and nonmalignant diseases; however, zoledronic acid is also most frequently associated with adverse events, such as bisphosphonate-related osteonecrosis of the jaw.

## Use of Bisphosphonates in Nonmalignant Diseases

### Bisphosphonates in Postmenopausal Osteoporosis

Osteoporosis poses a significant public health issue that greatly impacts morbidity and mortality, especially in postmenopausal women. Amino-bisphosphonates exert proven efficacy in reducing fracture risk at the spine, hip, and other nonvertebral skeletal sites and are the most frequently applied treatment strategy with the best cost-to-effectiveness ratio of all therapies for postmenopausal osteoporosis [9]. Women receiving bisphosphonates present decreased bone turnover and serum markers of bone turnover, such as cross-linked C-telopeptides of collagen type I [10]. In excess of their primary function of reducing skeletal-related events, bisphosphonates have also been associated with a significant decrease in morbidity and increase in survival in osteoporosis patients, which is not explainable by the mere effect of preventing fractures. The reasons for this observation are not yet fully understood. Possibly effects of bisphosphonates not directly related to the bone are jointly responsible for this observation, such as the inhibitory effect on the atherosclerotic process demonstrated by experimental evidence [11].

Intravenous zoledronic acid is the most effective bisphosphonate for treating osteoporosis with a 70 % fracture risk reduction, whereas the risk is reduced by 60 % using ibandronate. However, in osteoporosis patients, long-term treatment is frequently required, and oral applications, which are less frequently associated with adverse effects, are often preferred. The nitrogen-containing bisphosphonates alendronate and risedronate are eligible for oral application, are approximately equipotent, and exhibit a log-linear relationship between the dose and the increase in spine bone mineral density in the animal model [12]. Regarding duration of treatment, the benefits of continuing therapy probably outweigh the risk of harm in patients with bone mineral density in the osteoporosis range or previous history of fragility fracture. However, patients who are not at high risk for fracture are candidates for a "drug holiday" in order to minimize the risk of severe side effects [13]. Altogether, it is important to find a rational balance and give continued osteoporosis treatment to those in need, since bisphosphonates prevent many typical hip and vertebral compression fractures, particularly in elderly patients [4].

### Bisphosphonates in Chronic Kidney Disease and After Renal Transplantation

Indications for bisphosphonates in chronic kidney disease include hypercalcemia, treatment of low bone mineral density in all chronic kidney disease stages, and prevention of bone loss after renal transplantation. Renal transplant recipients are at high risk of developing osteoporosis and osteopenia due to underlying renal osteodystrophy, hypophosphatemia, and immunosuppression. Especially, the first year after renal transplantation often entails excessive bone loss, inter alia due to the application of high glucocorticoid doses. Additionally, persistent post-kidney transplant hyperparathyroidism may lead to or exacerbate preexisting bone and cardiovascular disease [14].

In chronic kidney disease, bone biopsy is mandatory before starting a bisphosphonate therapy in case suppressed bone turnover is suspected. Although it has been shown that bisphosphonates can safely be used in all chronic kidney disease stages, including dialysis patients, they must be carefully administered in these patients, because of their urinary elimination and potential renal toxicity. Renal toxicity is associated with infusion velocity and excessive dosage. Therefore, it is important to maintain the time of infusion, and in hemodialysis patients, administration during the hemodialysis session is recommended. A 50 % dose reduction is recommended in chronic kidney disease stage 4 and 5. Renal toxicity is less frequent when using oral bisphosphonate regimens [15]. Oral therapy regimens are also favorable and have been proven to be effective in patients after renal transplantation who are exposed to continuous immunosuppression and thus may have an especially high risk for side effects, such as bisphosphonate-related osteonecrosis of the jaw [16]. Low-dose alendronate or risedronate in addition to vitamin D supplementation given early after renal transplantation prevents early bone loss and is significantly correlated with increased lumbar, spine, and radius bone mineral density 6 months after transplantation when compared to vitamin D supplementation alone [17, 18].

## Other Indications

Glucocorticoid-induced osteoporosis is an important indication for bisphosphonate use in various diseases. As an example, Crohn's disease and its therapy affect bone health and result in a high prevalence of low bone mineral density disease such as osteoporosis and osteopenia, which may be ameliorated by bisphosphonate therapy [19]. Furthermore, bisphosphonates are first-choice treatment in Paget's disease, and their efficiency has been proven in osteogenesis imperfecta [20, 21].

Apart from their antiresorptive activity, bisphosphonates may also have specific analgesic or anti-inflammatory effects. Thus, rheumatic diseases associated with systemic and sometimes focal bone loss, such as rheumatoid arthritis, spondylarthritis, or SAPHO (synovitis, acne, pustulosis, hyperostosis, osteitis) syndrome, are candidates for bisphosphonate therapy. Also noninflammatory rheumatic diseases, such as aseptic osteonecrosis, neuropathic osteoarthropathy, algoneurodystrophy, and fibrous dysplasia, are associated with pain and increased focal bone remodeling. Several studies have shown promising therapeutic potential of bisphosphonates in these inflammatory or noninflammatory diseases where therapeutic options are often limited [21, 22].

Preliminary evidence exists that bisphosphonates may furthermore be useful to prevent vascular calcifications and as therapy of calciphylaxis, also known as calcific uremic arteriolopathy. Calciphylaxis is a rare but potentially life-threatening and difficultly treatable condition that almost exclusively affects patients with chronic kidney disease. In a small series of eight patients with calciphylaxis, progression of skin lesions stopped between 2 and 4 weeks after starting bisphosphonate therapy. Within 6 months, wound healing was complete in all patients without recurrence during at least 1 year follow-up [23].

## Use of Bisphosphonates in Malignancies

Bisphosphonates are the most common pharmaceutical intervention for prevention of skeletal-related events in patients with malignant skeletal involvement. In principle, bisphosphonates are probably beneficial in any tumor disease metastatic to the bone or in which the treatment causes loss in bone mineral density. Best described are bisphosphonate effects in patients with multiple myeloma, breast cancer, and prostate cancer, whereas data on the efficiency of bisphosphonate treatment in other malignancies is limited. Bisphosphonates significantly reduce the risk of skeletal complications in multiple myeloma and metastatic bone disease by 30–50 % and prevent cancer treatment-induced bone loss. Osteolytic metastases are primarily caused by excessive bone resorption through osteoclasts with concurrently impaired osteoblast function due to a variety of cytokines produced by metastatic cancer cells, influencing both osteoclast and osteoblast function [24, 25].

Beside the beneficial effects of bisphosphonates on pain and reduction of fractures [26], they also display antimyeloma and antitumor activity with prolonged overall survival reported for various malignancies [27–30]. Several mechanisms by which bisphosphonates exert antitumor effects are proposed. Firstly, bisphosphonates may preserve bone health and delay bone lesion progression by interrupting the vicious cycle of increased osteolysis coupled with increased tumor growth. Metastatic cells in bone secrete cytokines and growth factors, which may promote osteoclast function and survival and thus facilitate bone resorption. Osteoclasts, in turn, release bone-derived growth factors that possibly facilitate tumor cell survival and metastasis growth. Secondly, direct effects on cancer cells may contribute to the antitumor effect. Zoledronic acid inhibits growth, migration, and matrix-associated invasion of breast cancer cells [31]. In vitro, attenuated proliferation of breast cancer cells was demonstrated when treated with ibandronate. Especially, amino-bisphosphonates might have inherent anticancer activities independently of their direct effect on bone [32, 33], which depend on inhibition of protein prenylation through inhibition of the mevalonate pathway, a mechanism not shared by non-nitrogen-containing bisphosphonates [27, 33]. Amino-bisphosphonates inhibit the activity of small GTPases by preventing their posttranslational isoprenylation and thus promote the expression of proapoptotic genes and the upregulation of caspases [34], as activated RAS GTPases downregulate the expression of proapoptotic genes in malignant cells.

Thus, nitrogen-containing bisphosphonates may induce apoptosis in neoplastic cells via modulation of the activity of small GTPases [35]. Thirdly, bisphosphonates may stimulate innate antitumor immune mechanisms, such as $\gamma\delta$ T cells. In patients with prostate cancer, zoledronate therapy elicited a long-term shift of peripheral $\gamma\delta$ T cells towards an activated effector memory-like state associated with improved immune surveillance against transformed or malignant cells [36]. Furthermore, it is suggested that bisphosphonates effect angiogenesis and the stem cell niche by modulation of extracellular matrix gene expression. Hence, bisphosphonates provide more than just supportive care in patients with multiple myeloma or solid tumors with bone metastases.

## Bisphosphonates in Multiple Myeloma Patients

Multiple myeloma patients are often affected by pathological fractures early in their disease course but still have a long survival compared to other patients with bone metastases. Due to early and massive bone affection, potent intravenous bisphosphonate regimens are the preferred treatment strategy in multiple myeloma patients. However, the prolonged intravenous bisphosphonate use is probably the reason for a high incidence of bisphosphonate-related osteonecrosis of the jaw (up to 23 % [37]) in these patients. Furthermore, multiple myeloma patients often undergo aggressive high-dose chemotherapy followed by neutropenia and are mostly treated with multiple chemotherapy regimens during their disease course. Chemotherapy generally has immunosuppressant and antivasculogenic properties, and effects of stem cell depletion induced by high-dose chemotherapy on later wound healing capacity may further increase the risk of bisphosphonate-related osteonecrosis of the jaw. Therefore, the Mayo Clinic consensus statement and the IMWG guidelines recommend that bisphosphonate use should be reduced to 1 or 2 years in patients reaching a plateau phase or complete response. For patients with active disease, therapy frequency can be decreased to every

3 months after 2 years [38]. Despite a higher incidence of bisphosphonate-related osteonecrosis of the jaw in patients receiving zoledronic acid, it has to be taken into account that zoledronic acid has been demonstrated to be superior to pamidronate in preventing skeletal-related events at least in certain subsets of patients [39] and superior to non-nitrogen-containing clodronate not only in reducing skeletal-related events but also in improving event-free and overall survival in multiple myeloma patients [32, 40, 41]. Meta-regression analysis has suggested a borderline significant trend for overall survival based on the bisphosphonate potency, although overall survival does not seem to be different comparing zoledronic acid, pamidronate, and ibandronate in the meta-analysis [41]. Data clearly demonstrating the superiority of zoledronic acid compared to ibandronate in multiple myeloma patients is missing; however, ibandronate is not approved for use in multiple myeloma patients, although the incidence of bisphosphonate-related osteonecrosis of the jaw seems to be lower than with zoledronate treatment [37]. Thus, to date, intravenous zoledronate is the preferred bisphosphonate regimen for multiple myeloma patients.

## Bisphosphonates in Breast Cancer

Breast cancer is the most frequently diagnosed cancer in women of the western population, and bone loss is common throughout the disease course. About 70 % of patients with advanced breast cancer develop bone metastases, a complication that is often painful and potentially leads to debilitating skeletal-related events. In early breast cancer, accelerated bone mineral density loss frequently occurs in the wake of adjuvant therapy. Rate and extent of chemotherapy or endocrine cancer therapy-induced bone loss are often greater than decreases in bone mineral density during menopause. Bisphosphonates such as zoledronic acid are indicated for the treatment of breast cancer bone metastases and reduce the fracture risk by a third [42]. Zoledronate has been shown to also prevent cancer therapy-induced bone loss and improve bone mineral density in premenopausal women receiving adjuvant endocrine or chemotherapy for breast cancer [43].

The benefits of bisphosphonate therapy in breast cancer go beyond maintaining bone health and include potential anticancer effects [43], which are a desirable treatment quality for this patient population with a good prognosis, but a high risk of recurrent disease. In vitro, zoledronic acid displays a particularly strong antitumor effect on primary breast cancer cells, which may be equal or superior to commonly used chemotherapeutic regimens [44]. Preliminary clinical data suggest that bisphosphonate therapy may reduce circulating tumor cell numbers, which are a negative prognostic indicator of disease-free and overall survival in patients with advanced and metastatic disease [45]. Zoledronic acid demonstrated disease-free survival benefits and a 15 % improvement in overall survival in a meta-analysis including 9,518 breast cancer patients [42]. Notably, not all patient subgroups profit equally by bisphosphonate therapy, but the advantage seems to depend on hormone levels, age, and cancer stage. Especially, patients expected to have low estrogen levels, such as premenopausal patients undergoing ovarian suppression and postmenopausal women who were at least 5 years postmenopause, display significant improvement in overall survival. Thus, reproductive hormones seem to be a treatment modifier to take into account [46]. This might also be the reason for a stronger recurrence risk reduction in older patients (especially older than 60 years) compared to younger patients treated with zoledronate, ibandronate, or clodronate [45]. Patients with early-stage breast cancer clearly profit by zoledronate achieving a reduced risk of recurrence, which persists for years even after cessation of zoledronate treatment [45]. However, data in advanced breast cancer is conflicting, and zoledronate may even increase the risk of recurrence in this setting [42]. Generally, oral bisphosphonates do not seem to affect breast cancer recurrence in premenopausal women and yield inconsistent results in postmenopausal women. Thus, current clinical evidence is insufficient to support the use of oral bisphosphonates as a standard adjuvant breast cancer treatment.

In conclusion, zoledronic acid may be considered as standard of care in adjuvant breast cancer therapy, at least for certain patient subgroups as described above [47]. It stands to reason that an early start of bisphosphonate therapy during breast cancer disease course is advantageous. Treatment duration should not generally be restricted, as persistence with zoledronate therapy for more than 12 months is associated with a substantially greater reduction of skeletal-related events compared with zoledronate treatment for 1–3 months [48].

## Bisphosphonates in Prostate Cancer and Other Genitourinary Malignancies

In men, prostate cancer is the most frequent malignancy and the second most common cause of cancer death. Skeletal complications are numerous, either due to bone metastases or as a consequence of androgen deprivation therapy. Complications of bone metastases include bone pain, pathologic fractures, and spinal cord compression [49]. Less common genitourinary malignancies also have a predilection for metastases to the bone. Skeletal metastases have been reported in 20–40 % of patients with stage IV renal cell carcinoma or bladder cancer.

As seen in multiple myeloma and breast cancer patients, positive effects of bisphosphonate therapy in genitourinary malignancies do not only include reduction of skeletal-related events, but also improvement of overall survival. Preclinical studies in models of genitourinary cancers have shown that bisphosphonates can inhibit overall tumor progression, proliferation, invasion, and angiogenesis; activate the immune response against cancer cells; and produce synergistic anticancer effects with cytotoxic agents. Compared to other bisphosphonates, zoledronate demonstrated especially profound direct anticancer activity and synergy with cytotoxic chemotherapy in preclinical studies with prostate cancer cells. The anti-angiogenic effect of zoledronate is especially intriguing in the setting of renal cell carcinoma, characterized by extensive vascularization, and promises to increase the success of anti-angiogenic therapies in metastatic renal cell cancer [36].

Bisphosphonates are frequently used in prostate cancer with bone metastases, although current guidelines recommend their use only in castration-resistant prostate cancer [50]. There is little published guidance for the use of bisphosphonates in renal cell or bladder cancer. Both oral and intravenous bisphosphonates have palliative activity in genitourinary malignancies. Weekly oral alendronate prevents bone loss, increases bone mass, and decreases bone turnover in patients with androgen deprivation therapy for localized prostate cancer [51], and there is evidence that clodronate significantly improves overall survival in patients with prostate M1 disease beginning hormonal therapy. However, to date, zoledronate is the only bisphosphonate having demonstrated significant objective and durable benefits and to have received broad regulatory approval for preventing skeletal-related events in patients with bone metastases from castration-resistant prostate cancer or other genitourinary malignancies. Zoledronate reduces pain scores and proportion of patients with skeletal-related events, prolongs the time to the first skeletal-related event in genitourinary malignancies, and extends the time to disease progression with a trend for prolonged overall survival in renal cell cancer. In patients with bone metastases from bladder cancer, zoledronate increases the 1-year survival rate [36]. There is evidence to apply zoledronate early (i.e., before the first skeletal-related event) in prostate cancer metastatic to the bone, as this strategy is associated with a decreased risk of subsequent skeletal-related events compared to zoledronate treatment started after the first skeletal-related event [52]. Regarding the duration of bisphosphonate therapy, there is no clear recommendation, whether the therapy should be stopped after a finite length of time or extended for as long as it is tolerated. The suspected benefits for overall survival and increased fracture reduction with longer treatment duration revealed in retrospective database analyses argue against general treatment time restrictions in genitourinary malignancies.

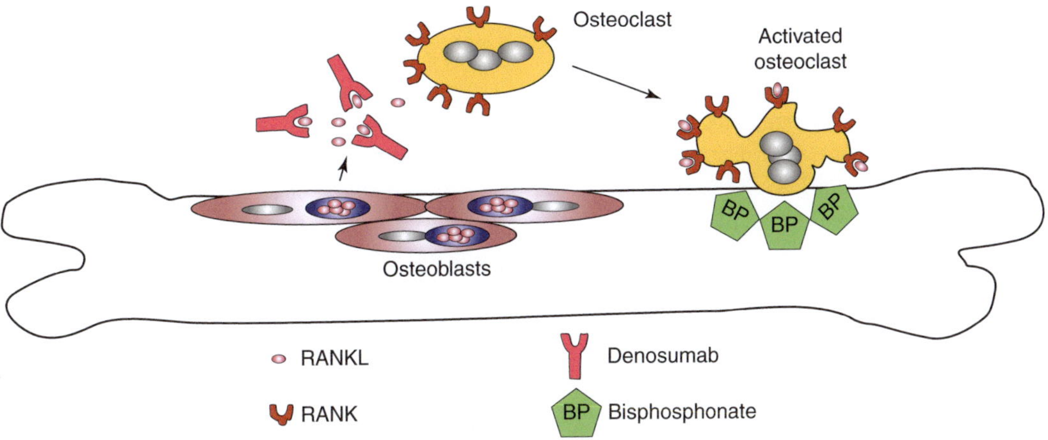


**Fig. 2.1** Mechanisms of action of denosumab and bisphosphonates. RANKL is secreted by osteoblasts and binds to the RANK receptor on osteoclasts, promoting osteoclast differentiation and activation. Denosumab binds RANKL and thereby inhibits the RANKL-RANK pathway. Bisphosphonates bind to the bone and enter and thus inhibit resorption by activated osteoclasts (Modified according to Yee and Raje [54] with kind permission of dove medical press)

## Denosumab as an Alternative to Bisphosphonate Therapy

Denosumab is a fully human monoclonal antibody that neutralizes the receptor activator of nuclear factor κB ligand (RANKL), a member of the tumor necrosis factor receptor superfamily. RANKL is produced by osteoblasts and activates the RANK receptor on osteoclast precursor cells and osteoclasts. The RANKL-RANK signaling pathway is essential for the differentiation, function, and survival of osteoclasts (Fig. 2.1) [53].

Denosumab is injected subcutaneously. Dosing ranges from 60 mg every 6 months in order to preserve bone density in postmenopausal women to 120 mg every 4 weeks in the setting of malignant disease metastatic to the bone. In contrast to bisphosphonates, denosumab does not accumulate in the bone and its effect is reversible after treatment discontinuation. The circulatory half-life is about 26 days [54].

The indications of denosumab are principally similar to bisphosphonates. However, certain aspects have to be taken into account for the therapeutic decision. The efficacy of denosumab in preventing skeletal-related events was demonstrated to be at least equal to zoledronate [55, 56] but seems to partly depend on the disease type. Denosumab treatment in postmenopausal osteoporosis results in a rapid and sustained reduction of bone turnover markers, a marked increase in bone mineral density and a decrease in fracture risk [57]. In breast [58] and prostate cancer [59] patients, suppression of bone turnover markers is greater than by zoledronic acid. In patients with cancer types other than breast or prostate (mainly lung and multiple myeloma) [55], denosumab was equipotent to zoledronate in preventing skeletal-related events.

The side effect profile of denosumab and bisphosphonates is partly overlapping. Especially adverse effects directly mediated by bone remodeling inhibition, namely, osteonecrosis of the jaw (ONJ), occur with similar frequency under treatment with denosumab and zoledronic acid [55, 56]. Acute-phase reactions, which are frequent after zoledronic acid application, occur rarely after denosumab [55]. Yet it has to be taken into account that the RANKL-RANK signaling pathway is not restricted to osteoclastogenesis: RANKL is a co-stimulatory cytokine for T cell activation [60] and lymphocyte development [61]. Concordantly, an increased infection rate was shown in patients with osteoporosis or early breast cancer treated with denosumab [62]. The interference with the immune system may also increase the risk of neoplasms [57]. Importantly, there is evidence hinting at a worse survival in patients with multiple myeloma treated with denosumab compared to zoledronate [55]. Thus, denosumab is thus currently not indicated in the setting of multiple myeloma. On the other hand, preclinical data from animal models of breast cancer and melanoma suggest a role of the RANKL-RANK signaling pathway in tumor genesis and metastasis [63, 64], and limited data indicates that denosumab may reduce disease progression in prostate cancer patients [54]. Furthermore, overall survival was not different in breast [58] and prostate cancer [59] patients treated with denosumab or zoledronic acid. Altogether, data concerning the possible anti-tumor effect of denosumab in comparison with bisphosphonates is still insufficient. The post-market period of denosumab is still comparably short and yet unknown side effects may emerge. Therefore, vigilance regarding adverse events related to possible effects of RANKL inhibition in tissues other than bone or to bone turnover over-suppression is mandatory [65].

In contrast to bisphosphonate clearance, denosumab clearance is largely independent of renal function, since, similarly to other monoclonal antibodies, denosumab is cleared by the reticuloendothelial system [66]. Subsequently, denosumab does not require dose reduction in case of renal dysfunction, is not contradicted in patients with renal failure [54], and thus seems to be the safest treatment option for patients with impaired renal function [65].

Denosumab is cost-effective compared to no treatment for fracture prevention in postmenopausal women with osteoporosis [57]. However, the estimation of the cost-effectiveness in comparison to bisphosphonates depends on the analytical perspective and model parameters and varies in different economic evaluations [67, 68].

Taken together, denosumab may be a suitable alternative to bisphosphonate therapy in certain settings, for example, for patients with postmenopausal osteoporosis or breast or prostate cancer, who suffer from renal impairment or are unable or refuse to take bisphosphonates.

## Conclusions

Bisphosphonates and denosumab are routinely used in the treatment of malignant and nonmalignant diseases with increased osteoclast activity. They effectively reduce skeletal-related events in patients suffering from osteoporosis and metastatic bone disease. Generally, side effects of bisphosphonate and denosumab treatment are infrequent, and they always have to be interpreted with regard to the underlying disease.

## References

1. Berenson JR, et al. American Society of Clinical Oncology clinical practice guidelines: the role of bisphosphonates in multiple myeloma. J Clin Oncol. 2002;20(17):3719–36.
2. Hillner BE, et al. American Society of Clinical Oncology guideline on the role of bisphosphonates in breast cancer. American Society of Clinical Oncology Bisphosphonates Expert Panel. J Clin Oncol. 2000; 18(6):1378–91.
3. Diel IJ, Bergner R, Grotz KA. Adverse effects of bisphosphonates: current issues. J Support Oncol. 2007;5(10):475–82.
4. Honig S, Chang G. Osteoporosis: an update. Bull NYU Hosp Jt Dis. 2012;70(3):140–4.
5. Shkolnikova J, Flynn J, Choong P. Burden of bisphosphonate-associated femoral fractures. ANZ J Surg. 2012;83(3):175–81.
6. Orozco C, Maalouf NM. Safety of bisphosphonates. Rheum Dis Clin North Am. 2012;38(4):681–705.
7. Marx RE. Pamidronate (Aredia) and zoledronate (Zometa) induced avascular necrosis of the jaws: a growing epidemic. J Oral Maxillofac Surg. 2003;61(9):1115–7.
8. Migliorati CA. Bisphosphanates and oral cavity avascular bone necrosis. J Clin Oncol. 2003;21(22): 4253–4.
9. Brandao CM, Machado GP, Acurcio FD. Pharmacoeconomic analysis of strategies to treat postmenopausal osteoporosis: a systematic review. Rev Bras Reumatol. 2012;52(6):924–37.
10. Kanterewicz E, et al. Distribution of serum betaCTX in a population-based study of postmenopausal women taking into account different anti-osteoporotic therapies (the FRODOS Cohort). J Bone Miner Metab. 2012;31(2):231–9.
11. Santos LL, Cavalcanti TB, Bandeira FA. Vascular effects of bisphosphonates-a systematic review. Clin Med Insights Endocrinol Diabetes. 2012;5:47–54.
12. Yates J. A meta-analysis characterizing the dose–response relationships for three oral nitrogen-containing bisphosphonates in postmenopausal women. Osteoporos Int. 2013;24(1):253–62.
13. McClung M, et al. Bisphosphonate therapy for osteoporosis: benefits, risks, and drug holiday. Am J Med. 2013;126(1):13–20.

14. Copley JB, Wuthrich RP. Therapeutic management of post-kidney transplant hyperparathyroidism. Clin Transplant. 2011;25(1):24–39.
15. Torregrosa JV, Ramos AM. Use of bisphosphonates in chronic kidney disease. Nefrologia. 2010;30(3):288–96.
16. Huang WH, et al. Use of alendronate sodium (fosamax) to ameliorate osteoporosis in renal transplant patients: a case–control study. PLoS One. 2012;7(11): e48481.
17. Abediazar S, Nakhjavani MR. Effect of alendronate on early bone loss of renal transplant recipients. Transplant Proc. 2011;43(2):565–7.
18. Torregrosa JV, et al. Open-label trial: effect of weekly risedronate immediately after transplantation in kidney recipients. Transplantation. 2010;89(12):1476–81.
19. Guo Z, et al. The efficacy and safety of bisphosphonates for osteoporosis or osteopenia in Crohn's disease: a meta-analysis. Dig Dis Sci. 2012;58(4): 915–22.
20. Hampson G, Fogelman I. Clinical role of bisphosphonate therapy. Int J Womens Health. 2012;4:455–69.
21. Abdelmoula LC, et al. Bisphosphonates: indications in bone diseases other than osteoporosis. Tunis Med. 2011;89(6):511–6.
22. Le Goff B, et al. Alternative use of bisphosphonate therapy for rheumatic disease. Curr Pharm Des. 2010;16(27):3045–52.
23. Torregrosa JV, et al. Successful treatment of calcific uraemic arteriolopathy with bisphosphonates. Nefrologia. 2012;32(3):329–34.
24. Ruggiero SL. Bisphosphonate-related osteonecrosis of the jaw: an overview. Ann N Y Acad Sci. 2011; 1218:38–46.
25. Coleman RE, McCloskey EV. Bisphosphonates in oncology. Bone. 2011;49(1):71–6.
26. Djulbegovic B, et al. Bisphosphonates in multiple myeloma. Cochrane Database Syst Rev. 2002;(3): CD003188.
27. Guenther A, et al. The bisphosphonate zoledronic acid has antimyeloma activity in vivo by inhibition of protein prenylation. Int J Cancer. 2010;126(1): 239–46.
28. Rennert G, et al. Use of bisphosphonates and reduced risk of colorectal cancer. J Clin Oncol. 2011;29(9): 1146–50.
29. Rennert G, Pinchev M, Rennert HS. Use of bisphosphonates and risk of postmenopausal breast cancer. J Clin Oncol. 2010;28(22):3577–81.
30. Chlebowski RT, et al. Oral bisphosphonate use and breast cancer incidence in postmenopausal women. J Clin Oncol. 2010;28(22):3582–90.
31. Dedes PG, et al. Expression of matrix macromolecules and functional properties of breast cancer cells are modulated by the bisphosphonate zoledronic acid. Biochim Biophys Acta. 2012;1820(12): 1926–39.
32. Morgan GJ, et al. First-line treatment with zoledronic acid as compared with clodronic acid in multiple myeloma (MRC Myeloma IX): a randomised controlled trial. Lancet. 2010;376(9757):1989–99.
33. Morgan GJ, et al. Effects of induction and maintenance plus long-term bisphosphonates on bone disease in patients with multiple myeloma: the Medical Research Council Myeloma IX Trial. Blood. 2012;119(23):5374–83.
34. Thaler R, et al. Ibandronate increases the expression of the pro-apoptotic gene FAS by epigenetic mechanisms in tumor cells. Biochem Pharmacol. 2012;85(2): 173–85.
35. Iguchi K. Effect of bisphosphonates on anticancer activity in prostate cancer cells. Yakugaku Zasshi. 2012;132(9):1025–30.
36. Aapro M, Saad F. Bone-modifying agents in the treatment of bone metastases in patients with advanced genitourinary malignancies: a focus on zoledronic acid. Ther Adv Urol. 2012;4(2):85–101.
37. Then C, et al. Incidence and risk factors of bisphosphonate-related osteonecrosis of the jaw in multiple myeloma patients having undergone autologous stem cell transplantation. Onkologie. 2012;35(11):658–64.
38. Lacy MQ, et al. Mayo clinic consensus statement for the use of bisphosphonates in multiple myeloma. Mayo Clin Proc. 2006;81(8):1047–53.
39. Rosen LS, et al. Zoledronic acid is superior to pamidronate for the treatment of bone metastases in breast carcinoma patients with at least one osteolytic lesion. Cancer. 2004;100(1):36–43.
40. Morgan GJ, et al. Effects of zoledronic acid versus clodronic acid on skeletal morbidity in patients with newly diagnosed multiple myeloma (MRC Myeloma IX): secondary outcomes from a randomised controlled trial. Lancet Oncol. 2011;12(8): 743–52.
41. Mhaskar R, et al. Bisphosphonates in multiple myeloma: a network meta-analysis. Cochrane Database Syst Rev. 2012;(5):CD003188.
42. Huang WW, et al. Zoledronic acid as an adjuvant therapy in patients with breast cancer: a systematic review and meta-analysis. PLoS One. 2012;7(7):e40783.
43. Aft R. Protection of bone in premenopausal women with breast cancer: focus on zoledronic acid. Int J Womens Health. 2012;4:569–76.
44. Fehm T, et al. Antitumor activity of zoledronic acid in primary breast cancer cells determined by the ATP tumor chemosensitivity assay. BMC Cancer. 2012; 12:308.
45. Aft R. Current perspectives on skeletal health and cancer progression across the disease continuum in breast cancer-the role of bisphosphonates. Ecancermedicalscience. 2012;6:265.
46. Coleman R, et al. Effects of bone-targeted agents on cancer progression and mortality. J Natl Cancer Inst. 2012;104(14):1059–67.
47. Gnant M. Adjuvant bisphosphonates: a new standard of care? Curr Opin Oncol. 2012;24(6):635–42.
48. Hatoum HT, et al. Treatment persistence with monthly zoledronic acid is associated with lower risk and frequency of skeletal complications in patients with breast cancer and bone metastasis. Clin Breast Cancer. 2011;11(3):177–83.

49. Berenson JR, et al. Prognostic factors and jaw and renal complications among multiple myeloma patients treated with zoledronic acid. Am J Hematol. 2011;86(1):25–30.
50. Heidenreich A, et al. Therapies used in prostate cancer patients by European urologists: data on indication with a focus on expectations, perceived barriers and guideline compliance related to the use of bisphosphonates. Urol Int. 2012;89(1):30–8.
51. Klotz LH, et al. A phase 3, double-blind, randomised, parallel-group, placebo-controlled study of oral weekly alendronate for the prevention of androgen deprivation bone loss in nonmetastatic prostate cancer: the Cancer and Osteoporosis Research with Alendronate and Leuprolide (CORAL) Study. Eur Urol. 2012;63(5):927–35.
52. Hatoum HT, et al. Zoledronic acid therapy impacts risk and frequency of skeletal complications and follow-up duration in prostate cancer patients with bone metastasis. Curr Med Res Opin. 2011;27(1):55–62.
53. Boyle WJ, Simonet WS, Lacey DL. Osteoclast differentiation and activation. Nature. 2003;423(6937):337–42.
54. Yee AJ, Raje NS. Denosumab, a RANK ligand inhibitor, for the management of bone loss in cancer patients. Clin Interv Aging. 2012;7:331–8.
55. Henry DH, et al. Randomized, double-blind study of denosumab versus zoledronic acid in the treatment of bone metastases in patients with advanced cancer (excluding breast and prostate cancer) or multiple myeloma. J Clin Oncol. 2011;29(9):1125–32.
56. Qi WX, et al. Risk of osteonecrosis of the jaw in cancer patients receiving denosumab: a meta-analysis of seven randomized controlled trials. Int J Clin Oncol. 2013;19(2):403–10.
57. Sutton EE, Riche DM. Denosumab, a RANK ligand inhibitor, for postmenopausal women with osteoporosis. Ann Pharmacother. 2012;46(7–8):1000–9.
58. Stopeck AT, et al. Denosumab compared with zoledronic acid for the treatment of bone metastases in patients with advanced breast cancer: a randomized, double-blind study. J Clin Oncol. 2010;28(35):5132–9.
59. Fizazi K, et al. Denosumab versus zoledronic acid for treatment of bone metastases in men with castration-resistant prostate cancer: a randomised, double-blind study. Lancet. 2011;377(9768):813–22.
60. Wong BR, et al. TRANCE is a novel ligand of the tumor necrosis factor receptor family that activates c-Jun N-terminal kinase in T cells. J Biol Chem. 1997;272(40):25190–4.
61. Kong YY, et al. OPGL is a key regulator of osteoclastogenesis, lymphocyte development and lymph-node organogenesis. Nature. 1999;397(6717):315–23.
62. Anastasilakis AD, et al. Efficacy and safety of denosumab in postmenopausal women with osteopenia or osteoporosis: a systematic review and a meta-analysis. Horm Metab Res. 2009;41(10):721–9.
63. Schramek D, et al. Osteoclast differentiation factor RANKL controls development of progestin-driven mammary cancer. Nature. 2010;468(7320):98–102.
64. Jones DH, et al. Regulation of cancer cell migration and bone metastasis by RANKL. Nature. 2006;440(7084):692–6.
65. Anastasilakis AD, et al. Long-term treatment of osteoporosis: safety and efficacy appraisal of denosumab. Ther Clin Risk Manag. 2012;8:295–306.
66. Baron R, Ferrari S, Russell RG. Denosumab and bisphosphonates: different mechanisms of action and effects. Bone. 2011;48(4):677–92.
67. Carter JA, Botteman MF. Health-economic review of zoledronic acid for the management of skeletal-related events in bone-metastatic prostate cancer. Expert Rev Pharmacoecon Outcomes Res. 2012;12(4):425–37.
68. Hiligsmann M, et al. Cost-effectiveness of denosumab in the treatment of postmenopausal osteoporotic women. Expert Rev Pharmacoecon Outcomes Res. 2013;13(1):19–28.

# Risk Factors for Medication-Related Osteonecrosis of the Jaw

**3**

Tae-Geon Kwon


**Abstract**

The clinician should attempt to determine the risk factors for a disease before treatment in order to prevent disease development. Even though numerous clinical case series have reported Medication-related osteonecrosis of the jaw (MRONJ) after intravenous or oral route administration of bisphosphonates (BPs), evidence-based research regarding risk factors is sparse. Currently, the route of administration, dose and duration of intake, nitrogen-containing BPs, and dental infection/dental invasive procedures can be suggested as risk factors for MRONJ. Recently, a human monoclonal antibody inhibiting osteoclasts, denosumab, has been introduced as an antiresorptive drug. The reported risk of denosumab-related osteonecrosis of the jaw (DRONJ) seems similar or slightly higher compared with intravenous intake of nitrogen-containing BPs. Dental extractions and oncological dosing could be related to an increased risk of DRONJ. There are also increasing reports of osteonecrosis of the jaw related with antiangiogenic chemotherapeutics.


## Terminology of Osteonecrosis of the Jaw

### Avascular/Ischemic Necrosis of the Jaw

Osteonecrosis usually refers to the death of bone resulting from a transient or permanent disruption of blood supply to the bone. An impaired blood supply causes avascular necrosis of the bone, which can be frequently found in long bones such as the femur head. In the orthopedic field, this is called "aseptic necrosis," "avascular necrosis," or "ischemic necrosis." In the oral and maxillofacial field, osteonecrosis of the jaw (ONJ) can frequently develop after radiation therapy. Radiation-induced osteoradionecrosis (ORN) is characterized by avascular necrosis with hypoxic, hypocellular, and hypovascular lesions [1]. Other conditions, such as local vascular insufficiency from thromboembolism or secondary to osteomyelitis and a pathological process after experiencing trauma, are also related to osteonecrosis [2, 3].

In 2003, a new type of ONJ was reported in relation to nitrogen-containing bisphosphonate


T.-G. Kwon, DDS, PhD
Department of Oral and Maxillofacial Surgery,
School of Dentistry, Kyungpook National University,
Samduck 2 Ga, Jungu, Daegu 700-412,
Republic of Korea
e-mail: kwondk@knu.ac.kr, taegeonkwon@gmail.com



S. Otto (ed.), *Medication-Related Osteonecrosis of the Jaws: Bisphosphonates, Denosumab, and New Agents*,
DOI 10.1007/978-3-662-43733-9_3, © Springer-Verlag Berlin Heidelberg 2015

(BP) administration, which has become known as "bisphosphonate-related osteonecrosis of the jaw" (BRONJ). Like avascular necrosis in the femoral head, this was first termed "avascular necrosis of the jaw" [4–6] because the etiological background was not completely understood at the time of the initial reports. Various clinical and experimental studies had already proved that BPs inhibit angiogenesis [7–10] or blood flow in bone [11]. However, if BRONJ is simply avascular necrosis, as in the hip or knee joint, it is difficult to explain why this necrosis develops almost exclusively in the jaw [12, 13]. Moreover, pathological specimens from BRONJ lesions are not completely avascular in humans [14] or animals [15]. Interestingly, there is various clinical and experimental evidence showing that BP administration is potentially beneficial for the treatment of femoral head avascular necrosis [16–18]. Nowadays, the term "avascular necrosis of the jaw" is no longer used for ONJ related to BP treatment.

## Bisphosphonate-Induced, -Related, or -Associated Jaw Necrosis

Osteonecrosis of the jaw after administration of bisphosphonates has been referred to in the literature by several different acronyms, including BIOJ (bisphosphonate-*induced* osteonecrosis of the jaw) [19], BAONJ (bisphosphonate-associated osteonecrosis of the jaw) [20, 21], or BRONJ (bisphosphonate-*related* osteonecrosis of the jaw) [22]. The term "*associated*" implies that BP is assumed to be the cause of the ONJ, whereas "*related*" implies that the BP was confirmed to be the cause of ONJ. The term "*induced*" represents a more direct cause–effect relationship. These three terms are widely used depending upon the authors' understanding of the pathogenesis of ONJ after bisphosphonate treatment. To emphasize the influence of immunity and infections, rather than being aseptic or avascular in origin, some reports insist on using the term "bisphosphonate-associated osteomyelitis of the jaw" [23]. In this chapter, the definition and staging system of ONJ after BP treatment followed the guideline of the AAOMS position paper [2], which uses the term "BRONJ."

In summary, although the term "bisphosphonate-*related* osteonecrosis of the jaw, BRONJ" can be changed if another pathophysiological background is elucidated, this is the most widely used term to reasonably characterize this disease. Since recent reports on the osteonecrosis of the jaw after administration of denosumab were published, the term "antiresorptive drug-induced osteonecrosis of the jaw (ARONJ)" has been proposed.

Recent AAOMS position paper 2014 suggested the term "medication-related osteonecrosis of the jaw (MRONJ)" [24]. This change reflects the increasing number of ONJ reports after antiresorptive (denosumab) and antiangiogenic agents (bevacizumab, sunitinib) administration. In this chapter, the risk factors for bisphosphonate-, denosumab- and antiangiogenic agent-related ONJ are discussed

## Risk Factors for BRONJ

### Introduction

Between 2003, when the initial scientific reports on BRONJ appeared [4, 5, 25], and 2009, more than 670 articles on BRONJ were published [26]. However, only a limited number of the reports were based on randomized and controlled trials. Additionally, there is not much evidence for the risk factors for BRONJ owing to the lack of an appropriate control group in many studies. Because of the low incidence and long-term incubation time of ONJ after bisphosphonate administration, it is nearly impossible to have a matched control group that is composed of patients receiving BPs owing to osteoporosis but without ONJ. At the same time, there are many confounding factors with regard to BRONJ development in elderly patients with systemic disease. Investigating the risk factors in elderly, osteoporotic patients is fundamentally difficult. Therefore, an analysis of the risk factors has been more frequently reported in patients who have taken intravenous bisphosphonates for malignant bone disease compared with oral bisphosphonates for osteoporosis. The determination of BRONJ risk factors has been largely dependent on data from cancer patients. However, it is difficult to discriminate between the complications that are attributed to BP administration itself and the morbidity of the cancer treatment process. To clarify risk factors, further investigation with adequate study design is needed to ensure an acceptable level of evidence. In this text, the proposed risk factors for BRONJ from previous articles are discussed, with a critical review (Table 3.1).

## Bisphosphonate Administration Itself: Type, Drug, Route, and Dose

The chemical structure of amino-bisphosphonates is characterized by the existence of nitrogen in the R-side chain, which ensures a stronger potency of the drug [3]. There is no doubt that these nitrogen-containing bisphosphonates predominantly cause BRONJ compared with non-nitrogen-containing bisphosphonates. Therefore, most of the studies on BRONJ focus on nitrogen-containing bisphosphonates (zoledronate, pamidronate, ibandronate, alendronate, risedronate, etc.) [27]. It has been reported that intravenous bisphosphonate administration (e.g., zoledronate and pamidronate) carries a higher risk of ONJ development compared with oral bisphosphonates [19, 28–32]. Bisphosphonates are actively prescribed to patients diagnosed with metastatic breast cancer, prostate cancer or multiple myeloma (MM), and the related hypercalcemia [33]. To inhibit osteolytic activity and treat the hypercalcemia from metastatic bone disease, bisphosphonates are widely used to prevent pathological fracture and pain from malignant bone disease. According to a review of previously published case series of 368 BRONJ patients (1966–2006), zoledronic acid comprised 35 % and pamidronate comprised 31 % of the total cases. Oral bisphosphonates (alendronate, risedronate, ibandronate) comprised only 4.8 % of the total cases [34]. The lower incidence of BRONJ by oral bisphosphonates could be attributed to differences in pharmacological efficiency between oral and intravenous bisphosphonates. Oral bisphosphonates have a low absorption rate (<1 %) in the gastrointestinal tract, whereas more than 50 % of the intravenous bisphosphonates are incorporated into the bone [35, 36]. The dose of bisphosphonates for cancer treatment is up to 12 times higher than for osteoporosis [37, 38].

## Intravenous Bisphosphonates

Many reports have revealed zoledronate to be associated with a high risk of osteonecrosis compared with pamidronate or other bisphosphonates [39–43]. Vahtsevanos et al. [44] and Hoff et al. [43] reported that having a history of zoledronic acid treatment increased 15-fold the relative risk of BRONJ. Pamidronate-related BRONJ data have shown that each additional year of administration increased the BRONJ risk up to 1.7 times [45]. This has been attributed to the more potent inhibitory action of zoledronate on bone turnover than that of pamidronate [46–48]. Zoledronate has an inhibitory effect on the bone turnover rate that is 10–100 times more powerful [46]. However, BP potency itself cannot explain all the reasons for the higher risk of BRONJ development after zoledronate treatment compared with pamidronate. For example, the relative inhibition of bone remodeling for ibandronate is ten times more than that of pamidronate [49]. However, ibandronate showed a 92 % reduced risk of BRONJ development in a longitudinal cohort study [44] or a very low incidence of BRONJ development when it was administered as a single medication [48]. Thumbigere-Math et al. [32] also reported that there was no significant difference in the cumulative dose of ibandronate in patients treated with ibandronate, whereas zoledronate and pamidronate had a significantly higher mean cumulative dose.

Among the patients exposed to intravenous bisphosphonates, around 1 % of the patients developed BRONJ at 1 year after treatment, which increased to 13 % at 4 years cumulatively [42]. Another report also showed that the cumulative danger of developing BRONJ reached 1 % after 1 year of administration and up to 20 % after 3 years [41]. Prolonged duration of BP administration [29, 32, 42, 43, 50] and an increased cumulative dose have been reported to be significant risk factors for BRONJ [32, 43, 48,

**Table 3.1** Significant risk factors for bisphosphonates-related osteonecrosis of the jaw (BRONJ). (Reprinted with kind permission of Springer Science + Business Media)

| Reference | Year | Type of study | Cause of BP treatment | No. of BRONJ patients | Control group | BP type in BRONJ | Risk factors significantly associated with BRONJ development |
|---|---|---|---|---|---|---|---|
| Sedghizadeh et al. [83] | 2013 | Retrospective study (population pharmacokinetic model) | Osteoporosis and cancer | 69 | 84 | A, 55 % Z, 20 % (Oral 71 %) | Longer duration BP, older age, and Asian race |
| Thumbigere-Math et al. [32] | 2012 | Retrospective study | Carcinoma (MM, breast and prostate carcinoma) | 18 | 558 | Z, 55.5 % P+Z, 39 % | High risk in zoledronate, hypothyroidism, smoking, diabetes, longer duration, and increased number of BP treatments |
| Vahtsevanos et al. [44] | 2009 | Longitudinal cohort (with vs without ONJ) | MM and cancer | 80 | 1,541 | Z, 97.5 % P, 20.0 % I, 3.8 % | Higher risk in dental extraction, denture use. More patients with MM than breast cancer, ibandronate and pamidronate showed a lower risk than zoledronate |
| Fehm et al. [50] | 2009 | Retrospective study | Breast carcinoma | 10 | 335 | Z, 70 % | Increased number and duration of BP |
| Mauri et al. [120] | 2009 | Meta-analysis from 15 RCT | Adjuvant breast carcinoma Tx. | 13 | 5312 | Z, 100 % | High risk in zoledronate |
| Boonyapakorn et al. [41] | 2008 | Prospective study | MM & carcinoma | 22 | 58 | Z, 64 %; P, 14 % | High risk in zoledronate (3.5 times higher than others), MM &and breast cancer, long-term use (>2.5 years) increases risk |
| Wessel et al. [66] | 2008 | Case–control | Carcinoma | 30 | 150 | | High risk in zoledronate, obesity, and smoking |
| Jadu et al. [45] | 2007 | Retrospective study (only P treatment) | MM | 24 | 120 | P, 100 % | Longer duration of BP, dental extractions, cyclophosphamide therapy, prednisone therapy, erythropoietin therapy, low hemoglobin levels, renal dialysis, and advanced age |
| Dimopoulos et al. [42] | 2006 | Prospective study | MM | 15 | 187 | Z, 47 % P+Z, 40 % | High risk in zoledronate |
| Bamias et al. [29] | 2005 | Retrospective study | Carcinoma (MM, breast, and prostate carcinoma) | 17 | 252 | Z, 41 % P+Z, 53 % | Total number and duration of BP exposure, high risk in zoledronate |

*BP* bisphosphonate; *A* alendronate; *P* pamidronate; *Z* zoledronate; *MM* multiple myeloma

50], especially for longer durations of zoledronate treatment [44]. The median exposure time for BRONJ development was 12–24 months for zoledronate, 19–30 months for pamidronate, and 13–21.5 months for ibandronate [32, 41–43]. It is unknown why BRONJ is more frequently reported in multiple myeloma and breast cancer patients than in prostate and renal cancer patients and in patients with Paget's disease. A possible explanation is the relatively longer duration and greater cumulative dose of bisphosphonate medication for multiple myeloma and breast cancer patients than that for the other diseases [43]. In general, development of BRONJ is associated with the combined effect of dose, duration, and potency of the bisphosphonates [43].

## Oral Bisphosphonates

The reported incidence of orally induced BRONJ is very low. According to the data from the Merck company, the estimated incidence of BRONJ after alendronate treatment was 0.7 cases per 100,000 person-years' exposure [51]. A population-based study from Australia [30] showed that weekly alendronate can possibly result in 0.01–0.04 % of cases developing BRONJ. A recent epidemiological investigation by a mail survey revealed a 0.1 % prevalence of BRONJ after oral bisphosphonate intake [52], which is higher than previously reported data from the company. Case–control studies have shown that oral treatment with BP is the definitive risk factor for ONJ [53, 54]. ONJ related to oral bisphosphonates comprised 15.3 % of the total number of BRONJ cases reported (a review of the literature 2003–2009 by Filleul et al. [55]) and was 7.8 % of the cases in an European multicenter study [56] and 39.5 % of the cases in a Japanese multicenter study [57]. Most of the BRONJ cases derived from oral BP treatment (oral BRONJ) were related to alendronate [52, 58–61].

Because the prevalence of oral BRONJ is quite low, it is difficult to determine significant risk factors. According to the American Association of Oral and Maxillofacial Surgeons (AAOMS) position paper [2], oral BRONJ risk increases when the duration of intake exceeds 3 years. However, there was no supporting scientific evidence for this notion. A nationwide survey in Japan [57] showed that the duration of bisphosphonate administration before ONJ onset was 33.2 months (0.2–135 months), whereas it was 23.6 months (1.2–103 months) for intravenous bisphosphonate intake. Fleisher et al. [62] reported a median 3 years for intravenous bisphosphonates and 5 years for oral bisphosphonates before the onset of ONJ. Other reports also showed similar periods of time before the onset of oral BRONJ: mean 48.8 months [53], 57.8 months [56], 66.5 months [60] or median 52.8 months [61]. Barasch et al. [54] reported that BRONJ risk begins within 2 years of bisphosphonate administration for both cancer and osteoporosis patients. This risk of BRONJ in non-cancer patients increased substantially after 5 years of BP treatment. These data reveal that oral BP-related ONJ was usually reported to develop between 2.5 and 5.5 years after BP treatment. This implies that oral BRONJ can also exist even without a long incubation time. Therefore, patients receiving oral BP for more than 2.5–3 years should be closely monitored.

Bisphosphonates have a long half-life. In particular, alendronate suppresses the bone turnover marker up to 5 years after cessation of the drug [63]. Patients without malignant bone disease receive BP for longer periods of time and may have a greater possibility of accumulating a higher dose of BP. If these BP-treated patients experience local risk factors, the number of BRONJ cases could be increased in the future.

## Systemic Risk Factors (Underlying Disease, Co-Morbidities, and Co-Medications)

### Intravenous Bisphosphonate Intake

Initial reports for case series of BRONJ showed that the medical comorbidities of the patients were chemotherapy, corticosteroid use, diabetes, smoking, alcohol abuse, low body weight, menopause, and old age [19]. Usually, chemotherapeutic agents and corticosteroids are commonly used for metastatic bone disease, with delayed wound healing being one of the inevitable adverse side effects of these treatments

[24]. According to Jadu et al. [45], antineoplastic drugs (cyclophosphamide) and corticosteroids increased the risk of BRONJ in multiple myeloma patients. In some reports, chemotherapy was significantly related to BRONJ development [32, 41, 48]. However, high-dose chemotherapy accompanies long-term BP treatment, and it is difficult to define delayed wound healing or bone exposure that would be attributed solely to the chemotherapy. Corticosteroid treatment has been reported to be one of the significant risk factors for BRONJ in a retrospective case–control study [45]. However, other reports have failed to find a statistical difference between the number of steroid users in BRONJ and the control group [29, 41, 43, 64–66]. The dose and duration of the corticosteroid treatment varies widely depending on the patients' disease and condition; thus, the contribution of corticosteroids to BRONJ development needs further investigation with a proper study design.

Other systemic risk factors are erythropoietin therapy [45], renal dialysis [45], and diabetes [32, 67]. Hypothyroidism was also reported to be associated with BRONJ development [32]. The exact mechanism of such risk factors in BRONJ onset needs to be investigated further. However, asthma, dyslipidemia, and hypertension have not been reported to be significant risk factors [36, 67].

### Oral Bisphosphonate Intake

It has been proven that oral BP increases ONJ risk [53, 54, 68]. However, in some reports, there was no significant effect of oral BP on ONJ development [66, 69]. This might be attributed to the limited number of cohort studies or case–control studies that can ensure an adequate level of scientific evidence. Therefore, the reported risk factor for BRONJ related to oral BP was based on the frequency of co-morbidity in a case series. Patients without systemic or local risk factors rarely develop BRONJ after oral bisphosphonate intake alone. A retrospective cohort study of 30 oral BRONJ patients [61] showed that diabetes (33 %) and systemic inflammatory disorders (20 %) involving long-term corticosteroid use (23 %) were the most common co-morbidities. A recent retrospective multicenter study showed that hypertension (40.2 %) and diabetes (9.2 %) were the major co-morbidities [58]. In some

reports, hypertension or cardiac disease was the most frequent systemic disease in oral BRONJ patients [70, 71]. Another report revealed that patients with BRONJ from oral BP who had comorbid conditions experienced prolonged healing times and reduced healing [61]. Therefore, systemic comorbidities need to be considered before treatment. However, these are "systemic comorbidities" and more scientific supporting data should be accumulated to confirm the "significant risk factors" related to oral BRONJ.

### Local Risk Factors (Infections, Extractions, Pressure Sores, etc.)

It has been clearly shown that dental risk factors such as invasive dental procedures (dental extraction), denture irritation, and periodontitis are related to BRONJ development [65]. Hoff et al. [43] reported that dental extraction increases the hazard ratio 9.9 times in multiple myeloma patients and 53.2 times in breast cancer patients. A longitudinal cohort study in cancer patients also showed an 18-fold elevated risk of BRONJ after extraction and a two-fold increase after denture irritation [44]. Dental surgical procedures increased the incidence of BRONJ as high as 5.3-fold [45] or seven-fold [64].

The healing process of a dental extraction site reflects the systemic wound healing capacity. Blood clot formation after extraction leads to granulated tissue and finally mineralization to an osseous structure. Because bisphosphonates accumulate in skeletal sites with high bone turnover, such as the maxilla or mandible [72], BP-bound osseous tissue resorbs slowly. This bacterially contaminated bone cannot be readily resorbed, and this prolonged open wound increases the risk of bacterial invasion. This can result in a favorable environment for the development of chronic osteomyelitis [73, 74].

Periodontal disease is one of the possible risk factors for BRONJ. Inflammation generally decreases the pH level and this acidic milieu leads to the protonated activation of nitrogen-containing BP [75, 76]. A recent investigation with a periodontitis-associated microbe showed that periodontitis is one of the significant risk factors for BRONJ in cancer patients [77].

The incidence of mandibular BRONJ is higher than that for maxillary BRONJ [19, 28, 41] and it is more common at sites with thin overlying mucosa, such as exostoses, the sharp mylohyoid ridge, and the mandibular torus [2, 78].

According to the literature, around 20 % [58], 28 % [59], 33 % [61], and 57 % [56] of oral BRONJ can be "spontaneous BRONJ," which means the absence of systemic or local risk factors or co-morbidities in BRONJ development. Further studies are needed for this type of BRONJ. Some authors have reported that osteonecrosis does not begin with aseptic necrosis, but is in fact "osteomyelitis from the very beginning" [79]. However, the presence of this spontaneous BRONJ supports the theory, at least in part, that osteonecrosis is primarily an aseptic process and that an infection develops afterward [80, 81].

## Host Factor

Age has been suggested to be one of the risk factors for BRONJ in malignant bone disease [29, 40, 45, 82]. Each additional year of life increases the risk by 1.1 times [45]. However, a report has shown that after statistical adjustment, old age did not increase the BRONJ risk in a cohort study [44]. Gender was not significantly associated with BRONJ [2]. Smoking has been proposed to be a significant risk factor [32, 66]. Obesity has also been suggested to be a risk factor [66]. Sedghizadeh et al. [83] carried out a pharmacokinetic study and showed that Asians are more susceptible to BRONJ than Caucasians, Hispanics, and African–Americans. The authors suggested that Asians have a lower body weight, and a smaller skeletal compartment that might result in drug accumulation and thereby, higher concentrations over time, as well as increased toxicity. However, there is no consensus on the reported risk factors related to these host factors.

## Genetic Risk Factors

Various factors have been suggested to be related to BRONJ development. A possible association with genetic factors has also been proposed by several investigators. Several genome-wide association studies [84, 85] have proposed that the single nucleotide polymorphism (SNP) of the cytochrome P450, the subfamily of the 2C polypeptide 8 (CYP2C8, rs1934951), in multiple myeloma patients, showed a significant association with BRONJ. CYP2C8 is mainly expressed in the liver and known to be related to drug metabolism and clearance [86]. However, other researchers could not find such a relationship between BRONJ and CYP2C8 SNP [87, 88]. This inconsistency might be attributed to the fundamental limitation in collecting homogeneous case and control groups. Another genetic polymorphism in the RBMS3 (rs17024608) gene was suggested to carry a high risk of BRONJ development [89]. Because these genetic investigations need a large amount of genotyping to increase the statistical power, further large genetic studies are needed to identify susceptible genes involved in BRONJ development.

## Surrogate Markers for BRONJ Risk

Bone remodeling is the combined process of bone resorption and bone formation. Prevention of skeletal-related events (SRE) of BP is attributed to reduced bone remodeling rather than bone formation [63]. Various bone turnover markers, such as CTX (C-terminal telopeptide), NTX (N-terminal telopeptide), PYD (pyridinoline), DPD (deoxypyridinoline), and P1NP (N-terminal propeptide of type 1 procollagen) are now widely used in clinical practice to diagnose specific bone diseases [90]. In particular, serum bone resorption markers have been utilized to determine the guidelines for osteoporosis treatment with BPs [91, 92]. BP treatment decreases bone turnover to 60–70 % below the baseline level [93].

It has been proposed that over-suppression of bone turnover may be related to the development of BRONJ [60] and bone turnover markers such as CTX have been recommended to determine the risk for BRONJ or to determine treatment options [60, 94]. Other reports also mentioned that CTX may be used for risk assessment [95]. However, these previous results were based on case series without a control group. Kunchur et al. [96] first reported the results of a case–control study. They reported that a CTX

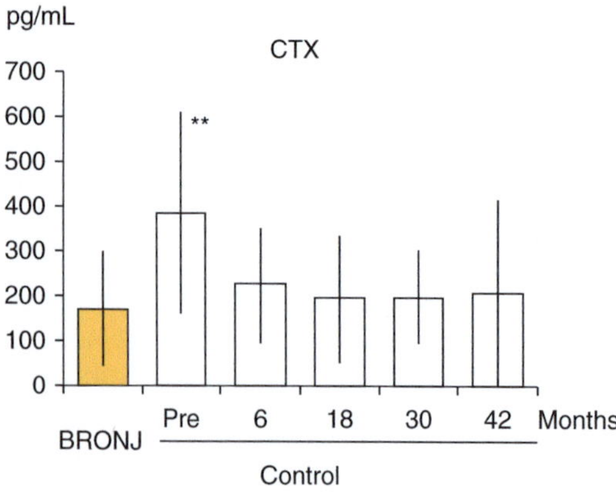

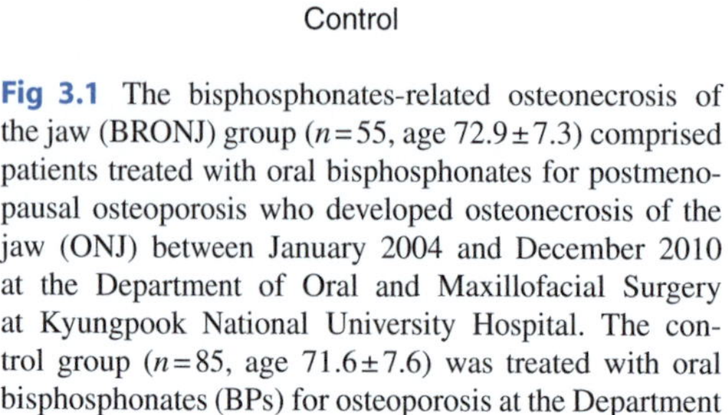

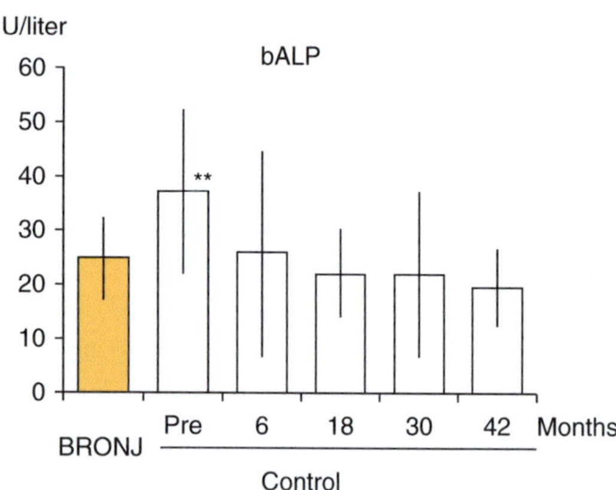

**Fig 3.1** The bisphosphonates-related osteonecrosis of the jaw (BRONJ) group ($n = 55$, age $72.9 \pm 7.3$) comprised patients treated with oral bisphosphonates for postmenopausal osteoporosis who developed osteonecrosis of the jaw (ONJ) between January 2004 and December 2010 at the Department of Oral and Maxillofacial Surgery at Kyungpook National University Hospital. The control group ($n = 85$, age $71.6 \pm 7.6$) was treated with oral bisphosphonates (BPs) for osteoporosis at the Department of Orthopedics, but did not have any signs or symptoms of jaw necrosis. Biochemical markers of BRONJ patients at the time of diagnosis (*yellow bar*) compared with the control patients before (Pre) and 6, 18, 30, and 42 months after oral bisphosphonate (alendronate, risedronate, pamidronate, and ibandronate) administration (*empty bars*). *CTX* C-terminal telopeptide of collagen type I, *bALP* bone-specific alkaline phosphatase. (** $p < 0.01$, Comparison between BRONJ patients and individual time points of the control group (Reprinted with kind permission of Springer Science + Business Media))

value of $< 150$ pg/ml did not correlate with the clinical risk factors of age, gender, co-morbidities, bone disease, or bisphosphonate duration, but stated that CTX can reflect a "risk zone ($<150–200$ pg/ml)" because the initial CTX values of BRONJ at the time of diagnosis were less than 200 pg/ml. If these are true, the CTX values can be used for assessing BRONJ risk and guidelines for a drug holiday, which may be beneficial in preventing BRONJ. However, various researchers greatly criticize the use of CTX as BRONJ marker, and their opinions have been expressed as 'letters to the editor' [97], case reports [98], or review articles [90, 99–101].

A recent case–control study with bisphosphonate patients reported that the serum CTX level has a limitation in showing BRONJ development [102, 103]. According to data from the author's hospital, CTX level after long-term BP treatment in the control patients was not statistically different from the BRONJ patients (Fig. 3.1). Kim et al. [102] carried out a case–control study that compared 37 BRONJ patients with 37 age- and gender-matched control patients (BP cover $> 24$ months, but without ONJ). Along with osteocalcin, DPD, NTX, and bone-specific alkaline phosphatase, CTX value did not show any differences between the case and control groups. The result revealed that it is discouraged to use bone turnover markers for BRONJ risk estimation.

Utilizing the surrogate markers of bone resorption to predict BRONJ risk has the following limitations. First, systemic bone turnover markers cannot readily reflect the maxillary and mandibular bone condition. Second, bone metastasis influences the CTX level in cancer patients. Therefore, the CTX level in these cancer patients covering BP is influenced by both factors; the BP administration itself and the bone metastasis condition [101, 104]. Third, according to histomorphometric analysis, some osteoporosis patients already show greatly suppressed bone remodeling before BP treatment [105]. Therefore, based on the current data, use of the CTX value as a predictor of BRONJ risk or disease progression cannot be supported.

In summary, nitrogen-containing bisphosphonates, intravenous route of administration, higher dose and longer duration of intake, and dental infections/dental surgical treatments can be regarded as "known" risk factors. However, other risk factors, particularly associated with oral BP-related ONJ, need further study with more sophisticated scientific investigation. Up to now, there has been no evidence for using bone resorption markers to predict BRONJ risk.

## Risk Factors for Denosumab-Related ONJ

Denosumab is a human monoclonal antibody against the receptor activator of nuclear factor kappa-B ligand (RANKL). Denosumab inhibits the RANKL, an important mediator of osteoclastic differentiation [106]. As an antiresorptive agent, denosumab reduces osteoclastogenesis and is widely used for the treatment of metastatic bone disease and osteoporosis [107–110]. It had been proposed that inhibition of RANK–RANKL interaction by denosumab may also influence monocyte migration and decrease cell survival [111], which may be related to ONJ development. However, the exact similarities and difference between the BRONJ and denosumab-related ONJ (DRONJ) have not yet been clearly understood.

Denosumab is usually administered via subcutaneous injection of 60 mg every 6 months (for osteoporosis or prevention of skeletal-related events (SRE)) or 120 mg monthly (for oncological conditions or bone metastasis). Unlike bisphosphonates, denosumab is not incorporated into the bone matrix and has a relatively short half life. Even though the denosumab shows the higher efficacy in preventing skeletally related events and a lower rate of renal complications in cancer patients, the occurrence of the ONJ was similar (zoledronate 1.3 %, denosumab 1.8 %) [112] or rather higher but not statistically significantly higher (zoledronate 1 %, denosumab 2 %) [107] than in zoledronate-treated patients.

The reported incidence of DRONJ ranges from 0 % to 4.7 % [112–116]. In a recent meta-analysis of seven randomized controlled trials for 8,963 patients with solid tumors, such as prostate or breast cancer, the overall incidence of DRONJ was 1.7 % (95 % CI, 0.9–3.1 %). Denosumab administration increased the risk of ONJ development compared with a control placebo group (RR 16.28, 95 % CI: 1.68–158.05, $p=0.017$), although the increase in risk between denosumab and bisphosphonates was not statistically significant (RR 1.48, 95 % CI: 0.96–2.29, $p=0.078$) [117]. However, denosumab (60 mg) treatment every 6 months for prostate cancer patients did not result in any ONJ development (DRONJ, $n=0/1,468$ patients) [115]. Another study also showed a very low incidence of ONJ ($n=2/2,207$) after 60 mg of denosumab every 6 months for 2 years in patients with postmenopausal osteoporosis [118].

According to the analysis of 37 cases of BRONJ (zoledronate) and 52 cases of DRONJ, related oral events were tooth extraction (64.9 % in BRONJ, 59.6 % in DRONJ) and oral infection (45.9 % in BRONJ, 50.0 % in DRONJ). The mandible carried a higher risk than the maxilla (mandible:maxilla=83.8 %:13.5 % in BRON, 65.4 %:28.8 % in DRONJ). The cumulative incidence of DRONJ was 0.8 % in the first year, 1.8 % in the second year, and 1.8 % in the third year, which was slightly higher but not statistically significantly higher than for BRONJ [116]. Denosumab for the treatment of giant cell tumors of the bone resulted in 1 % ($n=3/281$) ONJ, which occurred roughly 13–20 months after treatment initiation [119].

Based on the limited number of studies in the current literature, the oncological dose of denosumab (monthly 120 mg), the intraoral surgical trauma, and the local site (mandible) may be suggested to be risk factors related to DRONJ. Therefore, the related risk factors for DRONJ may not be significantly different from those for BRONJ. Further investigation is needed to clarify the risk factors related to these antiresorptive drugs to minimize ONJ after drug administration.

In the process of malignant tumor development, angiogenesis is critical for tumor growth, infiltration, and distant/regional metastasis [121]. Recently, angiogenic inhibitors targeting the vascular endothelial growth factors (VEGF) with tyrosine kinase inhibitors (TKIs), monoclonal antibody or mammalian target of rapamycin (mTOR) pathway are used for chemotherapeutic agents to treat advanced carcinoma or metastatic bone disease [122]. Recombinant monoclonal immunoglobulin antibody, bevacizumab, blocks the all isoforms of VEGF-A and can suppress cancer progression and bone metastasis [123]. Tyrosine kinas inhibitor such as sunitinib or sorafenib inhibits neoangiogenesis by targeting the VEGF receptors, platelet-derived growth factor receptors (PDGFR), macrophage colony-stimulating factor (M-CSF) and other signaling pathways [124]. Inhibitors of mTOR, sirolimus or everolimus, also suppress angiogenesis and are frequently used for advanced or metastatic carcinoma [125]. These antiangiogenic agents were approved for various cancers such as renal cell carcinoma with or without metastasis, gastrointestinal stromal tumors or metastatic colorectal carcinoma [126].

There are several clinical investigations and case reports of ONJ in patients treated with these antiangiogenic agents for chemotherapeutic medication. After first report of bevacizumab-related ONJ in 2008 [127], various case reports had been published ONJ after bevacizumab administration without association with BPs [128–131]. According to the randomized, prospective clinical trials from Guarneri et al. [128], the ONJ incidence were 0.2% in bevacizumab treatment and 0.9% in combined BP and bevacizumab administration for breast cancer patients. Other case series reported four ONJ cases after combined use of BPs with bevacizumab or sunitinib out of 22 patients who had been treated with this combination therapy (16% of incidence) [132]. It had been suggested increased incidence of ONJ after concomitant BP and sunitinib based on the clinical cases [133] or on retrospective review of 46 patients [122]. The ONJ incidence after combined BP and TKIs were 0% (n = 0/35) [134] to 10% (n = 5/52)[135]. ONJ development only after sunitinib application without BPs had also been reported [124, 136, 137]. mTOR inhibitor everolimus was also reported to be related with ONJ [138]. Therefore, recent AAOMS position paper on MRONJ (2014) suggested potential risk of TKIs and VEGF inhibitors in the development of ONJ without concomitant BP administration [24]. It had been suggested that these antiangiogenic agents can disrupt oral epithelium or suppress angiogenic signal-dependent osteoclast function [139]. Also, these agents possibly influence the host immune response and may interfere local immune response [126].

It is unclear to define the factors increasing the risk of ONJ after antiangiogenic agents because of the short survival rate and drug-administration period of the patients with advanced cancer. Therefore, increased or prolonged administration of antiangiogenic agents does not directly mean high risk of ONJ [128]. Patients with antiangiogenic agent-related frequently has a history of dental extraction [123, 132, 140]. However, dental examination had not been carried out before chemotherapy [135] or there was absence of dental predisposing factors in many patients [127–131]. In current, exact risk factors for antiangiogenic agent-relate ONJ cannot be accessible because of the lack of high level of evidence-based study in the literatures. Since the patients developed ONJ showed significantly higher survival than without ONJ after using these agents [122], the ONJ risk and survival benefit need to be considered in these advanced cancer patients.

## Conclusions

Dose, duration of intake, and intravenous route of administration of nitrogen-containing bisphosphonates as well as dental infections and dento-alveolar surgical procedures can be regarded as risk factors for MRONJ development. Oncological dosing, dental infections, and dento-alveolar surgeries also seem to be risk factors for the development of ONJ under denosumab treatment.

**Acknowledgements** This research was supported by the Basic Science Research Program through the National Research Foundation of Korea (NRF), funded by the Ministry of Education, Science, and Technology (NRF 2010-0011-445).

## References

1. Marx RE. Osteoradionecrosis: a new concept of its pathophysiology. J Oral Maxillofac Surg. 1983;41(5): 283–8.
2. Ruggiero SL, Dodson TB, Assael LA, Landesberg R, Marx RE, Mehrotra B. American Association of Oral and Maxillofacial Surgeons position paper on bisphos-

phonate-related osteonecrosis of the jaws–2009 update. J Oral Maxillofac Surg. 2009;67(5 Suppl): 2–12.

3. Sarin J, DeRossi SS, Akintoye SO. Updates on bisphosphonates and potential pathobiology of bisphosphonate-induced jaw osteonecrosis. Oral Dis. 2008;14(3):277–85.

4. Marx RE. Pamidronate (Aredia) and zoledronate (Zometa) induced avascular necrosis of the jaws: a growing epidemic. J Oral Maxillofac Surg. 2003;61(9): 1115–7.

5. Migliorati CA. Bisphosphanates and oral cavity avascular bone necrosis. J Clin Oncol. 2003;21(22):4253–4.

6. Bagan JV, Murillo J, Jimenez Y, Poveda R, Milian MA, Sanchis JM, et al. Avascular jaw osteonecrosis in association with cancer chemotherapy: series of 10 cases. J Oral Pathol Med. 2005;34(2):120–3.

7. Santini D, Vincenzi B, Avvisati G, Dicuonzo G, Battistoni F, Gavasci M, et al. Pamidronate induces modifications of circulating angiogenetic factors in cancer patients. Clin Cancer Res. 2002;8(5):1080–4.

8. Conte P, Coleman R. Bisphosphonates in the treatment of skeletal metastases. Semin Oncol. 2004; 31(5 Suppl 10):59–63.

9. Ferretti G, Fabi A, Carlini P, Papaldo P, CordialiFei P, Di Cosimo S, et al. Zoledronic-acid-induced circulating level modifications of angiogenic factors, metalloproteinases and proinflammatory cytokines in metastatic breast cancer patients. Oncology. 2005;69(1):35–43.

10. Metcalf S, Pandha HS, Morgan R. Antiangiogenic effects of zoledronate on cancer neovasculature. Future Oncol. 2011;7(11):1325–33.

11. Kapitola J, Zak J. Effect of pamidronate on bone blood flow in oophorectomized rats. Physiol Res. 1998;47(4):237–40.

12. Landesberg R, Woo V, Cremers S, Cozin M, Marolt D, Vunjak-Novakovic G, et al. Potential pathophysiological mechanisms in osteonecrosis of the jaw. Ann N Y Acad Sci. 2011;1218:62–79.

13. Reid IR. Osteonecrosis of the jaw: who gets it, and why? Bone. 2009;44(1):4–10.

14. Hansen T, Kunkel M, Weber A, James Kirkpatrick C. Osteonecrosis of the jaws in patients treated with bisphosphonates - histomorphologic analysis in comparison with infected osteoradionecrosis. J Oral Pathol Med. 2006;35(3):155–60.

15. Yamashita J, Koi K, Yang DY, McCauley LK. Effect of zoledronate on oral wound healing in rats. Clin Cancer Res. 2011;17(6):1405–14.

16. Little DG, Peat RA, McEvoy A, Williams PR, Smith EJ, Baldock PA. Zoledronic acid treatment results in retention of femoral head structure after traumatic osteonecrosis in young Wistar rats. J Bone Miner Res. 2003;18(11):2016–22.

17. Agarwala S, Jain D, Joshi VR, Sule A. Efficacy of alendronate, a bisphosphonate, in the treatment of AVN of the hip. A prospective open-label study. Rheumatology (Oxford). 2005;44(3):352–9.

18. Lai KA, Shen WJ, Yang CY, Shao CJ, Hsu JT, Lin RM. The use of alendronate to prevent early

collapse of the femoral head in patients with nontraumatic osteonecrosis. A randomized clinical study. J Bone Joint Surg Am. 2005;87(10):2155–9.

19. Marx RE, Sawatari Y, Fortin M, Broumand V. Bisphosphonate-induced exposed bone (osteonecrosis/osteopetrosis) of the jaws: risk factors, recognition, prevention, and treatment. J Oral Maxillofac Surg. 2005;63(11):1567–75.

20. Migliorati CA, Siegel MA, Elting LS. Bisphosphonate-associated osteonecrosis: a long-term complication of bisphosphonate treatment. Lancet Oncol. 2006;7(6): 508–14.

21. Khosla S, Burr D, Cauley J, Dempster DW, Ebeling PR, Felsenberg D, et al. Bisphosphonate-associated osteonecrosis of the jaw: report of a task force of the American Society for Bone and Mineral Research. J Bone Miner Res. 2007;22(10):1479–91.

22. AAOMS. American Association of Oral and Maxillofacial Surgeons position paper on bisphosphonate-related osteonecrosis of the jaws. J Oral Maxillofac Surg. 2007;65(3):369–76.

23. Wimalawansa SJ. Insight into bisphosphonate-associated osteomyelitis of the jaw: pathophysiology, mechanisms and clinical management. Expert Opin Drug Saf. 2008;7(4):491–512.

24. 2014 Position Paper on Medication Related Osteonecrosis of the Jaws, http://www.aaoms. org/docs/position_papers/mronj_position_paper. pdf?pdf=MRONJ-Position-Paper.

25. Wang J, Goodger NM, Pogrel MA. Osteonecrosis of the jaws associated with cancer chemotherapy. J Oral Maxillofac Surg. 2003;61(9):1104–7.

26. Kuhl S, Walter C, Acham S, Pfeffer R, Lambrecht JT. Bisphosphonate-related osteonecrosis of the jaws–a review. Oral Oncol. 2012;48(10):938–47.

27. Yamashita J, McCauley LK. Antiresorptives and osteonecrosis of the jaw. J Evid Based Dent Pract. 2012;12(3 Suppl):233–47.

28. Ruggiero SL, Mehrotra B, Rosenberg TJ, Engroff SL. Osteonecrosis of the jaws associated with the use of bisphosphonates: a review of 63 cases. J Oral Maxillofac Surg. 2004;62(5):527–34.

29. Bamias A, Kastritis E, Bamia C, Moulopoulos LA, Melakopoulos I, Bozas G, et al. Osteonecrosis of the jaw in cancer after treatment with bisphosphonates: incidence and risk factors. J Clin Oncol. 2005;23(34): 8580–7.

30. Mavrokokki T, Cheng A, Stein B, Goss A. Nature and frequency of bisphosphonate-associated osteonecrosis of the jaws in Australia. J Oral Maxillofac Surg. 2007;65(3):415–23.

31. Edwards BJ, Gounder M, McKoy JM, Boyd I, Farrugia M, Migliorati C, et al. Pharmacovigilance and reporting oversight in US FDA fast-track process: bisphosphonates and osteonecrosis of the jaw. Lancet Oncol. 2008;9(12):1166–72.

32. Thumbigere-Math V, Tu L, Huckabay S, Dudek AZ, Lunos S, Basi DL, et al. A retrospective study evaluating frequency and risk factors of osteonecrosis of the jaw in 576 cancer patients receiving intravenous

bisphosphonates. Am J Clin Oncol. 2012;35(4): 386–92.

33. Zavras AI. The impact of bisphosphonates on oral health: lessons from the past and opportunities for the future. Ann N Y Acad Sci. 2011;1218:55–61.

34. Woo SB, Hellstein JW, Kalmar JR. Narrative [corrected] review: bisphosphonates and osteonecrosis of the jaws. Ann Intern Med. 2006;144(10):753–61.

35. Ezra A, Golomb G. Administration routes and delivery systems of bisphosphonates for the treatment of bone resorption. Adv Drug Deliv Rev. 2000;42(3):175–95.

36. Yoneda T, Hagino H, Sugimoto T, Ohta H, Takahashi S, Soen S, et al. Bisphosphonate-related osteonecrosis of the jaw: position paper from the Allied Task Force Committee of Japanese Society for Bone and Mineral Research, Japan Osteoporosis Society, Japanese Society of Periodontology, Japanese Society for Oral and Maxillofacial Radiology, and Japanese Society of Oral and Maxillofacial Surgeons. J Bone Miner Metab. 2010;28(4):365–83.

37. Berenson JR, Rosen LS, Howell A, Porter L, Coleman RE, Morley W, et al. Zoledronic acid reduces skeletal-related events in patients with osteolytic metastases. Cancer. 2001;91(7):1191–200.

38. Reid IR, Brown JP, Burckhardt P, Horowitz Z, Richardson P, Trechsel U, et al. Intravenous zoledronic acid in postmenopausal women with low bone mineral density. N Engl J Med. 2002;346(9):653–61.

39. Zervas K, Verrou E, Teleioudis Z, Vahtsevanos K, Banti A, Mihou D, et al. Incidence, risk factors and management of osteonecrosis of the jaw in patients with multiple myeloma: a single-centre experience in 303 patients. Br J Haematol. 2006;134(6):620–3.

40. Estilo CL, Van Poznak CH, Wiliams T, Bohle GC, Lwin PT, Zhou Q, et al. Osteonecrosis of the maxilla and mandible in patients with advanced cancer treated with bisphosphonate therapy. Oncologist. 2008;13(8): 911–20.

41. Boonyapakorn T, Schirmer I, Reichart PA, Sturm I, Massenkeil G. Bisphosphonate-induced osteonecrosis of the jaws: prospective study of 80 patients with multiple myeloma and other malignancies. Oral Oncol. 2008;44(9):857–69.

42. Dimopoulos MA, Kastritis E, Anagnostopoulos A, Melakopoulos I, Gika D, Moulopoulos LA, et al. Osteonecrosis of the jaw in patients with multiple myeloma treated with bisphosphonates: evidence of increased risk after treatment with zoledronic acid. Haematologica. 2006;91(7):968–71.

43. Hoff AO, Toth BB, Altundag K, Johnson MM, Warneke CL, Hu M, et al. Frequency and risk factors associated with osteonecrosis of the jaw in cancer patients treated with intravenous bisphosphonates. J Bone Miner Res. 2008;23(6):826–36.

44. Vahtsevanos K, Kyrgidis A, Verrou E, Katodritou E, Triaridis S, Andreadis CG, et al. Longitudinal cohort study of risk factors in cancer patients of bisphosphonate-related osteonecrosis of the jaw. J Clin Oncol. 2009;27(32):5356–62.

45. Jadu F, Lee L, Pharoah M, Reece D, Wang L. A retrospective study assessing the incidence, risk factors and comorbidities of pamidronate-related necrosis of the jaws in multiple myeloma patients. Ann Oncol. 2007;18(12):2015–9.

46. Fleisch H. Bisphosphonates: mechanisms of action. Endocr Rev. 1998;19(1):80–100.

47. Rosen LS, Gordon D, Kaminski M, Howell A, Belch A, Mackey J, et al. Zoledronic acid versus pamidronate in the treatment of skeletal metastases in patients with breast cancer or osteolytic lesions of multiple myeloma: a phase III, double-blind, comparative trial. Cancer J. 2001;7(5):377–87.

48. Then C, Horauf N, Otto S, Pautke C, von Tresckow E, Rohnisch T, et al. Incidence and risk factors of bisphosphonate-related osteonecrosis of the jaw in multiple myeloma patients having undergone autologous stem cell transplantation. Onkologie. 2012; 35(11):658–64.

49. Lin JH. Bisphosphonates: a review of their pharmacokinetic properties. Bone. 1996;18(2):75–85.

50. Fehm T, Beck V, Banys M, Lipp HP, Hairass M, Reinert S, et al. Bisphosphonate-induced osteonecrosis of the jaw (ONJ): incidence and risk factors in patients with breast cancer and gynecological malignancies. Gynecol Oncol. 2009;112(3):605–9.

51. ADA. Dental management of patients receiving oral bisphosphonate therapy: expert panel recommendations. J Am Dent Assoc. 2006;137(8):1144–50.

52. Lo JC, O'Ryan FS, Gordon NP, Yang J, Hui RL, Martin D, et al. Prevalence of osteonecrosis of the jaw in patients with oral bisphosphonate exposure. J Oral Maxillofac Surg. 2010;68(2):243–53.

53. Fellows JL, Rindal DB, Barasch A, Gullion CM, Rush W, Pihlstrom DJ, et al. ONJ in two dental practice-based research network regions. J Dent Res. 2011;90(4):433–8.

54. Barasch A, Cunha-Cruz J, Curro FA, Hujoel P, Sung AH, Vena D, et al. Risk factors for osteonecrosis of the jaws: a case–control study from the CONDOR dental PBRN. J Dent Res. 2011;90(4):439–44.

55. Filleul O, Crompot E, Saussez S. Bisphosphonate-induced osteonecrosis of the jaw: a review of 2,400 patient cases. J Cancer Res Clin Oncol. 2010;136(8): 1117–24.

56. Otto S, Abu-Id MH, Fedele S, Warnke PH, Becker ST, Kolk A, et al. Osteoporosis and bisphosphonates-related osteonecrosis of the jaw: not just a sporadic coincidence–a multi-centre study. J Craniomaxillofac Surg. 2011;39(4):272–7.

57. Urade M, Tanaka N, Furusawa K, Shimada J, Shibata T, Kirita T, et al. Nationwide survey for bisphosphonate-related osteonecrosis of the jaws in Japan. J Oral Maxillofac Surg. 2011;69(11):e364–71.

58. Di Fede O, Fusco V, Matranga D, Solazzo L, Gabriele M, Gaeta GM, et al. Osteonecrosis of the jaws in patients assuming oral bisphosphonates for osteoporosis: a retrospective multi-hospital-based study of 87 Italian cases. Eur J Intern Med. 2013;11.

59. Manfredi M, Merigo E, Guidotti R, Meleti M, Vescovi P. Bisphosphonate-related osteonecrosis of the jaws: a case series of 25 patients affected by osteoporosis. Int J Oral Maxillofac Surg. 2011;40(3):277–84.

60. Marx RE, Cillo Jr JE, Ulloa JJ. Oral bisphosphonate-induced osteonecrosis: risk factors, prediction of risk using serum CTX testing, prevention, and treatment. J Oral Maxillofac Surg. 2007;65(12):2397–410.

61. O'Ryan FS, Lo JC. Bisphosphonate-related osteonecrosis of the jaw in patients with oral bisphosphonate exposure: clinical course and outcomes. J Oral Maxillofac Surg. 2012;70(8):1844–53.

62. Fleisher KE, Jolly A, Venkata UD, Norman RG, Saxena D, Glickman RS. Osteonecrosis of the jaw onset times are based on the route of bisphosphonate therapy. J Oral Maxillofac Surg. 2013;71(3):513–9.

63. Bone HG, Hosking D, Devogelaer JP, Tucci JR, Emkey RD, Tonino RP, et al. Ten years' experience with alendronate for osteoporosis in postmenopausal women. N Engl J Med. 2004;350(12):1189–99.

64. Badros A, Terpos E, Katodritou E, Goloubeva O, Kastritis E, Verrou E, et al. Natural history of osteonecrosis of the jaw in patients with multiple myeloma. J Clin Oncol. 2008;26(36):5904–9.

65. Durie BG, Katz M, Crowley J. Osteonecrosis of the jaw and bisphosphonates. N Engl J Med. 2005;353(1):99–102; discussion 99.

66. Wessel JH, Dodson TB, Zavras AI. Zoledronate, smoking, and obesity are strong risk factors for osteonecrosis of the jaw: a case–control study. J Oral Maxillofac Surg. 2008;66(4):625–31.

67. Khamaisi M, Regev E, Yarom N, Avni B, Leitersdorf E, Raz I, et al. Possible association between diabetes and bisphosphonate-related jaw osteonecrosis. J Clin Endocrinol Metab. 2007;92(3):1172–5.

68. Pazianas M, Miller P, Blumentals WA, Bernal M, Kothawala P. A review of the literature on osteonecrosis of the jaw in patients with osteoporosis treated with oral bisphosphonates: prevalence, risk factors, and clinical characteristics. Clin Ther. 2007;29(8):1548–58.

69. Cartsos VM, Zhu S, Zavras AI. Bisphosphonate use and the risk of adverse jaw outcomes: a medical claims study of 714,217 people. J Am Dent Assoc. 2008;139(1):23–30.

70. Malden N, Lopes V. An epidemiological study of alendronate-related osteonecrosis of the jaws.A case series from the south-east of Scotland with attention given to case definition and prevalence. J Bone Miner Metab. 2012;30(2):171–82.

71. Diniz-Freitas M, Lopez-Cedrun JL, Fernandez-Sanroman J, Garcia-Garcia A, Fernandez-Feijoo J, Diz-Dios P. Oral bisphosphonate-related osteonecrosis of the jaws: clinical characteristics of a series of 20 cases in Spain. Med Oral Patol Oral Cir Bucal. 2012;17(5):e751–8.

72. Allen MR, Burr DB. The pathogenesis of bisphosphonate-related osteonecrosis of the jaw: so many hypotheses, so few data. J Oral Maxillofac Surg. 2009;67(5 Suppl):61–70.

73. Bertoldo F, Santini D, Lo Cascio V. Bisphosphonates and osteomyelitis of the jaw: a pathogenic puzzle. Nat Clin Pract Oncol. 2007;4(12):711–21.

74. Abtahi J, Agholme F, Sandberg O, Aspenberg P. Bisphosphonate-induced osteonecrosis of the jaw in a rat model arises first after the bone has become exposed. No primary necrosis in unexposed bone. J Oral Pathol Med. 2012;41(6):494–9.

75. Otto S, Hafner S, Mast G, Tischer T, Volkmer E, Schieker M, et al. Bisphosphonate-related osteonecrosis of the jaw: is pH the missing part in the pathogenesis puzzle? J Oral Maxillofac Surg. 2010;68(5):1158–61.

76. Landesberg R, Cozin M, Cremers S, Woo V, Kousteni S, Sinha S, et al. Inhibition of oral mucosal cell wound healing by bisphosphonates. J Oral Maxillofac Surg. 2008;66(5):839–47.

77. Tsao C, Darby I, Ebeling PR, Walsh K, O'Brien-Simpson N, Reynolds E, et al. Oral health risk factors for bisphosphonate-associated jaw osteonecrosis. J Oral Maxillofac Surg. 2013;71(8):1360–6.

78. Pozzi S, Marcheselli R, Sacchi S, Baldini L, Angrilli F, Pennese E, et al. Bisphosphonate-associated osteonecrosis of the jaw: a review of 35 cases and an evaluation of its frequency in multiple myeloma patients. Leuk Lymphoma. 2007;48(1):56–64.

79. Aspenberg P. Osteonecrosis of the jaw: what do bisphosphonates do? Expert Opin Drug Saf. 2006;5(6):743–5.

80. Paparella ML, Brandizzi D, Santini-Araujo E, Cabrini RL. Histopathological features of osteonecrosis of the jaw associated with bisphosphonates. Histopathology. 2012;60(3):514–6.

81. Lesclous P, AbiNajm S, Carrel JP, Baroukh B, Lombardi T, Willi JP, et al. Bisphosphonate-associated osteonecrosis of the jaw: a key role of inflammation? Bone. 2009;45(5):843–52.

82. Wang EP, Kaban LB, Strewler GJ, Raje N, Troulis MJ. Incidence of osteonecrosis of the jaw in patients with multiple myeloma and breast or prostate cancer on intravenous bisphosphonate therapy. J Oral Maxillofac Surg. 2007;65(7):1328–31.

83. Sedghizadeh PP, Jones AC, LaVallee C, Jelliffe RW, Le AD, Lee P, et al. Population pharmacokinetic and pharmacodynamic modeling for assessing risk of bisphosphonate-related osteonecrosis of the jaw. Oral Surg Oral Med Oral Pathol Oral Radiol. 2013;115(2):224–32.

84. Sarasquete ME, Garcia-Sanz R, Marin L, Alcoceba M, Chillon MC, Balanzategui A, et al. Bisphosphonate-related osteonecrosis of the jaw is associated with polymorphisms of the cytochrome P450 CYP2C8 in multiple myeloma: a genome-wide single nucleotide polymorphism analysis. Blood. 2008;112(7):2709–12.

85. Zhong DN, Wu JZ, Li GJ. Association between CYP2C8 (rs1934951) polymorphism and bisphosphonate-related osteonecrosis of the jaws in patients

on bisphosphonate therapy: a meta-analysis. Acta Haematol. 2013;129(2):90–5.

86. Lai XS, Yang LP, Li XT, Liu JP, Zhou ZW, Zhou SF. Human CYP2C8: structure, substrate specificity, inhibitor selectivity, inducers and polymorphisms. Curr Drug Metab. 2009;10(9):1009–47.

87. Such E, Cervera J, Terpos E, Bagan JV, Avaria A, Gomez I, et al. CYP2C8 gene polymorphism and bisphosphonate-related osteonecrosis of the jaw in patients with multiple myeloma. Haematologica. 2011;96(10):1557–9.

88. English BC, Baum CE, Adelberg DE, Sissung TM, Kluetz PG, Dahut WL, et al. A SNP in CYP2C8 is not associated with the development of bisphosphonate-related osteonecrosis of the jaw in men with castrate-resistant prostate cancer. Ther Clin Risk Manag. 2010;6:579–83.

89. Nicoletti P, Cartsos VM, Palaska PK, Shen Y, Floratos A, Zavras AI. Genomewidepharmacogenetics of bisphosphonate-induced osteonecrosis of the jaw: the role of RBMS3. Oncologist. 2012;17(2):279–87.

90. Baim S, Miller PD. Assessing the clinical utility of serum CTX in postmenopausal osteoporosis and its use in predicting risk of osteonecrosis of the jaw. J Bone Miner Res. 2009;24(4):561–74.

91. Rosen HN, Moses AC, Garber J, Iloputaife ID, Ross DS, Lee SL, et al. Serum CTX: a new marker of bone resorption that shows treatment effect more often than other markers because of low coefficient of variability and large changes with bisphosphonate therapy. Calcif Tissue Int. 2000;66(2):100–3.

92. Nishizawa Y, Ohta H, Miura M, Inaba M, Ichimura S, Shiraki M, et al. Guidelines for the use of bone metabolic markers in the diagnosis and treatment of osteoporosis (2012 edition). J Bone Miner Metab. 2013;31(1):1–15.

93. Liberman UA, Weiss SR, Broll J, Minne HW, Quan H, Bell NH, et al. Effect of oral alendronate on bone mineral density and the incidence of fractures in postmenopausal osteoporosis. The Alendronate Phase III Osteoporosis Treatment Study Group. N Engl J Med. 1995;333(22):1437–43.

94. Kwon YD, Kim DY, Ohe JY, Yoo JY, Walter C. Correlation between serum C-terminal cross-linking telopeptide of type I collagen and staging of oral bisphosphonate-related osteonecrosis of the jaws. J Oral Maxillofac Surg. 2009;67(12):2644–8.

95. Lazarovici TS, Mesilaty-Gross S, Vered I, Pariente C, Kanety H, Givol N, et al. Serologic bone markers for predicting development of osteonecrosis of the jaw in patients receiving bisphosphonates. J Oral Maxillofac Surg. 2010;68(9):2241–7.

96. Kunchur R, Need A, Hughes T, Goss A. Clinical investigation of C-terminal cross-linking telopeptide test in prevention and management of bisphosphonate-associated osteonecrosis of the jaws. J Oral Maxillofac Surg. 2009;67(6):1167–73.

97. Khosla S, Burr D, Cauley J, Dempster DW, Ebeling PR, Felsenberg D, et al. Oral bisphosphonate-induced osteonecrosis: risk factors, prediction of risk using serum CTX testing, prevention, and treatment. J Oral Maxillofac Surg. 2008;66(6):1320–1; author reply 1–2.

98. Lehrer S, Montazem A, Ramanathan L, Pessin-Minsley M, Pfail J, Stock RG, et al. Bisphosphonate-induced osteonecrosis of the jaws, bone markers, and a hypothesized candidate gene. J Oral Maxillofac Surg. 2009;67(1):159–61.

99. Bilezikian JP, Matsumoto T, Bellido T, Khosla S, Martin J, Recker RR, et al. Targeting bone remodeling for the treatment of osteoporosis: summary of the proceedings of an ASBMR workshop. J Bone Miner Res. 2009;24(3):373–85.

100. Don-Wauchope AC, Cole DE. The (mis) use of bone resorption markers in the context of bisphosphonate exposure, dental surgery and osteonecrosis of the jaw. Clin Biochem. 2009;42(10–11):1194–6.

101. Cremers S, Farooki A. Biochemical markers of bone turnover in osteonecrosis of the jaw in patients with osteoporosis and advanced cancer involving the bone. Ann N Y Acad Sci. 2011;1218:80–7.

102. Kim JW, Kong KA, Kim SJ, Choi SK, Cha IH, Kim MR. Prospective biomarker evaluation in patients with osteonecrosis of the jaw who received bisphosphonates. Bone. 2013;57(1):201–5.

103. Choi SY, An CH, Kim SY, Kwon TG. Bone turnover and inflammatory markers of bisphosphonate-related osteonecrosis of the jaw in female osteoporosis patients. J Oral Maxillofac Surg Med Pathol. 2013;25:123–8.

104. Lopez-Carrizosa MC, Samper-Ots PM, Perez AR. Serum C-telopeptide levels predict the incidence of skeletal-related events in cancer patients with secondary bone metastases. Clin Transl Oncol. 2010;12(8):568–73.

105. Kimmel DB, Recker RR, Gallagher JC, Vaswani AS, Aloia JF. A comparison of iliac bone histomorphometric data in post-menopausal osteoporotic and normal subjects. Bone Miner. 1990;11(2):217–35.

106. Silva I, Branco JC. Rank/Rankl/opg: literature review. Acta Reumatol Port. 2011;36(3):209–18.

107. Fizazi K, Carducci M, Smith M, Damiao R, Brown J, Karsh L, et al. Denosumab versus zoledronic acid for treatment of bone metastases in men with castration-resistant prostate cancer: a randomised, double-blind study. Lancet. 2011;377(9768):813–22.

108. Anghel R, Bachmann A, Beksac M, Brodowicz T, Finek J, Komadina R, et al. Expert opinion 2011 on the use of new anti-resorptive agents in the prevention of skeletal-related events in metastatic bone disease. Wien Klin Wochenschr. 2013;125(15–16):439–47.

109. Body JJ. Inhibition of RANK Ligand to treat bone metastases. Bull Cancer. 2013;100(11):1207–13.

110. Silva I, Branco JC. Denosumab: recent update in postmenopausal osteoporosis. Acta Reumatol Port. 2012;37(4):302–13.

111. Pazianas M. Osteonecrosis of the jaw and the role of macrophages. J Natl Cancer Inst. 2011;103(3):232–40.

112. Lipton A, Fizazi K, Stopeck AT, Henry DH, Brown JE, Yardley DA, et al. Superiority of denosumab to zoledronic acid for prevention of skeletal-related events: a combined analysis of 3 pivotal, randomised, phase 3 trials. Eur J Cancer. 2012; 48(16):3082–92.

113. Fizazi K, Lipton A, Mariette X, Body JJ, Rahim Y, Gralow JR, et al. Randomized phase II trial of denosumab in patients with bone metastases from prostate cancer, breast cancer, or other neoplasms after intravenous bisphosphonates. J Clin Oncol. 2009;27(10):1564–71.

114. Lipton A, Steger GG, Figueroa J, Alvarado C, Solal-Celigny P, Body JJ, et al. Randomized active-controlled phase II study of denosumab efficacy and safety in patients with breast cancer-related bone metastases. J Clin Oncol. 2007;25(28):4431–7.

115. Smith MR, Egerdie B, Hernandez Toriz N, Feldman R, Tammela TL, Saad F, et al. Denosumab in men receiving androgen-deprivation therapy for prostate cancer. N Engl J Med. 2009;361(8):745–55.

116. Saad F, Brown JE, Van Poznak C, Ibrahim T, Stemmer SM, Stopeck AT, et al. Incidence, risk factors, and outcomes of osteonecrosis of the jaw: integrated analysis from three blinded active-controlled phase III trials in cancer patients with bone metastases. Ann Oncol. 2012;23(5):1341–7.

117. Qi WX, Tang LN, He AN, Yao Y, Shen Z. Risk of osteonecrosis of the jaw in cancer patients receiving denosumab: a meta-analysis of seven randomized controlled trials. Int J Clin Oncol. 2013;20.

118. Papapoulos S, Chapurlat R, Libanati C, Brandi ML, Brown JP, Czerwinski E, et al. Five years of denosumab exposure in women with postmenopausal osteoporosis: results from the first two years of the FREEDOM extension. J Bone Miner Res. 2012; 27(3):694–701.

119. Chawla S, Henshaw R, Seeger L, Choy E, Blay JY, Ferrari S, et al. Safety and efficacy of denosumab for adults and skeletally mature adolescents with giant cell tumour of bone: interim analysis of an open-label, parallel-group, phase 2 study. Lancet Oncol. 2013;14(9):901–8.

120. Mauri D, Valachis A, Polyzos IP, Polyzos NP, Kamposioras K, Pesce LL. Osteonecrosis of the jaw and use of bisphosphonates in adjuvant breast cancer treatment: a meta-analysis. Breast Cancer Res Treat. 2009;116(3):433–9.

121. Kerbel R, Folkman J. Clinical translation of angiogenesis inhibitors. Nat Rev Cancer. 2002;2(10): 727–39.

122. Smidt-Hansen T, Folkmar TB, Fode K, Agerbaek M, Donskov F. Combination of zoledronic Acid and targeted therapy is active but may induce osteonecrosis of the jaw in patients with metastatic renal cell carcinoma. J Oral Maxillofac Surg. 2013;71(9):1532–40.

123. Greuter S, Schmid F, Ruhstaller T, Thuerlimann B. Bevacizumab-associated osteonecrosis of the jaw. Ann Oncol. 2008;19(12):2091–2.

124. Koch FP, Walter C, Hansen T, Jager E, Wagner W. Osteonecrosis of the jaw related to sunitinib. Oral Maxillofac Surg. 2011;15(1):63–6.

125. Kneissel M, Luong-Nguyen NH, Baptist M, Cortesi R, Zumstein-Mecker S, Kossida S, et al. Everolimus suppresses cancellous bone loss, bone resorption, and cathepsin K expression by osteoclasts. Bone. 2004;35(5):1144–56.

126. Troeltzsch M, Woodlock T, Kriegelstein S, Steiner T, Messlinger K. Physiology and pharmacology of nonbisphosphonate drugs implicated in osteonecrosis of the jaw. J Can Dent Assoc. 2012;78:c85.

127. Estilo CL, Fornier M, Farooki A, Carlson D, Bohle G, 3rd, Huryn JM. Osteonecrosis of the jaw related to bevacizumab. J Clin Oncol. 2008 20;26(24): 4037–8.

128. Guarneri V, Miles D, Robert N, Dieras V, Glaspy J, Smith I, et al. Bevacizumab and osteonecrosis of the jaw: incidence and association with bisphosphonate therapy in three large prospective trials in advanced breast cancer. Breast Cancer Res Treat. 2010;122(1):181–8.

129. Disel U, Besen AA, Ozyilkan O, Er E, Canpolat T. A case report of bevacizumab-related osteonecrosis of the jaw: old problem, new culprit. Oral Oncol. 2012;48(2):e2–3.

130. Hopp RN, Pucci J, Santos-Silva AR, Jorge J. Osteonecrosis after administration of intravitreous bevacizumab. J Oral Maxillofac Surg. 2012;70(3):632–5.

131. Santos-Silva AR, Belizario Rosa GA, Castro Junior G, Dias RB, Prado Ribeiro AC, Brandao TB. Osteonecrosis of the mandible associated with bevacizumab therapy. Oral Surg Oral Med Oral Pathol Oral Radiol. 2013;115(6):e32–6.

132. Christodoulou C, Pervena A, Klouvas G, Galani E, Falagas ME, Tsakalos G, et al. Combination of bisphosphonates and antiangiogenic factors induces osteonecrosis of the jaw more frequently than bisphosphonates alone. Oncology. 2009;76(3): 209–11.

133. Hoefert S, Eufinger H. Sunitinib may raise the risk of bisphosphonate-related osteonecrosis of the jaw: presentation of three cases. Oral Surg Oral Med Oral Pathol Oral Radiol Endod. 2010;110(4):463–9.

134. Keizman D, Ish-Shalom M, Pili R, Hammers H, Eisenberger MA, Sinibaldi V, et al. Bisphosphonates combined with sunitinib may improve the response rate, progression free survival and overall survival of patients with bone metastases from renal cell carcinoma. Eur J Cancer. 2012;48(7):1031–7.

135. Beuselinck B, Wolter P, Karadimou A, Elaidi R, Dumez H, Rogiers A, et al. Concomitant oral tyrosine kinase inhibitors and bisphosphonates in advanced renal cell carcinoma with bone metastases. Br J Cancer. 2012;107(10):1665–71.

136. Fleissig Y, Regev E, Lehman H. Sunitinib related osteonecrosis of jaw: a case report. Oral Surg Oral Med Oral Pathol Oral Radiol. 2012;113(3):e1–3.

137. Nicolatou-Galitis O, Migkou M, Psyrri A, Bamias A, Pectasides D, Economopoulos T, et al. Gingival bleeding and jaw bone necrosis in patients with metastatic renal cell carcinoma receiving sunitinib: report of 2 cases with clinical implications. Oral Surg Oral Med Oral Pathol Oral Radiol. 2012;113(2): 234–8.

138. Kim DW, Jung YS, Park HS, Jung HD. Osteonecrosis of the jaw related to everolimus: a case report. Br J Oral Maxillofac Surg. 2013;51(8):e302–4.

139. Ayllon J, Launay-Vacher V, Medioni J, Cros C, Spano JP, Oudard S. Osteonecrosis of the jaw under bisphosphonate and antiangiogenic therapies: cumulative toxicity profile? Ann Oncol. 2009;20(3): 600–1.

140. Serra E, Paolantonio M, Spoto G, Mastrangelo F, Tete S, Dolci M. Bevacizumab-related osteneocrosis of the jaw. Int J Immunopathol Pharmacol. 2009 Oct-Dec;22(4):1121–3.

# Definition, Clinical Features and Staging of Medication-Related Osteonecrosis of the Jaw

**4**

Sven Otto, Tae-Geon Kwon, and Alexandre Th. Assaf


**Abstract**

Medication-related osteonecrosis of jaw (MRONJ) has become a well-known side effect of bisphosphonate therapy which predominantly occurs in patients suffering from malignant diseases who receive intravenous administrations of nitrogen-containing bisphosphonates. More recently, similar problems have been described after treatment with denosumab.

The majority of ONJ cases under bisphosphonate treatment occurred in the mandible (around 2/3 of the cases) with a predilection for the molar and premolar regions in both jaws. Besides exposed necrotic bone, pain and swelling of the surrounding soft tissues as well as intra- or extra-oral sinus tracts are typical signs of MRONJ. Furthermore, complications like abscess formation, pathological fractures, sinusitis and impairment of inferior alveolar nerve function might occur. Staging of MRONJ is usually performed according to the recommendations of the American Association of Oral and Maxillofacial Surgeons.



S. Otto, MD, DMD, FEBOMFS (✉)
Department of Oral and Maxillofacial Surgery,
Ludwig-Maximilians-University of Munich,
Munich, Germany
e-mail: Otto_Sven@web.de

T.-G. Kwon, DDS, PhD
Department of Oral and Maxillofacial Surgery,
Kyungpook National University,
Daegu, Korea

A.T. Assaf, MD, DMD, FEBOMFS
Department of Oral and Maxillofacial Surgery,
University Medical Center Hamburg Eppendorf,
Hamburg, Germany


## First Description

Bisphosphonates and denosumab are the most widely used classes of antiresorptive drugs in the management of osteoporosis and metastatic bone disease. Generally, they are well tolerated. However, in 2001 the first cases of jaw bone exposure that occurred after intravenous treatment with bisphosphonates were reported to the American Food and Drug Administration (FDA) by Ruggiero. In 2003 the first scientific publications emerged which initially described an avascular necrosis that occurred predominantly after intravenous treatment with nitrogen-containing bisphosphonates [1–3].


S. Otto (ed.), *Medication-Related Osteonecrosis of the Jaws: Bisphosphonates, Denosumab, and New Agents*,
DOI 10.1007/978-3-662-43733-9_4, © Springer-Verlag Berlin Heidelberg 2015

Notably the subtitle of one of these publications was "a growing epidemic" [1]. As soon as in 2004, a case series encompassing 63 cases of jaw bone osteonecrosis under bisphosphonate treatment in only one Department of Oral and Maxillofacial Surgery was published [4] and proofed that the abovementioned subtitle was true. This side effect of especially nitrogen-containing bisphosphonates was later referred to as bisphosphonate-related osteonecrosis of the jaws (BRONJ) and became a major problem of rising clinical importance around the world.

Soon after the market introduction of denosumab as an alternative antiresorptive drug, similar problems of exposed necrotic bone in the maxillofacial region occurred [5, 6]. Within the past few years, increasing numbers of ONJ cases under denosumab treatment have been reported [7, 8]. Seemingly, the prevalence rates of ONJ under intravenous nitrogen-containing bisphosphonates and denosumab treatment in the oncological setting are in a comparable order of magnitude [7, 9, 10]. Given the increasing number of denosumab applications for metastatic bone disease as well as osteoporosis, this has the potential to become a major clinical problem in the near future. Due to the fact that osteonecrosis of the jaws can occur under treatment with bisphosphonates as well as denosumab, the terminology medication-related ostenecrosis of the jaw has been introduced by the American Association of Oral and Maxillofacial Surgeons (AAOMS 2014) [11].

## Definition

According to the American Association of Oral and Maxillofacial Surgeons special commitee on medication-related osteonecrosis of the jaws, diagnosis is made by the following criteria [11, 12]:

(a) Presence of exposed bone (or bone that can be probed through an intraoral or extraoral fistula) in the maxillofacial region over a period of 8 weeks
(b) Current or previous treatment with antiresorptive (bisphosphonates or denosumab) or antiangiogenic agents
(c) No history of radiation therapy to the jaws or obvious metastatic disease to the jaws.

**Table 4.1** Definition: BRONJ (Bisphosphonate-Related Osteonecrosis of the Jaw) versus MRONJ (Medication-Related Osteonecrosis of the Jaw) [11] (Reprinted with kind permission of Elsevier)

| BRONJ (AAOMS 2009) definition | MRONJ (AAOMS 2014) definition |
|---|---|
| 1. Current or previous treatment with bisphosphonates | 1. Current or previous treatment with antiresorptive or antiangiogenic agents |
| 2. Exposed bone in the maxillofacial region that has persisted for more than 8 weeks | 2. Exposed bone *or bone that can be probed through an intraoral or extraoral fistula(e) in the maxillofacial region that has persisted for more than 8 weeks* |
| 3. No history of radiation therapy to the jaws | 3. No history of radiation therapy to the jaws *or obvious metastatic disease to the jaws* |

This reflects the criteria of the recently updated position paper of the AAOMS 2014. Table 4.1 provides a comparison between the definition of bisphonate-related osteonecrosis of the jaw (AAOMS 2009) and the updated definition of medication-related ostenecrosis of the jaw (AAOMS 2014).

However, histological criteria are not yet part of the definition, but histological investigation is strongly recommended whenever bone parts are resected and whenever the diagnosis is uncertain (see chapter 12 Histopathology of Medication-Related Osteonecrosis of the jaw). With regard to the fact that the vast majority of MRONJ patients suffer from a malignant underlying disease, exclusion of metastases in the jaw bone can be of crucial importance [13, 14].

## General Characteristics

In the vast majority of MRONJ cases, the administration of bisphosphonates or denosumab is due to a malignant underlying disease, especially breast cancer, prostate cancer and multiple myeloma [15–17]. However, depending on the underlying patient cohort, there is also a significant proportion of cases with osteoporosis being the underlying disease [17, 18]. The overwhelming majority of MRONJ cases occurred after long-term intravenous administration of nitrogen-containing bisphosphonates [19–21]. Less often MRONJ occurs after oral administration of nitrogen-containing bisphosphonates [18, 22, 23].

Due to the abovementioned underlying diseases, a lot of MRONJ patients suffer from comorbidities such as manifest bone metastasis (77.3 %) or metastases in organs other than bone. Therefore, a significant number of MRONJ patients have experienced chemotherapy or are currently under chemotherapy (72.7 %), or they receive co-medications such as steroids or anti-angiogenic drugs. Apart from that, there are also a significant proportion of cases with diabetes and vascular diseases [24]. All of these circumstances can contribute to a complication of the disease as well as interfere with the treatment modalities [16].

## Clinical Features

Exposed necrotic bone represents the clinical hallmark of the disease. It is present in the vast majority of MRONJ cases (up to 93.9 %) [16]. The extent of bone exposure can vary considerably – from only small bony edges (Fig. 4.1) over tooth sockets (Fig. 4.2) to whole parts of the jaw bone (Fig. 4.3). However, the extent of bone exposure is not directly related to the extent of underlying necrosis nor to the severity of the disease (Fig. 4.4).

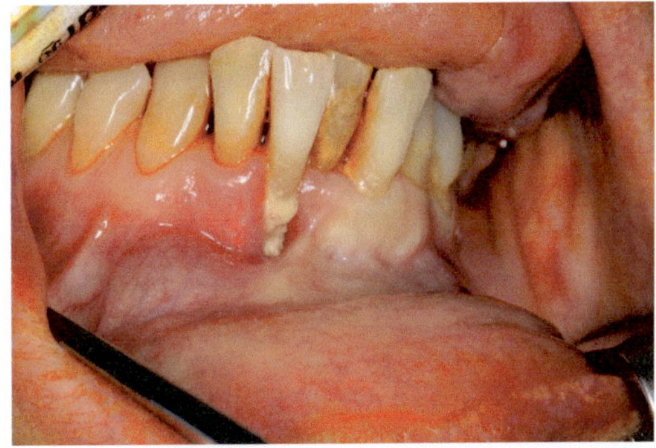

**Fig. 4.2** A 71-year-old male patient with an initial diagnosis of renal cancer, receiving monthly oral therapy of alendronate over a period of 34 months. Preoperative view on the affected area in the right side mandible in region 41 showing surrounding areas of the necrotic bone which were clinically accompanied by pain and signs of infection (MRONJ stage II)

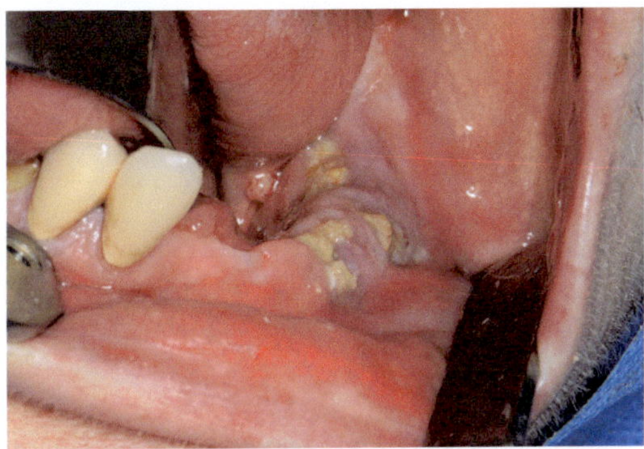

**Fig. 4.3** A 64-year-old female patient with an initial diagnosis of breast cancer, receiving monthly intravenous therapy of zoledronate over a period of 92 months. Preoperative view on the affected area in the left side mandible in region 035–037 showing extended areas of the necrotic bone. Besides, the patient had a second affected area of necrotic bone in the right side maxilla in region 011–014 (Fig. 4.8) (MRONJ stage II)

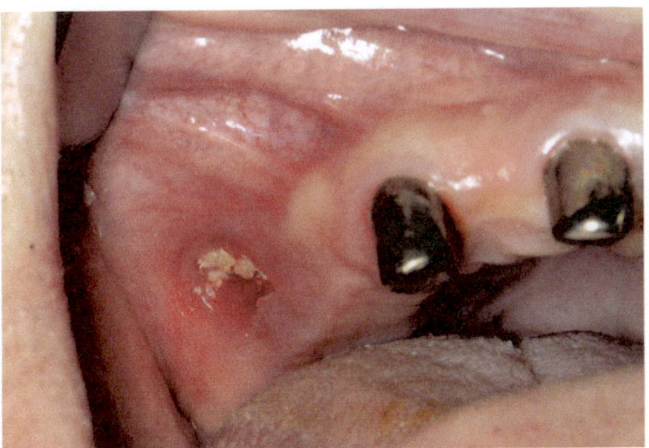

**Fig. 4.1** A 75-year-old male patient with an initial diagnosis of prostate cancer, receiving zoledronate every 4 weeks intravenously over a period of 25 months. Preoperative view on the affected area in the right side maxilla showing small bony edges of the necrotic bone (MRONJ stage I)

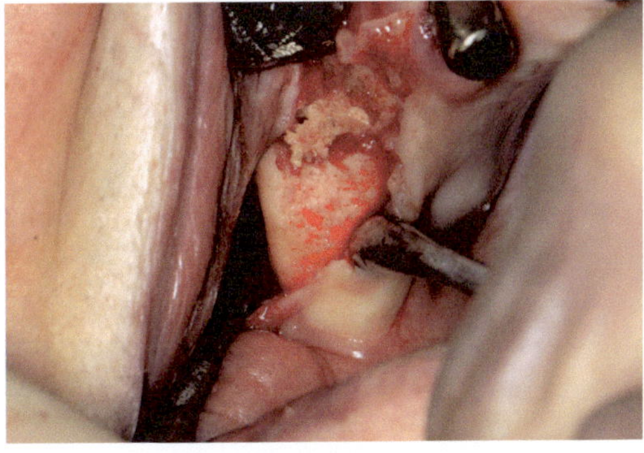

**Fig. 4.4** Same patient as in Fig. 4.1. Intraoperative view on the affected area in the right side maxilla showing the extension of the necrotic bone (MRONJ stage I)

Signs of infection such as soft tissue swelling, suppuration and intra- or extra-oral draining sinus tracts are often present and even local abscesses can occur (Table 4.2). When superinfection of the necrotic tissues occurs, patients can suffer from severe pain, although this condition is not obligatory, and interestingly a significant proportion of patients have no pain at all (Table 4.2). In severe cases local infections might develop into abscesses of the deep spaces of the head and neck with

potentially life-threatening characteristic [25, 26]. Even abscess formations in the brain secondary to MRONJ have been described. In rare cases, even septic systemic infections might occur [27].

A rare but typical symptom only occurring in the mandible is impairment of inferior alveolar nerve function due to MRONJ, often referred to as Vincent or numb chin symptom [28, 29]. Interestingly, this can be an early or even be the presenting symptom of the disease but can also occur in advanced stages of MRONJ [28, 29]. Depending on the affected area local inflammatory processes, sequestration or pathological fractures of the mandible might induce these symptoms showing up with numbness of the lower lip and chin, the gingiva and the teeth [29, 30]. However, as impairment of inferior alveolar nerve function can as well be a sign of metastatic infiltration (e.g. jaw bone metastasis), histological evaluation is strongly recommended [14, 28].

Severe functional and therapeutic problems can be caused by extended osteonecrosis of the jaws with pathological fractures of the mandible (see Fig. 4.5). It can occur due to structural weakening of the bone or following extensive resection of necrotic bone areas [31]. The frequency was observed to be 2.9–3.8 % of MRONJ cases, and it is by definition referred to stage 3 of MRONJ according to the AAOMS [11]. Treatment of pathological fractures due to MRONJ is particularly difficult and controversially discussed [31].

**Table 4.2** Clinical presentation of MRONJ

| Clinical presentation | Prevalence (n) | Percentage (%) |
| --- | --- | --- |
| Exposed bone | 62 | 93.9 |
| Pain | 52 | 78.8 |
| Wound healing disturbances | 45 | 68.2 |
| Swelling | 34 | 51.5 |
| Inflammation | 42 | 63.6 |
| Fistula formation | 27 | 40.9 |
| Pathological mandibular fractures | 3 | 4.5 |
| Impairment of inferior alveolar nerve | 6 | 9.1 |
| Involvement of maxillary sinus | 11 | 16.7 |
|   Sinusitis | (11) | (16.7) |
|   Oroantral fistula formation | (5) | (7.6) |

According to Otto et al. [16]

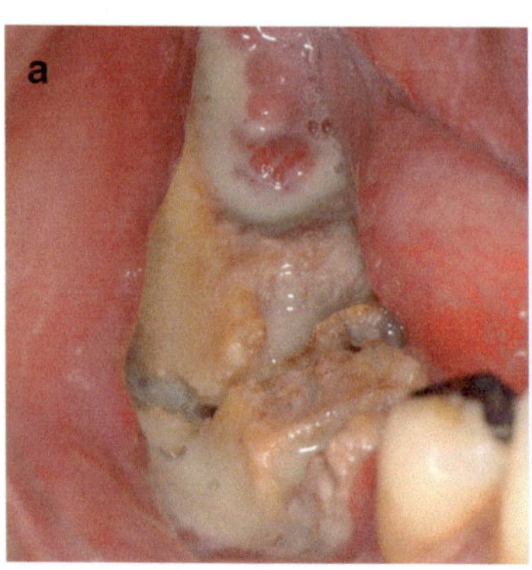
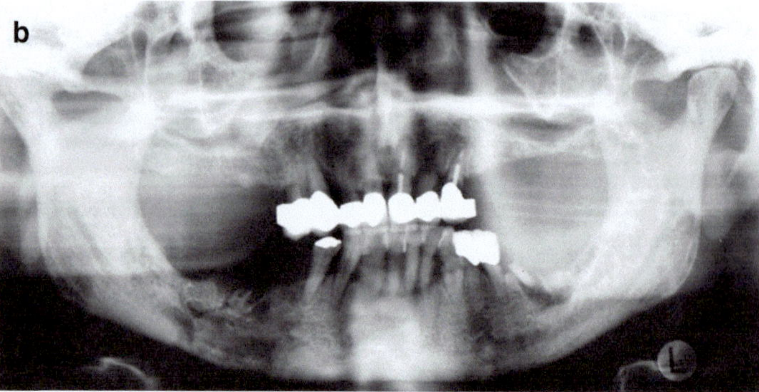

**Fig. 4.5** (**a, b**) Pathological fracture due to medication-related osteonecrosis of the jaw in a 65-year-old female patient suffering from metastatic breast cancer who was treated with intravenous administrations of nitrogen-containing bisphosphonates (zoledronate). (**a**) Intraoral view with a large area of exposed necrotic bone and sign of massive superinfection (swelling, pus) and a visible fracture of the mandible with mobile segments. (**b**) Panoramic radiograph of the patient with a mixed radiolucent and radiopaque appearance and a visible fracture line on the right mandibular body (Reprinted from Otto et al. [31] with kind permission of Thieme (© Georg Thieme Verlag KG.))

In the upper jaw which is involved in approximately 1/3 of the ONJ cases under bisphosphonate treatment [23, 24], the course of the disease can be complicated by maxillary sinusitis or oroantral and in rare cases even oronasal communications. Sinusitic complaints are described in up to 40 % of the MRONJ cases in the maxilla [32]. Oroantral communications can occur due to the disease itself or in the course of surgical treatment [24, 32] (Fig. 4.6).

Further symptoms, associated with MRONJ, are loosening of teeth, due to alterations inside necrotic bone areas [33, 34], and halitosis, due to bacterial inflammation [34, 35]. Loosening of teeth might be estimated as a cause for progress of the necrotic lesion.

Based on undergoing changes in necrotic bone areas and surrounding soft tissues, symptoms such as halitosis are commonly found in patients suffering from MRONJ [34, 36]. This might also be the result of bacterial colonisation of the affected regions, usually combined with a non-sterile infection of the bone and surrounding soft tissues. Pre-existing periodontitis as an inflammatory disease of the periodontium might be a contributory cause, occurring in 71–84 % of MRONJ cases [37–40]. In those cases, specific bacteria, such as *Porphyromonas gingivalis*, *Treponema denticola*, *Tannerella forsythia*, and *Aggregatibacter actinomycetemcomitans*, are found in smear test of oral polymicrobial biofilms [41].

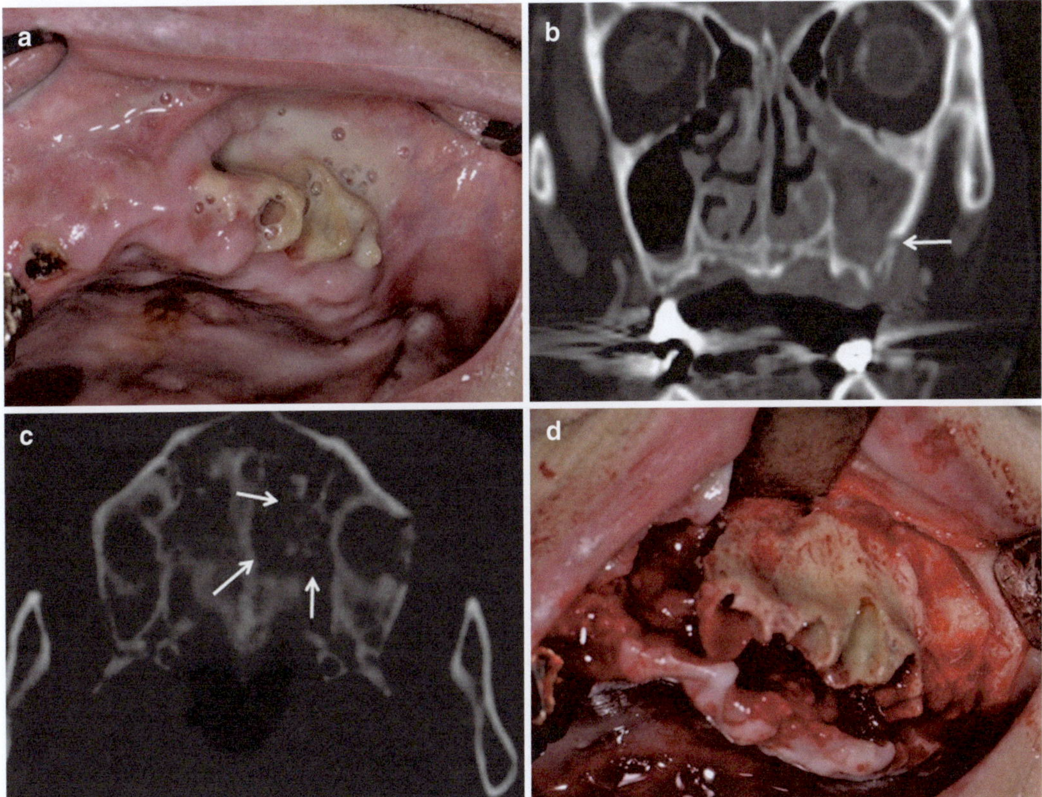

**Fig. 4.6** (**a**) Clinical presentation of a MRONJ stage III lesion in the left upper jaw of a 76-year-old female patient suffering from osteoporosis who was treated with alendronate (70 mg weekly) for 6 years and developed exposed necrotic bone after tooth extractions. (**b**, **c**) Preoperative coronal and axial sections of a cone beam CT showing signs of incomplete sequestration in the left upper jaw, palate and sinus wall (*white arrows*) as well as radiopacity of the left maxillary sinus. (**d**) Intraoperative view after exposure of the left upper jaw and before sequestrectomy and removal of necrotic bone parts

Dental, oral and maxillofacial complications found in patients with MRONJ are miscellaneous. They might arise from progression of the disease or as a consequence of treatment modalities, thus resulting in functional problems, such as impairment of chewing, loss of teeth sustaining bone areas and limited rehabilitation of chewing function. Besides, aesthetic restrictions might occur, e.g. tooth loss, impairment of facial contours due to extensive bone loss, deviation of the mandible after partly resections or permanently persistence of the oroantral fistula. Moreover, denture sore mouths, insufficient wound healing and drug-induced mucositis can occur [36].

Based on the accompanying occurrences due to osteonecrotic lesions, problems such as chewing disorders, ulcerated, painful and swollen oral mucosa; chronic sinus tracts and facial disfigurement; impaired speech, swallowing and eating; and/or frequent medical and dental evaluations as well as treatments may cause marked limitations in quality of life [42–45]. Recent studies have tried to analyze this potential negative impact on quality of life, caused by already mentioned complications in stages 1–3 [46–50]. Miksad et al. evaluated this on patients suffering from MRONJ and described significant reductions in quality of life. Especially in advanced stages, the quality of life can be markedly reduced [51].

## Staging According to the AAOMS 2007, 2009 and 2014 [11, 12]

In 2007 the American Association of Oral and Maxillofacial Surgeons introduced a staging of MRONJ cases (at this time called BRONJ) from stage 1 to stage 3 depending on bone exposure and absence or presence of signs of infection and stage 3 being the stage of complications [12]:

Stage 1: Exposed necrotic bone with no pain and no signs of infection

Stage 2: Exposed necrotic bone with pain and clinical evidence of infection

Stage 3: Exposed necrotic bone with pain, infection and one or more of the following:

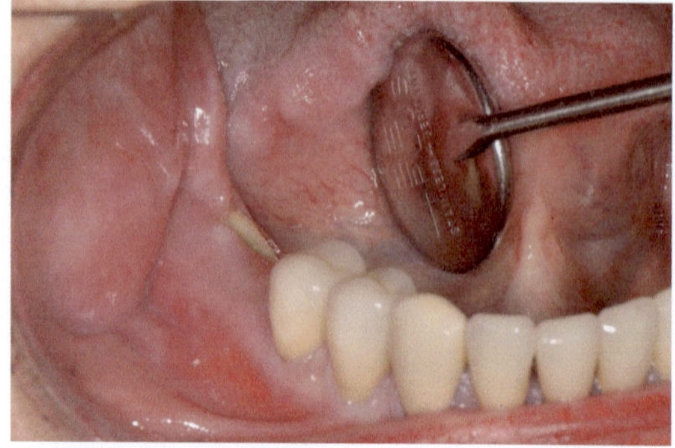

**Fig. 4.7** Stage 1 MRONJ lesion of the lingual aspect of the right mandible which occurred in an 81-year-old patient suffering from breast cancer which was treated with intravenous administrations of nitrogen-containing bisphosphonates (zoledronate)

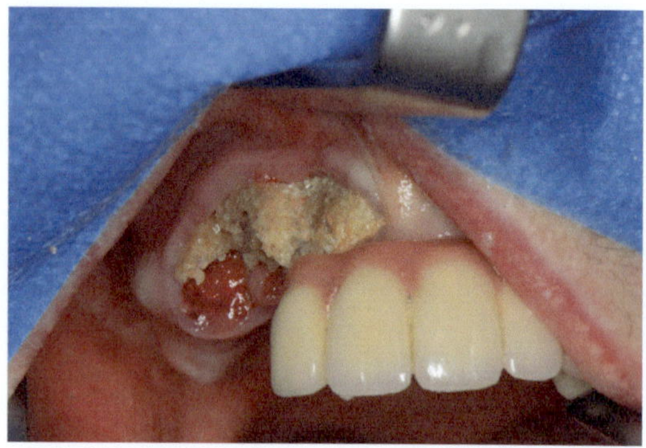

**Fig. 4.8** Same patient as in Fig. 4.3. Intraoperative view on the affected area in the right side maxilla in region 011–014 showing widely the necrotic bone (MRONJ stage II)

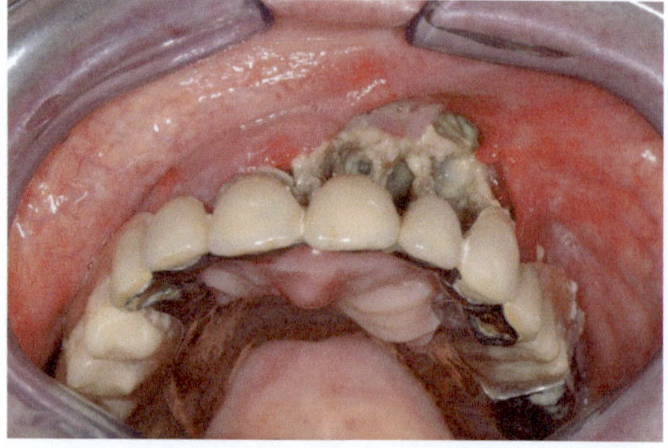

**Fig. 4.9** A 73-year-old patient suffering from breast cancer who received intravenous administrations of nitrogen-containing bisphosphonates (zoledronate) who presented with an osteonecrotic lesions with extension to the floor of the nose and involvement of the left maxillary sinus (MRONJ stage III). The lesion was so painful that the patient could not remove the prosthesis for several weeks

- Necrotic bone extending the alveolar bone to the inferior border or ramus in the mandible or to the maxillary sinus or zygoma
- Pathological fracture of the mandible
- Oroantral or oronasal communication
- Extraoral fistula formation (Fig. 4.7, 4.8 and 4.9)

## Stage 0

With regard to the fact that jaw bone necrosis can occur even when there is no bone exposure in 2009, a stage 0 was defined by the AAOMS which was confirmed in 2014. Stage 0 is defined as the presence of necrotic bone underneath normal epithelial coverage of the oral soft tissues [52]. As described by several authors, this type of MRONJ (at this time called BRONJ) combines clinical features and symptoms, such as jaw bone pain, gingival swelling, and bone enlargement, with the absence of dental disease and necrotic bone exposure [53–56]. Radiological signs of stage 0 might contain osteosclerosis in the symptomatic bone areas, periradicular radiolucencies, persisting alveolar sockets, and density confluence of cortical and cancellous bone [56]. Usually, surgical procedures at stage 0 are not indicated; nonetheless, some authors report surgical sequestrectomy and surgical debridement next to antibiotic therapy and antimicrobial rinse with the result of complete mucosal coverage [57] (Fig. 4.10) (Table 4.3) [11].

## Localisation

Approximately two thirds of all reported ONJ cases under bisphosphonate treatment occurred in the mandible, whereas only one third were localised in the maxilla [5, 16, 17, 23]. Potential reasons for this predisposition of the mandible might be the different vascularity of the mandible and maxilla and the different relation between cortical and spongious bone. Up to now there is no such data with regard to the distribution of ONJ cases under denosumab treatment available.

But there is also a characteristic distribution of MRONJ lesions within the jaws with a predilection for the molar and premolar region (Fig. 4.11) in the mandible as well as in the maxilla [16, 17]. With regard to the potential role of local infections in the pathogenesis of the disease (see chapter 13 Pathogenesis of Medication-Related Osteonecrosis of the Jaw), this might be due to larger root surfaces in these areas and the likelihood of local dental (endodontic or periodontal) infections and the frequency of dentoalveolar surgeries in these areas. Besides that there seems to be a predisposition for MRONJ in areas with thin mucosal layers, especially in the lingual aspects of the mandible and in the area of tori (Fig. 4.12).

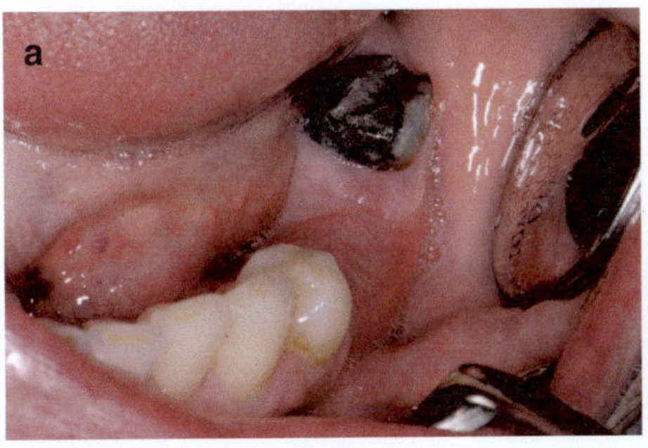
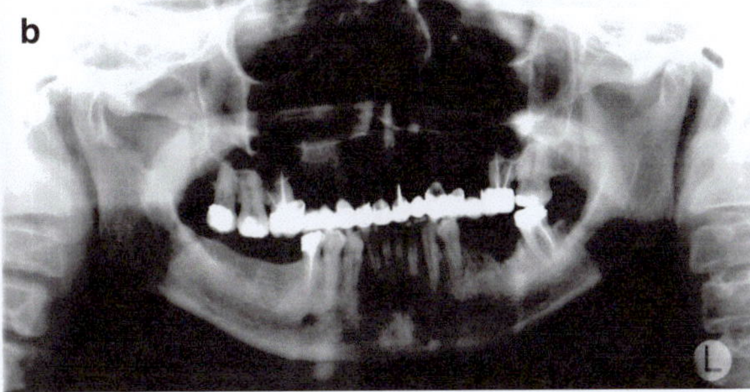

**Fig. 4.10** (**a**) Clinical presentation of a 51-year-old female patient suffering from breast cancer after intravenous treatment with nitrogen-containing bisphosphonates (zoledronate) who developed complaints (pain) in the left mandible without bone exposure after a tooth extraction (referring to stage 0 of the AAOMS 2009 and 2014). (**b**) Panoramic radiograph of the same patient showing bone sclerosis in the left mandible (region 36/37) and an incomplete remodelling of the extraction alveolus region 36

**Table 4.3** Staging of BRONJ/MRONJ according to AAOMS 2009 and 2014 update [11] (Reprinted with kind permission of Elsevier)

|  | 2009 AAOMS staging | 2014 AAOMS staging |
|---|---|---|
| At risk | No apparent necrotic bone in patients who have been treated with either oral or IV BP | No changes |
| Stage 0 | No clinical evidence of necrotic bone, but nonspecific clinical findings and symptoms | No changes |
| Stage 1 | Exposed and necrotic bone in asymptomatic patients without evidence of infection | Exposed and necrotic bone, *or fistulae that probes to bone*, in patients who are asymptomatic and have no evidence of infection |
| Stage 2 | Exposed and necrotic bone associated with infection as evidenced by pain and erythema in region of exposed bone with or without purulent drainage | Exposed and necrotic bone, *or fistulae that probes to bone*, associated with infection as evidenced by pain and erythema in the region of the exposed bone with or without purulent drainage |
| Stage 3 | Exposed and necrotic bone in patients with pain, infection, and one or more of the following: exposed and necrotic bone extending beyond the region of alveolar bone, (i.e., inferior border and ramus in the mandible, maxillary sinus and zygoma in the maxilla) resulting in pathologic fracture, extraoral fistula, oral antral/oral nasal communication, or osteolysis extending to the inferior border of the mandible or the sinus floor | Exposed and necrotic bone *or a fistula that probes to bone* in patients with pain, infection, and one or more of the following: exposed and necrotic bone extending beyond the region of alveolar bone, (i.e., inferior border and ramus in the mandible, maxillary sinus and zygoma in the maxilla) resulting in pathologic fracture, extra-oral fistula, oral antral/oral nasal communication, or osteolysis extending to the inferior border of the mandible of sinus floor |

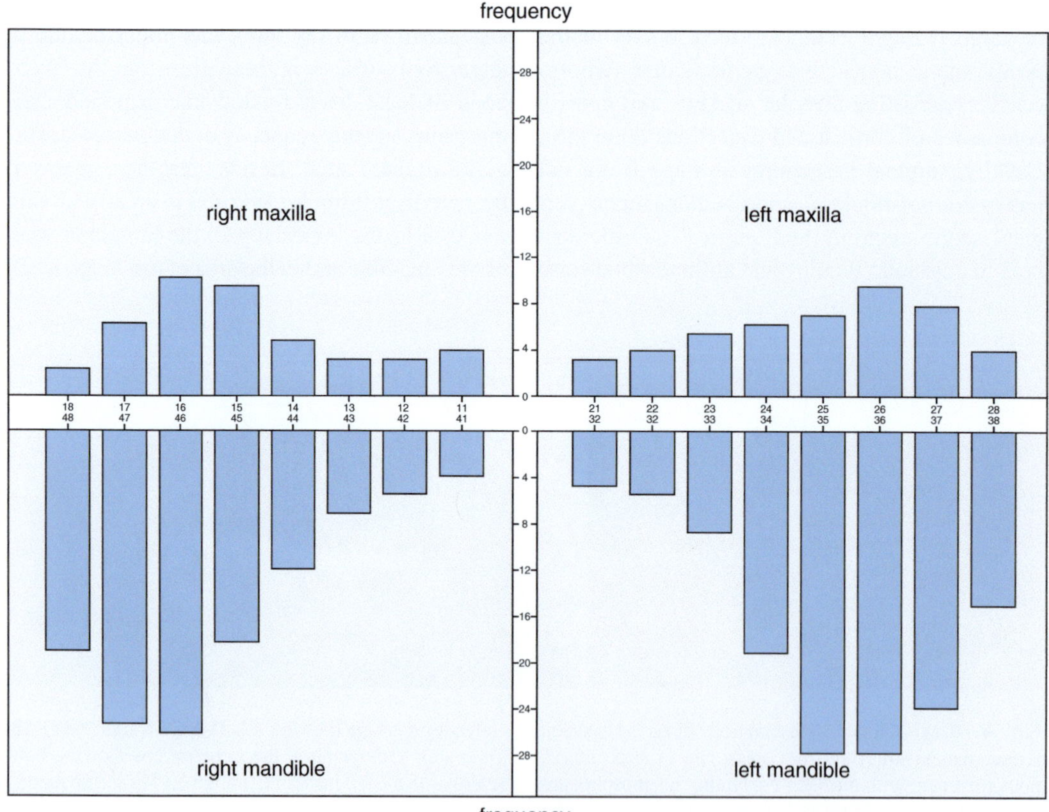


**Fig. 4.11** Distribution of MRONJ lesions in the jaw bones (Reprinted from Otto et al. [16] with kind permission of Elsevier)

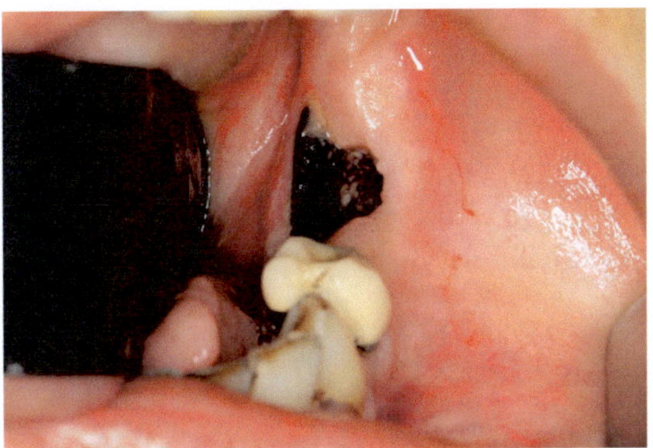

**Fig. 4.12** A 50-year-old female patient with an initial diagnosis of breast cancer, receiving monthly intravenous therapy of zoledronate over a period of 35 months. Preoperative view on the affected area in the left side mandibular angle, showing widely the necrotic bone (MRONJ stage II)

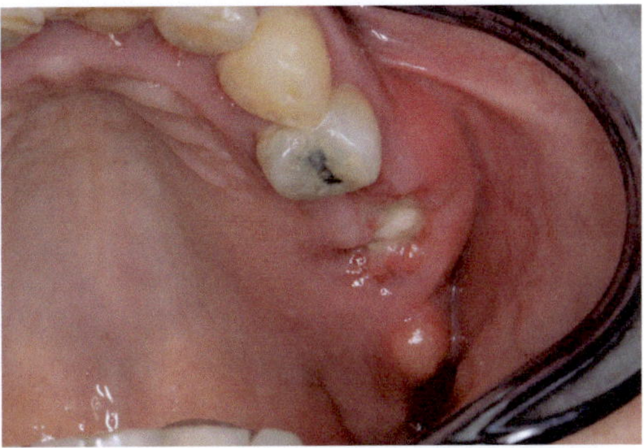

**Fig. 4.13** A 76-year-old female patient suffering from metastatic breast cancer who received monthly subcutaneous administrations of denosumab 120 mg and developed exposed necrotic bone of the left upper jaw and sign of infection (pain, swelling, pus on palpation) after teeth extraction

## Medication-Related Osteonecrosis Occurring Outside the Oral Cavity

In literature only few cases have been described, where osteonecrosis occurred in other locations outside the oral cavity. One case reports about a 64-year-old male patient, treated with zoledronic acid due to multiple myeloma, who presented painful, non-healing sockets after left-sided tooth extractions with periodontal necrosis and formation of a sequestrum. During re-examination after 6 months, the same patient revealed painless ulceration of the left auditory canal, and further radiological examinations and local debridement verified the diagnosis of medication-related osteonecrosis of the auditory canal [58]. The second case described was a 79-year-old female patient receiving oral bisphosphonates due to osteoporosis. This patient also developed an osteonecrosis inside the left auditory canal, verified by CT scans and surgical debridement with histological examination [59].

## Osteonecrosis of the Jaw due to RANKL Inhibitor (Denosumab) Treatment

In recent years, osteoporosis and metastatic bone disease have mostly been treated using nitrogen-containing bisphosphonates. But since 2010, an alternative drug called denosumab (Prolia®) has been approved for treatment in Europe (*Committee for Medicinal Products for Human Use* (CHMP) by the *European Medicines Agency* (EMA)) and in the United States (*Food and Drug Administration* (FDA)). Interestingly, denosumab as a subcutaneously dosed monoclonal antibody against RANK ligand (RANKL) shows similar side effects to zoledronic acid. One of the major complications is the comparable "denosumab-related osteonecrosis of the jaws" (DRONJ). Almost identical effects have been described for the treatment of breast and prostate cancers and multiple myeloma [7, 8, 60]. The complication of osteonecrosis of the jaws related to denosumab seems radiologically, clinically and histologically comparable. Results of a comparative study from 2013 could show that even the risk of development of MRONJ (zoledronic acid = 1.1 %) and DRONJ (denosumab = 0.8 %) is approximately identical [61]. Intraoral affections of DRONJ appear in similar regions as in DRONJ (Fig. 4.13). Therefore, the special committee of the AAOMS 2014 favors the term medication-related osteonecrosis of the jaws [11].

> **Conclusions**
> Osteonecrosis of the jaw due to bisphosphonate and denosumab treatment has become a well-known and clinically important entity which predominantly occurs in patients suffering from malignant underlying diseases who received intravenous administrations

of nitrogen-containing bisphosphonates or subcutaneous administrations of denosumab. Exposed necrotic bone in the maxillofacial region is the clinical hallmark of the disease. In the majority of cases, it is accompanied by signs of infection such as pain, swelling of surrounding soft tissues or draining fistulas. Further complications such as involvement of the maxillary sinus or pathological fractures of the mandible might occur in the course of the disease.

**Acknowledgements** The authors like to thank Rudolf Herzig and Gerhard Poetzel for their support in the preparation of the clinical images.

# References

1. Marx RE. Pamidronate (Aredia) and zoledronate (Zometa) induced avascular necrosis of the jaws: a growing epidemic [Letter]. J Oral Maxillofac Surg. 2003;61:1115.
2. Wang J, Goodger NM, Pogrel MA. Osteonecrosis of the jaw associated with cancer chemotherapy. J Oral Maxillofac Surg. 2003;61:1104–7.
3. Migliorati CA. Bisphosphonates and oral cavity avascular bone necrosis. J Clin Oncol. 2003;21(22):4253–4.
4. Ruggiero SL, Mehrotra B, Rosenberg TJ, Engroff SL. Osteonecrosis of the jaws associated with the use of bisphosphonates: a review of 63 cases. J Oral Maxillofac Surg. 2004;62(5):527–34.
5. Aghaloo TL, Felsenfeld AL, Tetradis S. Osteonecrosis of the jaw in a patient on denosumab. J Oral Maxillofac Surg. 2010;68(5):959–63.
6. Stopeck AT, Lipton A, Body JJ, Steger GG, Tonkin K, de Boer RH, et al. Denosumab compared with zoledronic acid for the treatment of bone metastases in patients with advanced breast cancer: a randomized, double-blind study. J Clin Oncol. 2010;28(35):5132–9.
7. Henry DH, Costa L, Goldwasser F, Hirsh V, Hungria V, Prausova J, et al. Randomized, double-blind study of denosumab versus zoledronic acid in the treatment of bone metastases in patients with advanced cancer (excluding breast and prostate cancer) or multiple myeloma. J Clin Oncol. 2011;29(9):1125–32.
8. Saad F, Brown JE, Van Poznak C, Ibrahim T, Stemmer SM, Stopeck AT, et al. Incidence, risk factors, and outcomes of osteonecrosis of the jaw: integrated analysis from three blinded active-controlled phase III trials in cancer patients with bone metastases. Ann Oncol. 2012;23(5):1341–7.
9. Lipton A, Fizazi K, Stopeck AT, Henry DH, Brown JE, Yardley DA, et al. Superiority of denosumab to zoledronic acid for prevention of skeletal-related events: a combined analysis of 3 pivotal, randomised, phase 3 trials. Eur J Cancer. 2012;48(16):3082–92.
10. Van den Wyngaert T, Wouters K, Huizing MT, Vermorken JB. RANK ligand inhibition in bone metastatic cancer and risk of osteonecrosis of the jaw (ONJ): non bis in idem? Support Care Cancer. 2011;19(12):2035–40.
11. Ruggiero SL, Dodson TB, Fantasia J, Goodday R, Aghaloo T, Mehrotra B, et al. American Association of Oral and Maxillofacial Surgeons Special Committee Position Paper on Medication-Related Osteonecrosis of the Jaw. J Oral and Maxillofac Surg 2014; 72(10):1938–56.
12. Advisory Task Force on Bisphosphonate-Related Osteonecrosis of the Jaws. American Association of Oral and Maxillofacial Surgeons position paper on bisphosphonate-related osteonecrosis of the jaws. J Oral Maxillofac Surg. 2007;65:369–76.
13. Otto S, Schuler K, Ihrler S, Ehrenfeld M, Mast G. Osteonecrosis or metastases of the jaw or both? Case report and review of the literature. J Oral Maxillofac Surg. 2010;68(5):1185–8.
14. Bedogni A, Saia G, Ragazzo M, Bettini G, Capelli P, D'Alessandro E, et al. Bisphosphonate-associated osteonecrosis can hide jaw metastases. Bone. 2007; 41(6):942–5.
15. Bamias A, Kastritis E, Bamia C, Moulopoulos LA, Melakopoulos I, Bozas G, et al. Osteonecrosis of the jaw in cancer after treatment with bisphosphonates: incidence and risk factors. J Clin Oncol. 2005;23(34): 8580–7.
16. Otto S, Schreyer C, Hafner S, Mast G, Ehrenfeld M, Stürzenbaum S, et al. Bisphosphonate-related osteonecrosis of the jaws - characteristics, risk factors, clinical features, localization and impact on oncological treatment. J Craniomaxillofac Surg. 2012;40(4):303–9.
17. Abu-Id MH, Warnke PH, Gottschalk J, Springer I, Wiltfang J, Acil Y, et al. "Bis-phossy jaws" – high and low risk factors for bisphosphonate-induced osteonecrosis of the jaw. J Craniomaxillofac Surg. 2008;36(2):95–103.
18. Otto S, Abu-Id MH, Fedele S, Warnke PH, Becker ST, Kolk A, et al. Osteoporosis and bisphosphonates-related osteonecrosis of the jaw: not just a sporadic coincidence–a multi-centre study. J Craniomaxillofac Surg. 2011;39(4):272–7.
19. Rugani P, Luschin G, Jakse N, Kirnbauer B, Lang U, Acham S. Prevalence of bisphosphonate-associated osteonecrosis of the jaw after intravenous zoledronate infusions in patients with early breast cancer. Clin Oral Investig. 2013;18(2):401–7.
20. Hoff AO, Toth BB, Altundag K, Johnson MM, Warneke CL, Hu M, et al. Frequency and risk factors associated with osteonecrosis of the jaw in cancer patients treated with intravenous bisphosphonates. J Bone Miner Res. 2008;23:826–36.
21. Walter C, Al-Nawas B, Frickhofen N, Gamm H, Beck J, Reinsch L, et al. Prevalence of bisphosphonate associate osteonecrosis of the jaws in multiple myeloma patients. Head Face Med. 2010;6:11. doi:10.1186/1746-160X-6-11.

22. Yarom N, Yahalom R, Shoshani Y, Hamed W, Regev E, Elad S. Osteonecrosis of the jaw induced by orally administered bisphosphonates: incidence, clinical features, predisposing factors and treatment outcome. Osteoporos Int. 2007;18(10):1363–70.

23. Assaf AT, Zrnc TA, Riecke B, Wikner J, Zustin J, Friedrich RE, et al. Intraoperative efficiency of fluorescence imaging by Visually Enhanced Lesion Scope (VELscope®) in patients with bisphosphonate related osteonecrosis of the jaw (MRONJ). J Craniomaxillofac Surg. 2013;42(5):e157–64. doi:10.1016/j.jcms.2013.07.014. pii: S1010-5182(13)00212-6.

24. Assaf AT, Smeets R, Riecke B, Weise E, Gröbe A, Blessmann M, et al. Incidence of bisphosphonate-related osteonecrosis of the jaw in consideration of primary diseases and concomitant therapies. Anticancer Res. 2013;33(9):3917–24.

25. Mehanna P, Goddard R. Bisphosphonate associated osteonecrosis: an unusual case. Aust Dent J. 2010;55(3): 311–3.

26. Soda T, Fukumoto R, Hayashi T, Oka D, Fujimoto N, Koide T. A case of prostate cancer associated with bisphosphonate-related osteonecrosis of the jaw followed by retropharyngeal abscess. Hinyokika Kiyo. 2013;59(9):587–91.

27. Matsushita A, Kamigaki S, Nakamura Y. A case of brain abscess secondary to bisphosphonate-related osteonecrosis of the jaws in metastatic bone lesions from breast carcinoma. Gan To Kagaku Ryoho. 2013;40(5):631–3.

28. Otto S, Hafner S, Grötz KA. The role of inferior alveolar nerve involvement in bisphosphonate-related osteonecrosis of the jaw. J Oral Maxillofac Surg. 2009;67(3):589–92. doi:10.1016/j.joms.2008.09.028.

29. Assaf AT, Jürgens TP, Benecke AW, Riecke B, Blessmann M, Zrnc TA, et al. Numb chin syndrome. A rare and often overlooked symptom. J Orofac Pain. 2014;28(1):80–90. 01/2014 Date accepted: 2013-07-19.

30. Sierra-Hidalgo F, de Pablo-Fernández E, Correas-Callero E, Villarejo-Galende A. Numb chin syndrome caused by bisphosphonates-induced osteonecrosis of the jaw. Rev Neurol. 2009;49(4):190–2.

31. Otto S, Pautke C, Hafner S, Hesse R, Reichardt LF, Mast G, et al. Pathologic fractures in bisphosphonate-related osteonecrosis of the jaw—review of the literature and review of our own cases. Craniomaxillofac Trauma Reconstr. 2013;6(3):147–54.

32. Mast G, Otto S, Mücke T, Schreyer C, Bissinger O, Kolk A, et al. Incidence of maxillary sinusitis and oro-antral fistulae in bisphosphonate-related osteonecrosis of the jaw. J Craniomaxillofac Surg. 2012;40(7):568–71.

33. Piesold JU, Al-Nawas B, Grötz KA. Osteonecrosis of the jaws by long term therapy with bisphosphonates. Mund Kiefer Gesichtschir. 2006;10(5):287–300.

34. Saldanha S, Shenoy VK, Eachampati P, Uppal N. Dental implications of bisphosphonate-related osteonecrosis. Gerodontology. 2012;29(3):177–87.

35. Di Fede O, Fusco V, Matranga D, Solazzo L, Gabriele M, Gaeta GM, et al. Osteonecrosis of the jaws in patients assuming oral bisphosphonates for osteoporosis: a retrospective multi-hospital-based study of 87 Italian cases. Eur J Intern Med. 2013;24(8):784–90. pii: S0953-6205(13)00139-8.

36. Grötz KA, Piesold JU, Al-Nawas B. Bisphosphonat-assoziierte Kiefernekrose (BPONJ) und andere Medikamenten-assoziierte Kiefernekrosen 1e18. http://www.awmf.org. 2012, (007/091).

37. Jadu F, Lee L, Pharoah M, Reece D, Wang L. A retrospective study assessing the incidence, risk factors and comorbidities of pamidronate-related necrosis of the jaws in multiple myeloma patients. Ann Oncol. 2007;18(12):2015–9.

38. Marx RE, Sawatari Y, Fortin M, Broumand V. Bisphosphonate-induced exposed bone (osteonecrosis/osteopetrosis) of the jaws: risk factors, recognition, prevention, and treatment. J Oral Maxillofac Surg. 2005;63(11):1567–75.

39. Saussez S, Javadian R, Hupin C, Magremanne M, Chantrain G, Loeb I, et al. Bisphosphonate-related osteonecrosis of the jaw and its associated risk factors: a Belgian case series. Laryngoscope. 2009;119(2):323–9.

40. Thumbigere-Math V, Michalowicz BS, Hodges JS, Tsai ML, Swenson KK, Rockwell L, et al. Periodontal disease as a risk factor for bisphosphonate-related osteonecrosis of the jaw. J Periodontol. 2013;85(2):226–33.

41. Tsao C, Darby I, Ebeling PR, Walsh K, O'Brien-Simpson N, Reynolds E, et al. Oral health risk factors for bisphosphonate-associated jaw osteonecrosis. J Oral Maxillofac Surg. 2013;71(8):1360–6.

42. Ficarra G, Beninati F, Rubino I, Vannucchi A, Longo G, Tonelli P, et al. Osteonecrosis of the jaws in periodontal patients with a history of bisphosphonates treatment. J Clin Periodontol. 2005;32(11):1123–8.

43. Merigo E, Manfredi M, Meleti M, Corradi D, Vescovi P. Jaw bone necrosis without previous dental extractions associated with the use of bisphosphonates (pamidronate and zoledronate): a four-case report. J Oral Pathol Med. 2005;34(10):613–7.

44. Mignogna MD, Fedele S, Lo Russo L, Ciccarelli R, Lo Muzio L. Case 2. Osteonecrosis of the jaws associated with bisphosphonate therapy. J Clin Oncol. 2006;24(9):1475–7.

45. Vannucchi AM, Ficarra G, Antonioli E, Bosi A. Osteonecrosis of the jaw associated with zoledronate therapy in a patient with multiple myeloma. Br J Haematol. 2005;128(6):738.

46. Gutta R, Louis PJ. Bisphosphonates and osteonecrosis of the jaws: science and rationale. Oral Surg Oral Med Oral Pathol Oral Radiol Endod. 2007;104(2): 186–93.

47. Hewitt C, Farah CS. Bisphosphonate-related osteonecrosis of the jaws: a comprehensive review. J Oral Pathol Med. 2007;36(6):319–28.

48. Lam DK, Sandor GK, Holmes HI, Evans AW, Clokie CM. A review of bisphosphonate-associated osteonecrosis of the jaws and its management. J Can Dent Assoc. 2007;73(5):417–22.

49. Mariotti A. Bisphosphonates and osteonecrosis of the jaws. J Dent Educ. 2008;72(8):919–29.

50. Migliorati CA, Siegel MA, Elting LS. Bisphosphonate-associated osteonecrosis: a long-term complication of bisphosphonate treatment. Lancet Oncol. 2006;7(6):508–14.
51. Miksad RA, Lai KC, Dodson TB, Woo SB, Treister NS, Akinyemi O, et al. Quality of life implications of bisphosphonate-associated osteonecrosis of the jaw. Oncologist. 2011;16(1):121–32.
52. Patel S, Choyee S, Uyanne J, Nguyen AL, Lee P, Sedghizadeh PP, et al. Non-exposed bisphosphonate-related osteonecrosis of the jaw: a critical assessment of current definition, staging, and treatment guidelines. Oral Dis. 2012;18(7):625–32.
53. Junquera L, Gallego L. Nonexposed bisphosphonate-related osteonecrosis of the jaws: another clinical variant? J Oral Maxillofac Surg. 2008;66(7):1516–7.
54. Fedele S, Porter SR, D'Aiuto F, Aljohani S, Vescovi P, Manfredi M, et al. Nonexposed variant of bisphosphonate-associated osteonecrosis of the jaw: a case series. Am J Med. 2010;123(11):1060–4.
55. Vescovi P, Nammour S. Bisphosphonate-related osteonecrosis of the jaw (MRONJ) therapy. A critical review. Minerva Stomatol. 2010;59(4):181–203. 204–13.
56. Hutchinson M, O'Ryan F, Chavez V, Lathon PV, Sanchez G, Hatcher DC, et al. Radiographic findings in bisphosphonate-treated patients with stage 0 disease in the absence of bone exposure. J Oral Maxillofac Surg. 2010;68(9):2232–40.
57. Mawardi H, Treister N, Richardson P, Anderson K, Munshi N, Faiella RA, et al. Sinus tracts–an early sign of bisphosphonate-associated osteonecrosis of the jaws? J Oral Maxillofac Surg. 2009;67(3):593–601.
58. Polizzotto MN, Cousins V, Schwarer AP. Bisphosphonate-associated osteonecrosis of the auditory canal. Br J Haematol. 2006;132(1):114.
59. Salzman R, Hoza J, Perina V, Stárek I. Osteonecrosis of the external auditory canal associated with oral bisphosphonate therapy: case report and literature review. Otol Neurotol. 2013;34(2):209–13.
60. Fizazi K, Carducci M, Smith M, Damião R, Brown J, Karsh L, et al. Denosumab versus zoledronic acid for treatment of bone metastases in men with castration-resistant prostate cancer: a randomised, double-blind study. Lancet. 2011;377(9768):813–22.
61. Henry D, Vadhan-Raj S, Hirsh V, von Moos R, Hungria V, Costa L, et al. Delaying skeletal-related events in a randomized phase 3 study of denosumab versus zoledronic acid in patients with advanced cancer: an analysis of data from patients with solid tumors. Support Care Cancer. 2013;22(3):679–87.

# Epidemiology of Medication-Related Osteonecrosis of the Jaw



Towy Sorel Lazarovici and Tal Yoffe


**Abstract**

Osteonecrosis of the jaw is a devastating side effect of long-term bisphosphonate (BP) use. We investigated epidemiological aspects of Bisphosphonate-related osteonecrosis of the jaws (BRONJ/MRONJ).

The epidemiology of BRONJ/MRONJ was divided according to the type of BPs and the route of administration: specifically, osteoporotic patients who are often administered oral BPs and cancer patients who predominantly receive intravenous BPs.

The prevalence of BRONJ/MRONJ with oral BP use was estimated as being between 0.01 and 0.05 %, and it was higher after dental extraction. The prevalence of BRONJ/MRONJ with intravenous BP administration reached as high as 10 %, with the highest prevalence observed among multiple myeloma patients and the lowest prevalence measured among breast cancer patients.


## Introduction

Bisphosphonates (BPs) are antiresorptive agents that have been used for decades. BPs are recommended mainly for the treatment of metabolic bone diseases, such as osteoporosis and osteopenia [1], and for controlling skeletal complications associated with multiple myeloma and metastases of solid tumors to the bone [2–5]. However, the devastating side effect of osteonecrosis of the jaw in association with their use has been documented in the literature over the last decade [6–15].

The mechanisms of action of BPs are discussed into detail in the pharmacology (see Chap. 1). Their main effect is inhibition of bone resorption by suppressing osteoclast activation and inducing osteoclast apoptosis [15, 16]. Theories dealing with the pathogenesis of osteonecrosis of the jaw (see pathogenesis chapter 13) are also discussing the anti-angiogenic nature of BPs, expressed by interference with endothelial cell proliferation [17]. Although no general agreement has yet been reached regarding the mecha-


T.S. Lazarovici, DMD (✉) • T. Yoffe, DMD
Department of Oral and Maxillofacial Surgery,
Sheba Medical Center, Israel
e-mail: towy_lazarovici@yahoo.com;
yorota@gmail.com



S. Otto (ed.), *Medication-Related Osteonecrosis of the Jaws: Bisphosphonates, Denosumab, and New Agents*, 55
DOI 10.1007/978-3-662-43733-9_5, © Springer-Verlag Berlin Heidelberg 2015

nism leading to osteonecrosis of the jaw, it is well recognized that the overall effect of BPs is reduced bone turnover. BPs are also known to cause delayed wound healing by the inhibition of proliferation of fibroblasts and keratinocytes [18].

Bisphosphonate-related osteonecrosis of the jaws (BRONJ) can develop either spontaneously or after triggering events, such as a dentoalveolar surgery in the form of tooth extraction and placement of dental implants or a predispoding condition in the form of periodontitis, dentoalveolar abscess, or a poorly fitted denture [7–12]. Given that a bone heavily laden with BPs has limited capabilities to cope with bone remodeling, which is required for the above-mentioned conditions affecting the oral osseous structure, raises the likelihood that they would be associated with a higher prevalence of BRONJ.

This chapter will describe the differences of prevalence of BRONJ depending on bisphosphonate type and route of administration as well as differences between so-called "spontaneous" development of BRONJ and after "triggering events" such as dentoalveolar surgical procedures and local infections. First of all, a clear distinction must be made between those two patient populations. The former group is comprised of patients diagnosed as having osteoporosis or osteopenia who ingest mainly oral BPs (alendronate or risedronate) on a weekly basis. The latter group is comprised of oncologic patients that are either in an advanced stage of disease in which bone metastases have occurred and need to be controlled or, alternatively, in patients with multiple myeloma, all of whom receive intravenous (IV) BPs (e.g., zoledronic acid or pamidronate) on a monthly basis. The major differences between the bioavailability of these drugs lead to the different prevalence of BRONJ. Specifically, the bioavailability of the oral BPs is markedly lower than that of the IV BPs, and the prevalence of BRONJ reflects this difference [19]. As such, the prevalence of BRONJ in each of these two groups of patients will be dealt with separately.

Unfortunately, currently available information on the overall prevalence of BRONJ is relatively limited because it is mostly derived from anecdotal reports, case series from single institutions, sporadic reports to the Food and Drug Administration, and drug manufacturers' data. The diagnosis of BRONJ is often not confirmed by oral health care specialists. Moreover, these data are distorted by inconsistencies in definitions as well by incomplete and possibly biased reporting.

It is safe to assume that there is major underreporting of the development of BRONJ, whether it might be due to the mildness of symptoms in cases of early stages of the disease and the subsequent failure of patients to seek medical consult or to the misdiagnosis by health providers who had not encountered BRONJ before. This feature is especially relevant for patients who are taking oral BPs and are not being monitored on a regular basis in medical centers, unlike patients who are receiving IV BPs and are routinely screened for side effects before each session of drug administration. Thus, given the nature of the current sources of information, it is not possible to accurately determine the prevalence or incidence rates of BRONJ development, and only estimations can be provided.

## BRONJ Among Osteoporotic Patients on Oral Bisphosphonates

Elderly people comprise the fastest growing population in the world. About 20 % of the general population is over the age of 60 years in western countries [20]. Life expectancy is ~20 years for women aged 65 years and 17.5 years for men aged 65 years, and these figures of life expectancy are continuously rising. Overall, 20–30 % of women and 5–20 % of men aged 50 years or older in the western population have osteoporosis, and approximately 70 % of them will be treated at some point with oral BPs [21–23]. This increasing exposure to oral BPs place more people at risk to develop BRONJ, making it a potential major public health issue.

The accumulation of data on the prevalence of BRONJ began with the first reports of BRONJ in the late 2003 [7] and were mainly derived from information supplied by the manufacturer of alendronate, the most common oral BP (Merck, Whitehouse Station, NJ, USA). Merck's first report on the prevalence of BRONJ emerged after 3 years' accumulation of dozens of reports in the published literature: the reported prevalence was 0.7:100,000 cases per drug patient-years in 2006 [24]. The first large non-commercially associated study that addressed the issue of BRONJ prevalence was performed in Australia and reported in 2007. BRONJ cases that had emerged between 2004 and 2005 were identified primarily by a postal survey of the Australian Oral and Maxillofacial Surgeons, with additional cases from other dental specialists and the Commonwealth of Australia Adverse Drug Reaction Committee. The frequency of BRONJ in osteoporotic patients, mainly those on weekly oral alendronate, was between 0.01 and 0.04 % patients, and the calculated frequency rose to 0.09–0.34 % among those who underwent dental extractions [11]. A similar association between a higher BRONJ prevalence and triggering events was found in further studies. One intra-institutional study from South Korea found 24 cases of BRONJ out of a total of 12,752 patients on oral BPs: the prevalence of BRONJ was calculated as being 0.05 %, and only 20 % had developed spontaneously [25]. Another survey performed in south east Scotland was based on data that were accumulated between 2004 and 2009. Those authors concluded that the prevalence of spontaneous development of BRONJ was 0.017 % and that the prevalence of BRONJ after dental extraction was 0.03 % [26]. Other studies, however, were not able to confirm the conclusion of there being a higher prevalence after triggering events. A large postal survey was conducted on patients with a history of chronic oral BP exposure within a large integrated health care delivery system in northern California. Responders with oral symptoms were either examined or their medical records were inspected. A total of 8,572 patients were surveyed, and a 0.055 % prevalence of spontaneous emergence of BRONJ was calculated, with only 0.044 % of the responders reporting a recent history of a dental extraction [27].

One large retrospective cohort study from the USA identified members via health insurance claim diagnosis codes and identified potential cases of BRONJ that were confirmed by a medical record review. Only 2 out of 8468 oral BPs consumers developed BRONJ, resulting in a prevalence of only 0.023 % [28]. In contrast, a small retrospective study that was performed at the University of Southern California between 2002 and 2006 found 9 patients who were diagnosed as having BRONJ out of a total of 208 patients being treated with oral BPs [29]. Those authors estimated a BRONJ prevalence of 4 % after a tooth extraction, representing one of the highest reported occurrence rates of BRONJ: that, however, was probably due to the small study group and to the institution's being a referral center. The prevalence of BRONJ is apparently somewhere between 0.01 and 0.05 %. It is also apparent that it is higher when the patient who is administered with either oral or IV BPs undergoes oral surgery, such as dental extraction or placement of dental implants.

## BRONJ Among Oncologic Patients on Intravenous Bisphosphonates

The data on side effects, including those on BRONJ, seem to be more reliable with regard to cancer patients since they are screened routinely in medical centers prior to each administration of IV BPs and have greater access to oral and maxillofacial consultations.

Some of the relevant publications combined patients with all types of cancer who receive IV BPs, and those studies addressed the issue of BRONJ prevalence in general, while others differentiated between several types of cancer. The data presented in Table 5.1 clearly show that the incidence of BRONJ among cancer patients on IV BPs (1.2–9.9 %) is between 10- and 100fold more than the incidence among osteoporotic patients on a regimen of oral BPs. It is also evident that the incidence of BRONJ among multiple myeloma patients is higher than that among breast or prostate cancer patients. A very large American cohort study concluded that the standardized incidence per 1,000 person-years was 9.9 for patients with multiple myeloma. Specifically, they had an almost 4.5-fold higher incidence than that of breast cancer patients, while breast cancer patients had an almost 2.7-fold higher risk than patients with prostate cancer [28]. Bamias et al. found more than a

**Table 5.1** Epidemiology of bisphosphonate-related osteonecrosis of the jaws (BRONJ) in cancer patients receiving intravenous bisphosphonates

| Author | Type of study | Number | Diagnosis | BRONJ prevalence | Precipitating factor |
|---|---|---|---|---|---|
| Boonyapakorn et al. [30] | Prospective | 80 | Cancer | 3.1 % | 77 % after tooth extractions<br>23 % spontaneous |
| Vahtsevanos et al. [31] | Retrospective | 1621 | Cancer | 8.5 % of MM<br>3.1 % of BCA<br>4.9 % of PCA | |
| Bamias et al. [32] | Prospective | 252 | Cancer | 9.9 % of MM<br><br>2.9 % of BCA<br>6.5 % of PCA | Almost all after dental procedures or dentures |
| Dimopoulos et al. [33] | Prospective | 202 | MM | 7.4 % | |
| Wang et al. [34] | Retrospective | 447 | Cancer | 3.8 % of MM<br>2.5 % of BCA<br>2.9 % of PCA | |
| Hoff et al. [35] | Retrospective | 1888 | Cancer | 2.4 % of MM<br>1.2 % of BCA | |
| Thumbigere-Math et al. [36] | Retrospective | 576 | Cancer | 7.2 % of MM<br><br>4.2 % of BCA<br>2.4 % of PCA | 59 % s/p tooth extraction<br>41 % spontaneous |
| Assaf et al. [37] | Retrospective | 169 | Cancer | 8.9 % | |
| Rugani et al. [38] | Retrospective | 63 | BCA | 10.4 % | |
| Walter et al. [39] | Prospective | 43 | PCA | 18.6 % | All patients after tooth extractions or denture pressure sore |
| Walter et al. [40] | Retrospective | 75 | BCA | 5.3 % | 50 % after tooth extraction |

*MM* multiple myeloma, *BCA* breast cancer, *PCA* prostate cancer

triple incidence of BRONJ in multiple myeloma patients when compared to breast cancer patients. Those authors conducted a prospective study on 252 patients who were receiving IV BPs and reported an incidence of 9.9 % among multiple myeloma patients, 2.9 % among breast cancer and 6.5 % among prostate cancer patients. As expected, most of the affected patients had a history of dental procedures or of using dentures [32]. Thumbigere-Math et al. reported similar findings in a retrospective study on 576 cancer patients: their figures showed a prevalence of 7.2 % among multiple myeloma patients, 4.2 % among breast cancer patients, and 2.4 % among prostate cancer patients. As expected, most of their cases developed after tooth extractions [36].

Likewise, Vahtsevanos et al.'s retrospective study on 1621 cancer patients found an incidence of 8.5 % among multiple myeloma patients, 3.1 % among breast cancer patients, and 4.9 % among prostate cancer patients [31]. Wang et al. did not report triple odds for multiple myeloma patients: their findings were a BRONJ prevalence of 3.8 % among multiple myeloma patients, 2.5 % among breast cancer patients, and 2.9 % among prostate cancer patients [34]. A higher incidence of BRONJ rates among multiple myeloma patients was also reported in non-comparative studies. Dimopoulos et al.'s prospective study on multiple myeloma patients found an incidence of 7.4 % for BRONJ development [33]. Although there are also studies that report a high incidence

**Table 5.2** Epidemiology of osteonecrosis in cancer patients treated with denosumab

| Author | Year | Drug | Osteonecrosis ($n$ patients) |
| --- | --- | --- | --- |
| Stopeck et al. [46] | 2010 | Zoledronic acid vs. denosumab | 14/1013 vs. 20/1020 |
| Fizazi et al. [47] | 2011 | Zoledronic acid vs. denosumab | 12/945 vs. 22/943 |
| Henry et al. [48] | 2011 | Zoledronic acid vs. denosumab | 11/878 vs. 10/878 |
| Smith et al. [49] | 2012 | Denosumab | 33/716 |
| Papapoulos et al. [50] | 2012 | Denosumab | 2/2206 |
| Lipton et al. [51] | 2012 | Zoledronic acid vs. denosumab | 37/2836 vs. 52/2841 |

of BRONJ among breast cancer patients [38] and prostate cancer patients [39], they are the exception rather than the rule and are probably due to small study populations. Taken together, these published data indicate a lower prevalence of BRONJ for patients with breast carcinoma (2–3 %), a higher prevalence in patients with prostate carcinoma, and the highest prevalence for patients with multiple myeloma (up to 10 %).

## Osteonecrosis of the Jaw and New Antiresorptive Drugs (Denosumab)

There have been recent reports of osteonecrosis of the jaws developing after exposure to drugs other than BPs [41, 42]. The most alarming results were associated with denosumab, which is a fully human monoclonal antibody that inhibits the maturation of osteoclasts. The first reports of osteonecrosis developing after exposure to denosumab appeared in 2010 [43, 44], with the most extensive study having been prospectively conducted on 5,723 cancer patients [45]. Those patients were randomly assigned to receive either denosumab or zoledronic acid. Oral adverse events were determined by an independent blinded committee of dental experts. The overall incidence of osteonecrosis was 1.6 % (89 patients), most of whom (52 vs. 37) developed under denosumab. Again, as expected, tooth extraction was reported in 61.8 % of the affected patients [45]. The conclusion that can be drawn from the comparative studies listed in Table 5.2 is that osteonecrosis related to the administration of denosumab might be similar or even more prevalent than with intravenous BPs and that comparable or even higher incidence rates of MRONJ development after exposure to denosumab might be expected.

> **Conclusion**
>
> The prevalence of BRONJ is higher after intravenous BPs compared to oral BPs, and even higher among the latter after oral surgical procedures and local infections. This should also be borne in mind in the development of new drugs that carry the risk of medication-related osteonecrosis of the jaw (MRONJ).

## References

1. Kanis JA, Gertz BJ, Singer F, et al. Rationale for the use of alendronate in osteoporosis. Osteoporos Int. 1995;5:1–13.
2. Glover D, Lipton A, Keller A, et al. Intravenous pamidronate disodium treatment of bone metastases in patients with breast cancer. A dose-seeking study. Cancer. 1994;74:2949–55.
3. Body JJ, Lortholary A, Romieu G, et al. A dose-finding study of zoledronate in hypercalcemic cancer patients. J Bone Miner Res. 1999;14:1557–61.
4. Rogers MJ, Watts DJ, Russell R. Overview of bisphosphonates. Cancer. 1997;80(8 Suppl):1652–60.
5. Boissier S, Ferreras M, Peyruchaud O, et al. Bisphosphonates inhibit breast and prostate carcinoma cell invasion, an early event in the formation of bone metastases. Cancer Res. 2000;60:2949–54.
6. Wang J, Goodger NM, Pogrel MA. Osteonecrosis of the jaws associated with cancer chemotherapy. J Oral Maxillofac Surg. 2003;61:1104–7.
7. Marx RE. Pamidronate (Aredia) and zoledronate (Zometa) induced avascular necrosis of the jaws: a growing epidemic. J Oral Maxillofac Surg. 2003;61:1115–7.
8. Ruggiero SL, Mehrotra B, Rosenberg TJ, et al. Osteonecrosis of the jaws associated with the use of bisphosphonates: a review of 63 cases. J Oral Maxillofac Surg. 2004;62:527–34.
9. Marx RE, Sawatari Y, Fortin M, et al. Bisphosphonate-induced exposed bone (osteonecrosis/osteopetrosis) of the jaws: risk factors, recognition, prevention, and treatment. J Oral Maxillofac Surg. 2005;63:1567–75.
10. Migliorati CA, Casiglia J, Epstein J, et al. Managing the care of patients with bisphosphonate-associated osteonecrosis: an American Academy of Oral Medicine position paper. J Am Dent Assoc. 2005;136:1658–68.

11. Mavrokokki T, Cheng A, Stein B, et al. Nature and frequency of bisphosphonate-associated osteonecrosis of the jaws in Australia. J Oral Maxillofac Surg. 2007;65:415–23.

12. Yarom N, Yahalom R, Shoshani Y, et al. Osteonecrosis of the jaw induced by orally administered bisphosphonates: incidence, clinical features, predisposing factors and treatment outcome. Osteoporos Int. 2007;18:1363–70.

13. Lazarovici TS, Yahalom R, Taicher S, et al. Bisphosphonate-related osteonecrosis of the jaws: a single-center study of 101 patients. J Oral Maxillofac Surg. 2009;67:850–5.

14. Lazarovici TS, Yahalom R, Taicher S, et al. Bisphosphonate-related osteonecrosis of the jaws associated with dental implants. J Oral Maxillofac Surg. 2010;68:790–6.

15. Hellstein JW, Marek CL. Bisphosphonate osteochemonecrosis (bis-phossy jaw): is this phossy jaw of the 21st century? J Oral Maxillofac Surg. 2005;63:682–9.

16. Russell RG, Watts NB, Ebetino FH, et al. Mechanisms of action of bisphosphonates: similarities and differences and their potential influence on clinical efficacy. Osteoporos Int. 2008;19:733–59.

17. Allegra A, Oteri G, Nastro E, et al. Patients with bisphosphonates-associated osteonecrosis of the jaw have reduced circulating endothelial cells. Hematol Oncol. 2007;25:164–9.

18. Landesberg R, Cozin M, Cremers S. Inhibition of oral mucosal cell wound healing by bisphosphonates. J Oral Maxillofac Surg. 2008;66:839–47.

19. Watts NB, Diab DL. Long-term use of bisphosphonates in osteoporosis. J Clin Endocrinol Metab. 2010; 95:1555–65.

20. Population Division of the Department of Economic and Social Affairs of the United Nations Secretariat: World Population Prospects: The 2012 Revision. New York: United Nations; 2013

21. Bleibler F, Konnopka A, Benzinger P, et al. The health burden and costs of incident fractures attributable to osteoporosis from 2010 to 2050 in Germany–a demographic simulation model. Osteoporos Int. 2013;24: 835–47.

22. Cauley JA. Public health impact of osteoporosis. J Gerontol A Biol Sci Med Sci. 2013;68:1243–51.

23. Pazianas M, Miller P, Blumentals WA, et al. A review of the literature on osteonecrosis of the jaw in patients with osteoporosis treated with oral bisphosphonates: prevalence, risk factors, and clinical characteristics. Clin Ther. 2007;29:1548–58.

24. American Dental Association Council on Scientific Affairs. Dental management of patients receiving oral bisphosphonate therapy: expert panel recommendations. J Am Dent Assoc. 2006;137:1144–50.

25. Hong JW, Nam W, Cha IH, et al. Oral bisphosphonate-related osteonecrosis of the jaw: the first report in Asia. Osteoporos Int. 2010;21:847–53.

26. Malden N, Lopes V. An epidemiological study of alendronate-related osteonecrosis of the jaws. A case series from the South-East of Scotland with attention given to case definition and prevalence. J Bone Miner Metab. 2012;30:171–82.

27. Lo JC, O'Ryan FS, Gordon NP, et al. Predicting Risk of Osteonecrosis of the Jaw with Oral Bisphosphonate Exposure (PROBE) Investigators: prevalence of osteonecrosis of the jaw in patients with oral bisphosphonate exposure. J Oral Maxillofac Surg. 2010; 68:243–53.

28. Tennis P, Rothman KJ, Bohn RL, et al. Incidence of osteonecrosis of the jaw among users of bisphosphonates with selected cancers or osteoporosis. Pharmacoepidemiol Drug Saf. 2012;21:810–7.

29. Sedghizadeh PP, Stanley K, Caligiuri M, et al. Oral bisphosphonate use and the prevalence of osteonecrosis of the jaw: an institutional inquiry. J Am Dent Assoc. 2009;140:61–6.

30. Boonyapakorn T, Schirmer I, Reichart PA, et al. Bisphosphonate-induced osteonecrosis of the jaws: prospective study of 80 patients with multiple myeloma and other malignancies. Oral Oncol. 2008;44:857–69.

31. Vahtsevanos K, Kyrgidis A, Verrou E, et al. Longitudinal cohort study of risk factors in cancer patients of bisphosphonate-related osteonecrosis of the jaw. J Clin Oncol. 2009;27:5356–62.

32. Bamias A, Kastritis E, Bamia C, et al. Osteonecrosis of the jaw in cancer after treatment with bisphosphonates: incidence and risk factors. J Clin Oncol. 2005; 23:8580–7.

33. Dimopoulos MA, Kastritis E, Anagnostopoulos A, et al. Osteonecrosis of the jaw in patients with multiple myeloma treated with bisphosphonates: evidence of increased risk after treatment with zoledronic acid. Haematologica. 2006;91:968–71.

34. Wang EP, Kaban LB, Strewler GJ, et al. Incidence of osteonecrosis of the jaw in patients with multiple myeloma and breast or prostate cancer on intravenous bisphosphonate therapy. J Oral Maxillofac Surg. 2007;65:1328–31.

35. Hoff AO, Toth BB, Altundag K, et al. Frequency and risk factors associated with osteonecrosis of the jaw in cancer patients treated with intravenous bisphosphonates. J Bone Miner Res. 2008;23:826–36.

36. Thumbigere-Math V, Tu L, Huckabay S, et al. A retrospective study evaluating frequency and risk factors of osteonecrosis of the jaw in 576 cancer patients receiving intravenous bisphosphonates. Am J Clin Oncol. 2012;35:386–92.

37. Assaf AT, Smeets R, Riecke B, et al. Incidence of bisphosphonate-related osteonecrosis of the jaw in consideration of primary diseases and concomitant therapies. Anticancer Res. 2013;33:3917–24.

38. Rugani P, Luschin G, Jakse N, et al. Prevalence of bisphosphonate-associated osteonecrosis of the jaw after intravenous zoledronate infusions in patients with early breast cancer. Clin Oral Investig. 2014;18:401–7.

39. Walter C, Al-Nawas B, Grötz KA, et al. Prevalence and risk factors of bisphosphonate-associated osteonecrosis of the jaw in prostate cancer patients with advanced disease treated with zoledronate. Eur Urol. 2008;54:1066–72.

40. Walter C, Al-Nawas B, du Bois A, et al. Incidence of bisphosphonate-associated osteonecrosis of the jaws in breast cancer patients. Cancer. 2009;115:1631–7.

41. Troeltzsch M, Woodlock T, Kriegelstein S, et al. Physiology and pharmacology of nonbisphosphonate drugs implicated in osteonecrosis of the jaw. J Can Dent Assoc. 2012;78:c85.

42. Sivolella S, Lumachi F, Stellini E, et al. Denosumab and anti-angiogenetic drug-related osteonecrosis of the jaw: an uncommon but potentially severe disease. Anticancer Res. 2013;33:1793–7.

43. Taylor KH, Middlefell LS, Mizen KD. Osteonecrosis of the jaws induced by anti-RANK ligand therapy. Br J Oral Maxillofac Surg. 2010;48:221–3.

44. Aghaloo TL, Felsenfeld AL, Tetradis S. Osteonecrosis of the jaw in a patient on Denosumab. J Oral Maxillofac Surg. 2010;68:959–63.

45. Saad F, Brown JE, Van Poznak C, et al. Incidence, risk factors, and outcomes of osteonecrosis of the jaw: integrated analysis from three blinded active-controlled phase III trials in cancer patients with bone metastases. Ann Oncol. 2012;23:1341–7.

46. Stopeck AT, Lipton A, Body JJ, et al. Denosumab compared with zoledronic acid for the treatment of bone metastases in patients with advanced breast cancer: a randomized, double-blind study. J Clin Oncol. 2010;28:5132–9.

47. Fizazi K, Carducci M, Smith M, et al. Denosumab versus zoledronic acid for treatment of bone metastases in men with castration-resistant prostate cancer: a randomised, double-blind study. Lancet. 2011;377:813–22.

48. Henry DH, Costa L, Goldwasser F, et al. Randomized, double-blind study of denosumab versus zoledronic acid in the treatment of bone metastases in patients with advanced cancer (excluding breast and prostate cancer) or multiple myeloma. J Clin Oncol. 2011;29:1125–32.

49. Smith MR, Saad F, Coleman R, et al. Denosumab and bone-metastasis-free survival in men with castration-resistant prostate cancer: results of a phase 3, randomised, placebo-controlled trial. Lancet. 2012;379:39–46.

50. Papapoulos S, Chapurlat R, Libanati C, et al. Five years of denosumab exposure in women with post-menopausal osteoporosis: results from the first two years of the FREEDOM extension. J Bone Miner Res. 2012;27:694–701.

51. Lipton A, Fizazi K, Stopeck AT, et al. Superiority of denosumab to zoledronic acid for prevention of skeletal-related events: a combined analysis of 3 pivotal, randomised, phase 3 trials. Eur J Cancer. 2012;48:3082–92.

# Imaging Modalities and Characteristics in Medication-Related Osteonecrosis of the Jaw

Florian A. Probst, Monika Probst, and Sotirios Bisdas


**Abstract**

Though diagnosis itself is based on anamnesis and clinical presentation, imaging occupies an integral part of the management of medication-related osteonecrosis of the jaws (MRONJ). Various radiographic signs may be seen on panoramic radiographs, cone-beam computed tomography (CBCT), or multislice CT (MSCT) like sclerosis, persisting alveolar sockets, and lack of bone filling in extractions sites, osteolysis, and sequestration. While panoramic radiographs serve as a baseline diagnostic tool, computed tomography (CT) or cone-beam computed tomography (CBCT) and magnetic resonance imaging (MRI) provide three-dimensional information of osteonecrotic lesions and may aid in assessing the extent of necrosis, monitoring the disease, and detecting early lesions. Anyway, no imaging modality is able to reliably depict the margins of a necrosis so far. CT and MRI offer a wide spectrum of findings but those are often not very specific. In the future, nuclear medicine imaging like combined SPECT/CT or PET/CT may further improve the diagnosis of MRONJ by combining functional and anatomical information.



F.A. Probst, MD, DDS (⊠)
Department of Oral and Maxillofacial
Surgery, University Hospital Munich (LMU),
Lindwurmstr. 2a, Munich 80337, Germany
e-mail: florian.probst@med.uni-muenchen.de

M. Probst, MD
Department of Neuroradiology,
Klinikum rechts der Isar, Technical University
Munich, Ismaningerstr. 22, Munich 81675, Germany
e-mail: Monika.probst@tum.de

S. Bisdas, MD, PhD, MSc
Department of Neuroradiology, Eberhard Karls
University Tübingen, Hoppe-Seyler-Str. 3,
Tübingen 72076, Germany
e-mail: sotirios.bisdas@med.uni-tuebingen.de


## Introduction

According to AAOMS criteria and some early reports, the diagnosis of BRONJ is traditionally based on anamnesis and clinical examination [1]. The criteria that have to be fulfilled in order to establish diagnosis of BRONJ are already mentioned in the previous chapters, including clinically exposed bone in the oral cavity for 8 weeks or more [2]. Therefore, imaging techniques are not a prerequisite for the diagnosis itself. However, they play an important role for assessment of the extent of a necrosis and possible side effects


S. Otto (ed.), *Medication-Related Osteonecrosis of the Jaws: Bisphosphonates, Denosumab, and New Agents*,
DOI 10.1007/978-3-662-43733-9_6, © Springer-Verlag Berlin Heidelberg 2015

**Table 6.1** Summary of radiographic findings in MRONJ

| Radiopacity | Radiolucency | Findings in advanced disease/complications |
| --- | --- | --- |
| Sclerosis, focal/diffuse | Impaired healing of extraction sites, lack of bone filling, persisting alveolar sockets | Sequestra |
| Thickening of the lamina dura | Osteolysis of cortical/spongious bone | Pathological fractures |
| Prominent mandibular canal | Focal cortical disruption | Signs of sinusitis |
| Periosteal reaction | Periradicular lucency | |

like accompanying inflammatory soft-tissue involvement or for the detection of pathological fractures. Furthermore, imaging can help to monitor disease progression and to differentiate between osteonecrosis and neoplastic lesion like metastasis. Additionally, imaging is of special interest concerning the detection of early stages of BRONJ, which do not present with clinically exposed bone, corresponding to stage 0 of the disease [3, 4].

While panoramic radiographs serve as valuable basic tools in MRONJ imaging, radiologic tomographic techniques like computed tomography (CT) or cone-beam computed tomography (CBCT) can provide three-dimensional information of the region of interest. Furthermore, magnetic resonance imaging (MRI) is increasingly becoming the focus of attention, as it is assumed that it might aid in early detection and assessment of a lesion's dimension. Last but not least, functional imaging techniques like scintigraphy, bone single-photon emission computed tomography (SPECT), or positron emission tomography with computed tomography (PET/CT) have the potential to complement the radiologic spectrum of MRONJ imaging. In the following, the relevant radiographic, MR, and nuclear medicine imaging techniques for the MRONJ imaging will be pictorially presented.

an initial imaging modality for patients with suspicion of MRONJ [1, 5, 6]. Panoramic radiographs provide information not only about signs of osteonecrosis but also about coexisting dental aspects like apical osteolysis, periodontal lesions, or carious lesions. Furthermore, plain radiographs are pricy and available in almost every dental clinic and maxillofacial surgery unit.

There are various typical signs of BRONJ on panoramic radiographs (Table 6.1). Alterations of the bone structure may appear mainly with osteolysis, sclerosis, or a combination [6–10]. Sclerosis is a highly frequent sign, seen at all stages of the disease, especially in the early stage [3–5, 11]. Sclerose-like areas can vary from a distinct focal sclerosis of the alveolar process to a diffuse and wide range involvement of greater parts of the mandible or maxilla [3, 11]. Further frequently reported signs are thickening of the alveolar margins, the lamina dura, or the cortical borders and narrowing of the mandibular canal [3, 5, 11, 12]. Also radiolucent appearance with osteolysis, disturbance of the cortical bone, and delayed healing of extraction sockets or even persisting alveolar sockets can be observed (Fig. 6.1) [3, 5, 6, 11, 13]. In advanced stages of BRONJ, sequestra are another typical finding. Moreover, widening of the periodontal ligament space and periapical lucencies may be apparent [11].

## Panoramic Radiographs

Conventional dentomaxillofacial diagnostic x-ray supplied by periapical and panoramic radiographs allows for baseline MRONJ imaging. Especially panoramic radiographs enable a prompt overview of teeth and mandibular and maxillary bones. They should be considered as

## Radiologic Tomographic Techniques (CT, CBCT)

In contrast to conventional radiographs, including panoramic radiographs, tomographic techniques like computed tomography (CT) or cone-beam computed tomography (CBCT) allow for three-dimensional evaluation of the jaws.

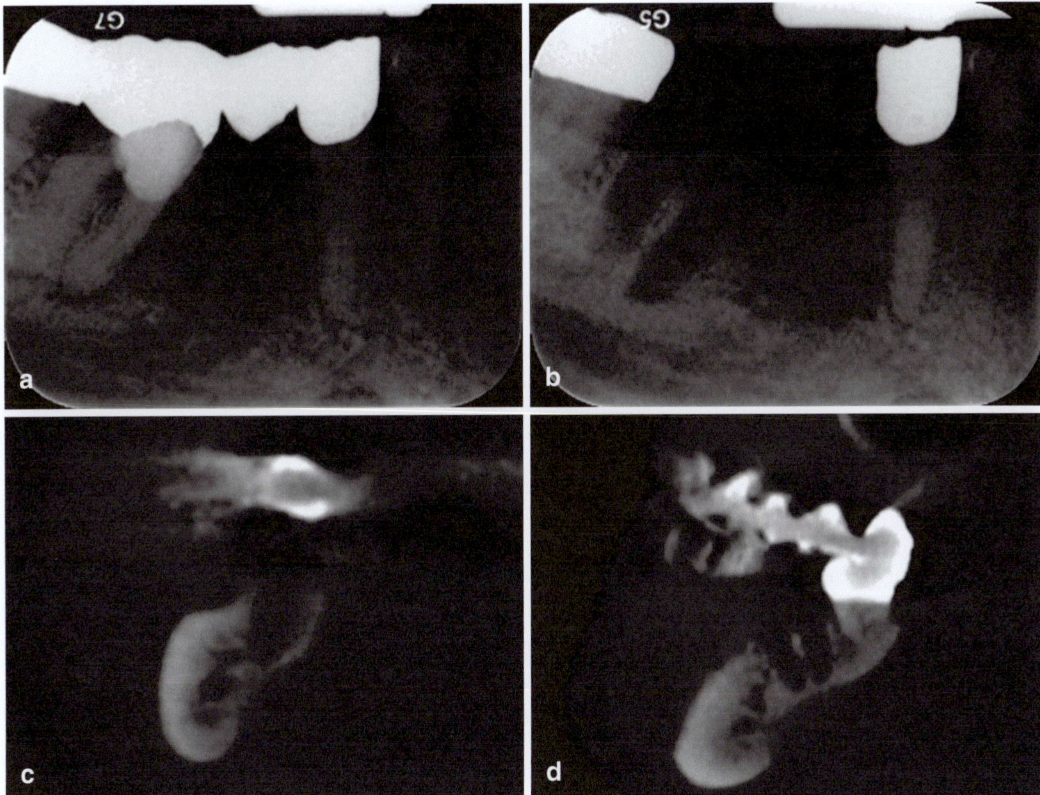

**Fig. 6.1** A 70-year-old male presented clinically with a non-healing extraction wound and exposed bone and putrid exudate in the right mandible in region 45–46. Extraction of tooth 46 had been performed 3 months before. The patient received intravenous bisphosphonate therapy with zoledronate (4 mg/month) since 3 and 1/2 years, due to osseous metastases from prostate carcinoma. (**a**) Plain film radiograph prior to extraction. (**b**) Plain film radiograph 3 month after extraction of tooth 46. Lack of bone filling and persisting alveolar sockets are obvious. (**c**) Coronal/(**d**) sagittal sections derived from CBCT data showing lack of bone filling

The radiographic signs of BRONJ on panoramic radiographs, which were described above, can be seen in CT images in an analogous way (Table 6.1).

Based on bisphosphonate-induced disorganized bone homeostasis, the affected bone is often associated with sclerosis [14, 15], and consequently, it is a frequent sign seen in radiologic imaging in BRONJ cases (Table 6.1). Sclerosis can range from focal to extended involvement and may have a flocculent or more dense character with irregular trabeculation (Figs. 6.2, 6.4, and 6.6). In advanced lesions, osteonecrosis can present as an inhomogeneous bone density with "cotton-wool" appearance. Dealing with diffuse sclerosis, buccal and lingual cortical bone was reported to be thickened with reduced contrast to the spongious bone [3]. The mandibular canal can present prominently when sclerosis affects the margins of the canal (Figs. 6.3 and 6.4) [3, 5]. Thickening of the alveolar margins and lamina dura is described as well [3, 5].

On the other side, osteonecrotic areas feature a loss in bone mineralization and fragmentation and often present with radiolucent areas on panoramic radiographs and lowered attenuation in CT (Table 6.1) (Fig. 6.6) [3, 5, 6, 11, 16].

Several reports suggest significant advantages of CT imaging when compared to panoramic radiographs [5, 6, 9, 13, 17–19]. Location and extension of a lesion may be assessed more exactly by tomography. The dimension of a

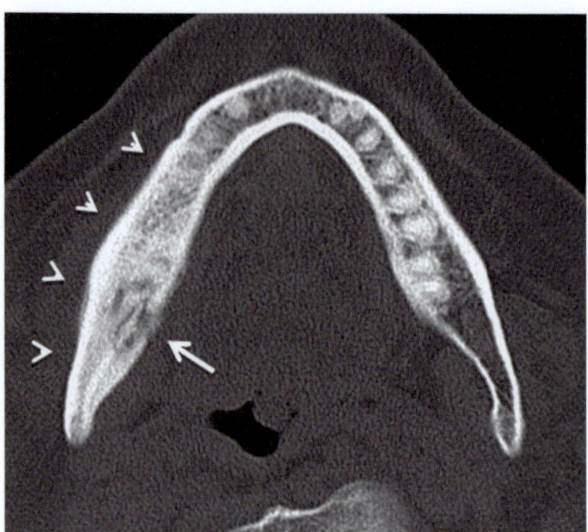

**Fig. 6.2** Multislice computed tomography (MSCT). Extended sclerotic changes of the right mandibular corpus and ramus (*arrowheads*). Sequestration and lingual cortical disruption (*large arrow*)

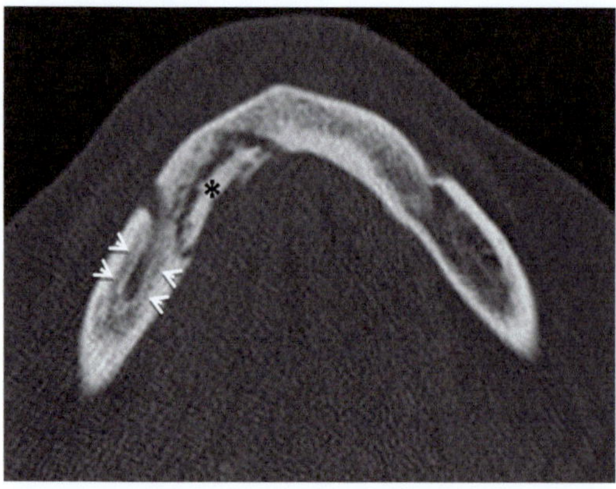

**Fig. 6.3** BRONJ in the right mandible. Multislice CT depicting a large lingual mandibular sequestration (*black asterisk*) and prominent mandibular canal (*white arrowheads*) as sclerosis affects the margins of the canal

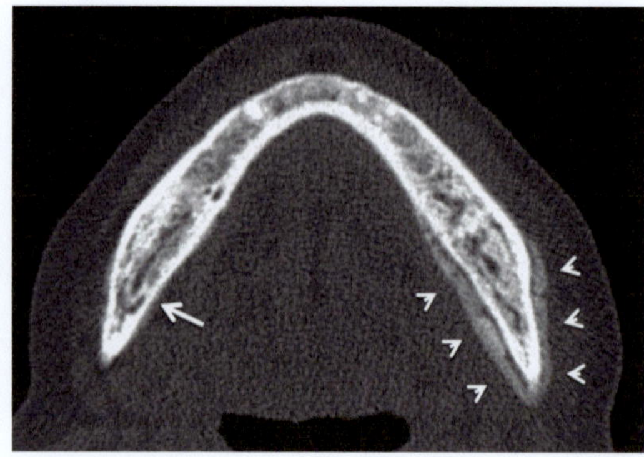

**Fig. 6.4** Multislice computed tomography (MSCT). Mandible affected by BRONJ. Extended left perimandibular periosteal reaction (*arrowheads*). Osteosclerosis with disorganized irregular medullary trabeculation throughout the complete mandible. Prominent mandibular canal can be seen at the right mandible (*large arrow*)

lesion was proved to be larger on CT and MRI as well as in histopathology than the area of clinically exposed bone [20]. Panoramic radiographs seem to underestimate the dimension of a lesion compared to CT imaging, and the existence of smaller sequestra may be overlooked more easily in panoramic radiographs (Fig. 6.6) [17].

Preoperative knowledge about the extension of a bisphosphonate-related necrosis is valuable for surgical planning. Up to now, there is paucity of available data in this concern. In a study of 24 patients suffering from different stages of

BRONJ, panoramic radiographs, CT, and MRI were performed. While detectability of CT and MRI exceeded that of panoramic radiographs by far, it was obvious that CT and MRI presented with difficulties in evaluating the exact extent of the lesions, and so it was concluded that the precision of these both modalities, displaying the extension of osteonecrosis, is limited [9]. Guggenberger et al. (2013) compared extension of bisphosphonate-related lesions in ten patients undergoing PET/CT, contrast-enhanced MRI, panoramic views derived from CBCT, and pre-operative and intraoperative assessment. PET/CT and contrast-enhanced MRI were able to display more extensive changes compared with panoramic views derived from CBCT and clinical examination. It was reported that preoperative examination detected smaller extension of the disease than the other examinations. All in all, PET/CT and contrast-enhanced MRI detected more extensive involvement of BRONJ compared with panoramic views from CBCT and clinical examinations [21]. Nonetheless, the latter two studies demonstrate the current limitations of all modalities in order to assess the exact extension of lesion in BRONJ cases. While MRI and PET-CT may overestimate the real lesion dimensions, CBCT imaging as well as preoperative and intraoperative estimations may underestimate the real extension. For the surgeon it is worthwhile to note that for preoperative work-up, these differences between the imaging modalities should be taken into consideration [21]. Further studies are needed and may include precise histopathological assessment and intraoperative assessment with the aid of fluorescence imaging as described in brief in the treatment chapter [22, 23].

Recently, imaging focus also headed toward the possibility to detect MRONJ in an early stage, when there is no presence of clinically exposed bone in the oral cavity. Sclerosis is reported to be a consistent finding in imaging of early disease [3, 16]. In contrast to low-grade or sclerosing osteomyelitis however, periosteal response seems not to be characteristic in early stages (Fig. 6.4) [3, 10].

In a cohort of 32 patients with BRONJ, a cluster analysis was performed on the basis of different radiologic features. Patients were grouped in 4 categories based on CT findings. The authors found a positive correlation with the clinical extension analysis [17]. In contrast, a staging based solely on panoramic radiographs was judged not to be reliable because lesions tend to be underestimated and because of a missing correlation between clinical extension and dental panoramic radiograph clusters [16]. Purulent secretion and sequestration are correlating with the size of osteonecrotic lesions and demonstrated the value of CT imaging in patients with BRONJ [24].

Quantification of imaging features may be promising in order to assess the presence of a bisphosphonate-related bony disorder in an objective manner. CT imaging and consecutive work-up of bone matrix density were performed in patients with confirmed BRONJ and compared with samples from cadaveric controls. Unfortunately, higher bone tissue density was evident only in a subset of BRONJ patients, suggesting that density may have limitations as a biomarker for early detection of this condition [25].

In a retrospective pilot study, different techniques were tested in order to analyze cortical bone dimensional changes caused by bisphosphonates based on CBCT imaging. The evaluation of the mandibular cortical bone at the site of the mental foramen seems to be helpful for the detection of cortical bone dimensional changes. Alterations in the bone architecture were even evident in areas of the mandible, which were not affected by clinical bone exposure. It was concluded that the technique described may aid in detecting early bone alterations helping to predict BRONJ in individuals. However, further longitudinal studies were proposed to verify this technique [12].

Cone-beam computed tomography (CBCT) is a tomographic imaging technique that has become increasingly popular in dentomaxillofacial imaging over the last decade. Within a short imaging time, high-resolution three-dimensional datasets of the head and neck region can be generated. Software applications allow displaying panoramic views as well as multiplanar reconstructions [26]. Furthermore, CBCT imaging comes along with considerably reduced radiation exposure compared to multislice CT protocols [27, 28]. Accordingly, this technique is of increased importance in the setting of BRONJ [10, 12, 29–33].

Radiographic findings (Table 6.1) can be similarly found in CBCT and multidetector CT (Fig. 6.6). However, it hast to be considered that CBCT attenuation measurements are less reliable compared with those in multidetector CT and soft-tissue contrast is lower compared with multidetector CT [34].

Inflammatory affection of soft tissues like cervical lymphadenopathy, mass-like thickening of the masticator muscles, and abscess formation are addressed more properly with multidetector CT imaging or MRI, especially if imaging is contrast enhanced.

Further radiographic findings in advanced disease that should be kept in mind are sequestra, pathological fractures, and maxillary sinus affection (Figs. 6.2, 6.3, 6.5, and 6.6) [35, 36]. These findings should be given special attention and three-dimensional imaging modalities are strongly recommended in this context. For example, panoramic radiographs seem to underestimate the dimension of a lesion compared to CT imaging, and the existence of smaller sequestra may be overlooked more easily in panoramic radiographs (Fig. 6.6) [17, 35].

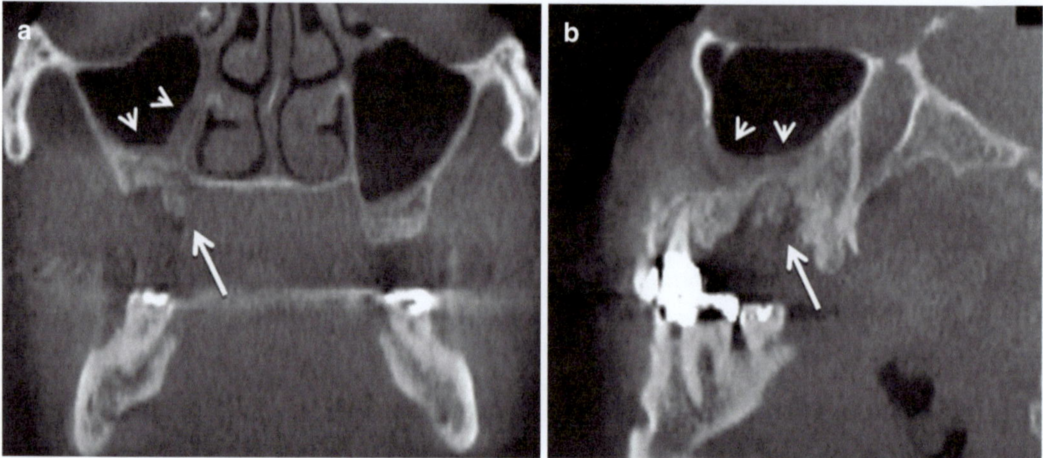

**Fig. 6.5** A 73-year-old male clinically presenting with signs of sinusitis and exposed bone in the right posterior maxilla. (**a**) Coronal and (**b**) sagittal sections derived from CBCT data. *Large arrows* are depicting a sequestrum. *Arrowheads* show mucosal thickening in the right maxillary sinus as radiologic correlate to maxillary sinusitis due to BRONJ

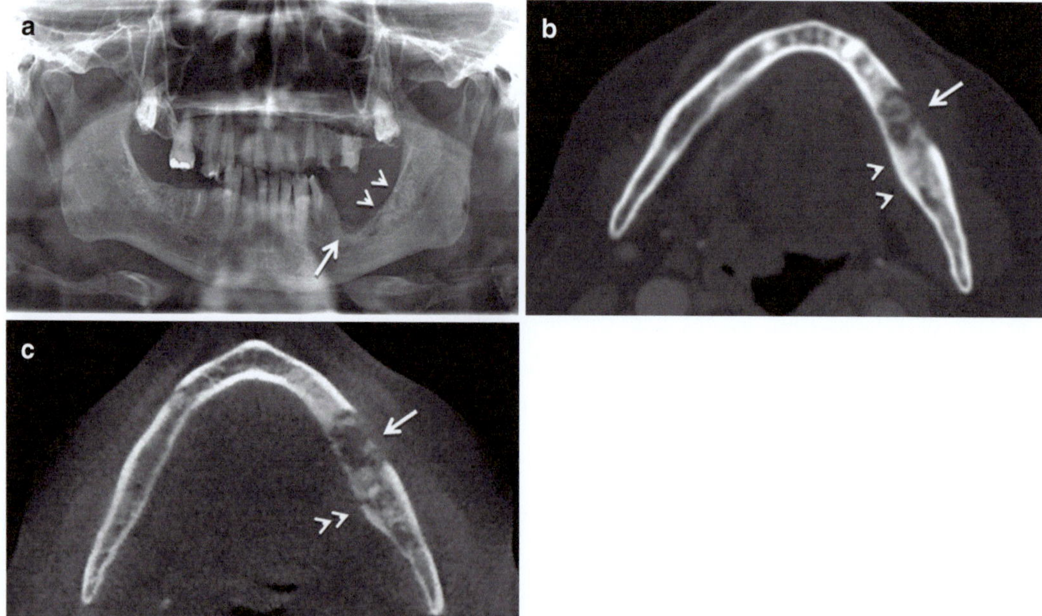

**Fig. 6.6** A 69-year-old male patient received intravenous bisphosphonate therapy with zoledronate (4 mg/month) due to osseous metastases from prostate carcinoma. (**a**) Panoramic radiograph. *Large arrow* is showing a radiolucent area corresponding to alveolar margin osteolysis. Posterior to the osteolysis, the *two arrowheads* depict osteosclerosis with disorganized medullary trabeculation and "cotton-wool"-like appearance. (**b**) Multislice computed tomography (MSCT). The *large arrow* indicates the osteolytic area; the *two arrowheads* indicate the osteosclerosis. In contrast to the panoramic radiograph, sequestration is visible as well (within the osteolytic area). (**c**) Cone-beam computed tomography (CBCT). Osteolytic area can be seen as well (*large arrow*). Additionally, lingual cortical disruption becomes evident in the shown layer (*consecutive arrowheads*)

## Magnetic Resonance Imaging (MRI)

Free from ionizing radiation, MR imaging should be preferentially performed in 1.5 T or 3 T MR units, which may use the full spectrum of the modern sequences that provide "state-of-the-art" 2D and 3D T1- and T2-weighted imaging [9, 16, 21]. New MR scanners are also offered with multiple channel head/neck coils (up to 32 channels) that enable superior spatial resolution (in submillimeter range) in reasonable acquisition time for the patient. Besides the conventional morphological imaging, which has to be enhanced by contrast agent administration and suitable saturation of the fat planes in extracranial head, new functional MR imaging techniques (i.e., perfusion, diffusion) are available and may facilitate early disease diagnosis or monitoring in the future. Nonetheless, preliminary studies failed to demonstrate any strong supporting evidence in clinically manifested cases [37] as well as in the early stage of non-traumatic osteonecrosis models [38].

MR imaging of BRONJ is complementary to CT imaging revealing signal intensity alterations in a homogeneous pattern or affecting the periphery of the lesion in a band-like pattern [16], which has also a close correlation to the "bone-within-bone" appearance often seen in CT [16, 39]. In general, BRONJ is typically associated with decreased signal intensity on T1-weighted images and variable signal intensity changes on T2-weighted or short inversion time inversion-recovery (STIR) images and contrast-enhanced images [6, 7, 16, 40]. Typically, low T1 signal (reflecting low water content) in open wounds is associated with intermediate or slightly increased signal intensity on T2-weighted images (reflecting edema and inflammation) (Figs. 6.7, 6.8, and 6.9). Rather than T1-weighted images, the T2 signal intensity of the abnormalities, possibly associated with the disease stage including early cases with intermediate symptoms, is not variable, thus not pathognomonic and should be meticulously appreciated together with the CT findings, which may reveal subtle changes (i.e., focal hyperdensity) [6, 16, 40]. Generally, little information has been published about the early stages of BRONJ because they are not typically imaged with MR imaging or because the unexposed bone does not raise the suspicion of BRONJ. In doubtful cases (i.e., ambivalent signal on T1- and T2-weighted images), signal changes in gingival region, inferior alveolar nerve, and neighboring soft-tissue MR imaging, not readily appreciated, even in the contrast-enhanced CT also due to metal artifacts that may obscure the lesions in CT, may suggest BRONJ (Fig. 6.10). The involvement in MRI may appear more extensive after contrast enhancement than in CT [9, 41], but imaging-based disease quantification should preferably encounter native T1- and T2-weighted findings though the latter usually overestimate the disease extent compared to intraoperative findings [9, 21] or offer no significant additional information for the resection margins [42]. Up to now and partly due to study design problems, there are no longitudinal studies reporting on the clinical fate of "silent" changes seen in CT or MRI not concordant to the classical BRONJ appearance.

In late stages or chronic cases, the reported signal intensity on T2-weighted images is also variable with predominating low T2 signal (or STIR-signal) indicating non-viable bone as reported in cases with uncontrollable pain unresponsive to conventional treatment before surgical resection [20]. Areas with unexposed bone may demonstrate increased, sometimes peripheral, signal intensity on T2-weighted or STIR images [6, 20] (Figs. 6.8 and 6.9). This signal intensity pattern implies probably a chronic osteomyelitis and is often accompanied by avid contrast enhancement. This corroborates the notion of the additive value of intravenous contrast for disease detection and quantification. However, contrast-enhanced MRI alone fails to distinguish between necrotic bone, osteomyelitis, and reactive signal changes of bone marrow secondary to surrounding inflammation of soft tissue. The bone marrow enhancement correlates with the degree of fatty marrow replacement and decreased signal intensity on T1-weighted images and typically spares the low T2 signal bony sequestrum (Figs. 6.8 and 6.9) [7, 9, 16]. In general, contrast enhancement may extend to the cortical bone, bone marrow, adjacent soft tissues

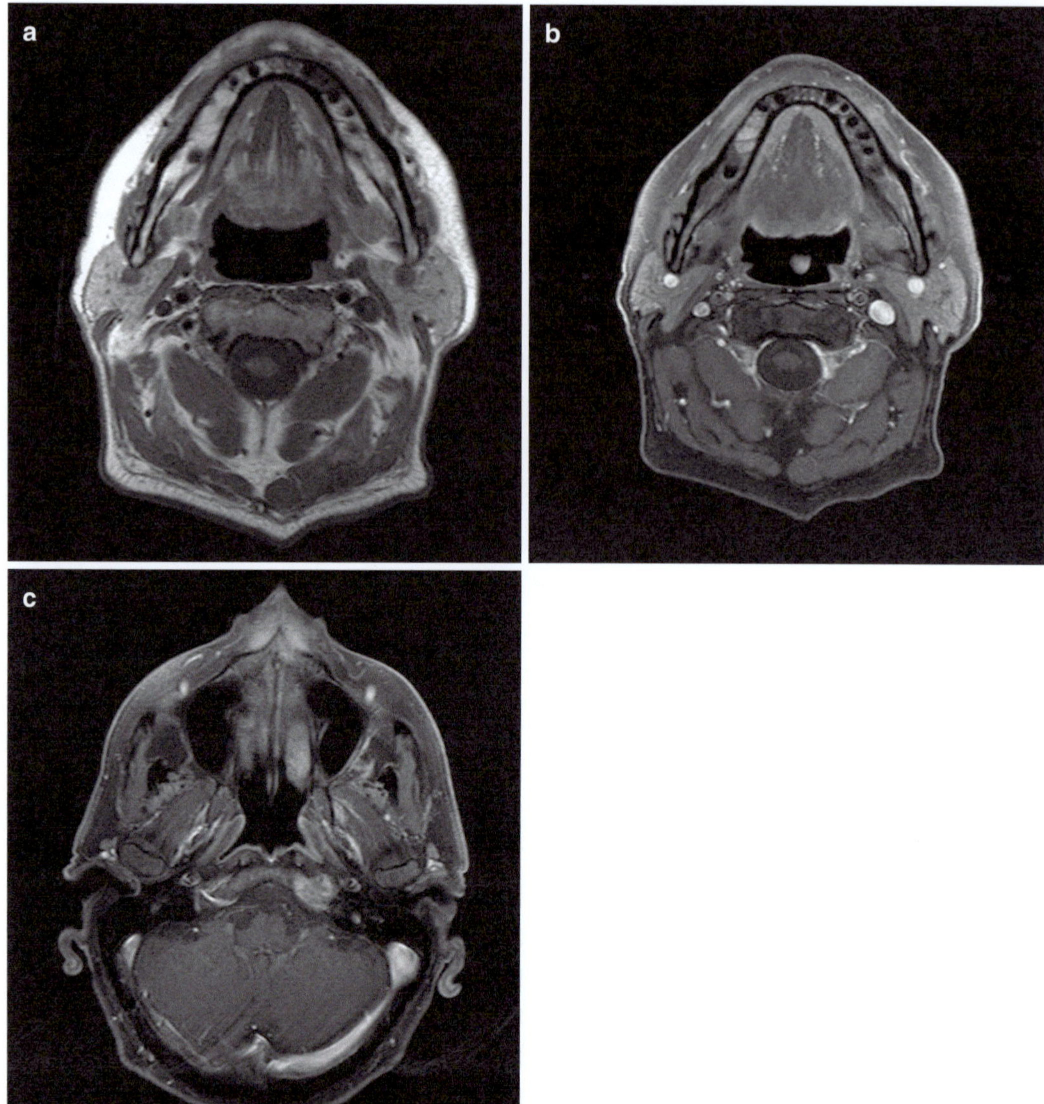

**Fig. 6.7** (**a–c**) A 61-year-old woman with breast cancer and symptomatic osteonecrosis. Axial T1-weighted image (**a**) shows focal lesion of osteonecrosis in the left mandible as hypointense zone without cortical affection. After gadolinium administration and fat saturation (**b**), the lesion does not demonstrate significant enhancement. Adjacent fat-saturated, post-contrast T1-weighted MR image shows enhancing metastatic lesion in the left middle skull base (**c**)

(including mylohyoid ridge, buccinator muscle, orbicular muscle, and masticator space), paranasal sinuses, inferior alveolar and mandibular canal, and in the locoregional lymph nodes (Fig. 6.11). The commonly seen focal mass-like thickening of the adjacent soft tissue as well as cervical lymphadenopathy may clinically mimic neoplastic disease, either relapsing tumors or metastases (Fig. 6.11). The mass-like tissue changes are frequently located submandibular followed by the submandibular angle and jugulodigastric chains and should be encountered in the differential diagnosis [16, 37].

When we compare side-by-side the different imaging techniques, the overall detectability of BRONJ lesions in MR imaging is very high,

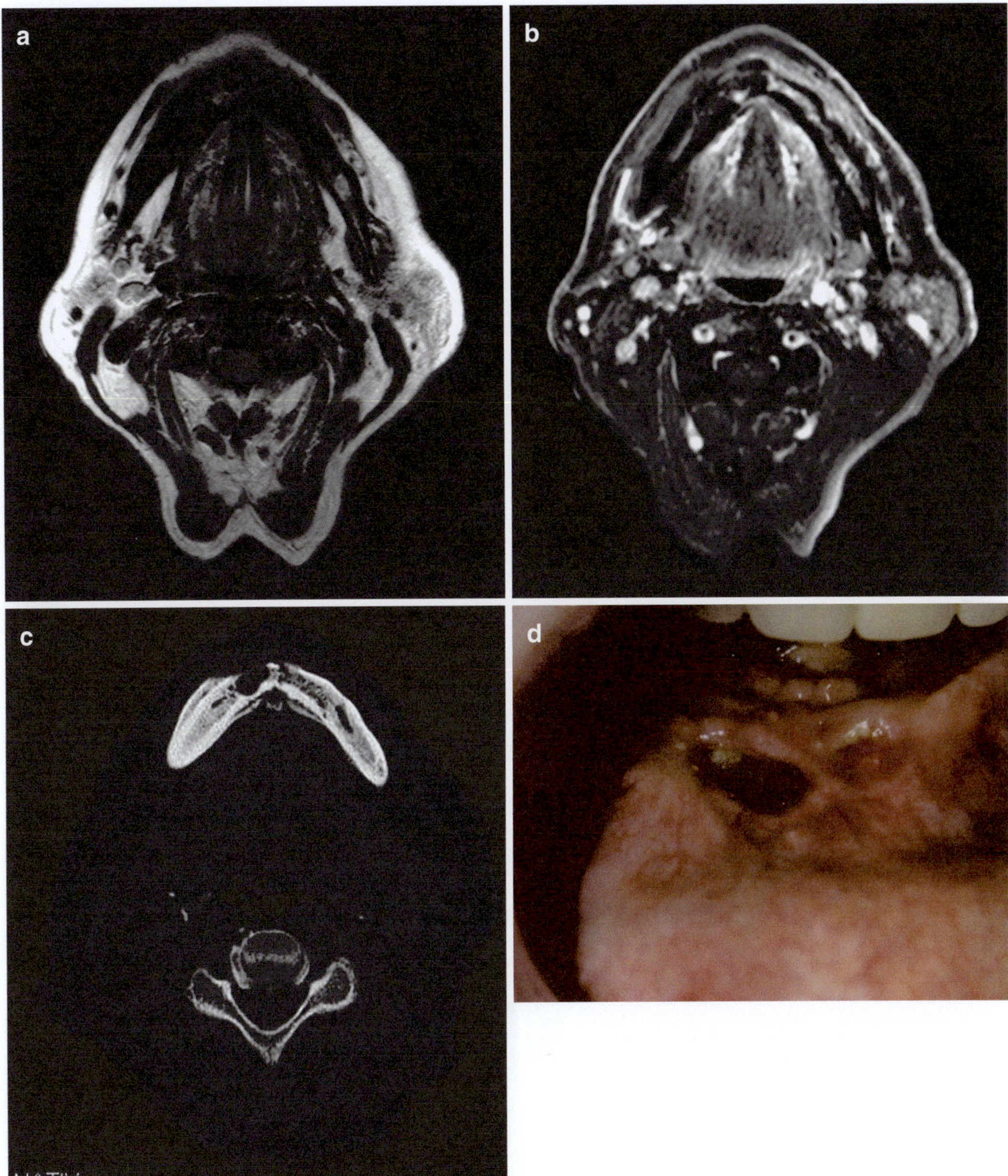

**Fig. 6.8** (**a–d**) A 50-year-old woman with breast cancer. Axial T2-weighted image (**a**) shows pathologic mesial fracture in the mandible as well as decreased marrow signal intensity with cortical affection and hyperostosis on the right side, accompanied by soft-tissue changes in the labial and buccal premandibular region. The soft-tissue changes and the affected bone marrow, especially on the left side, show avid enhancement in fat-saturated T1-weighted image (**b**). The corresponding axial CT image (**c**) demonstrates cortical thickening, medullary sclerosis, pathologic fracture, and non-healing socket, the latter being also evident in the clinical examination (**d**)

justifying its application as a preoperative and monitoring tool [20]. However, a close correlation between intraoperative and MR imaging findings is not always evident [9, 21]. The sensitivity of MRI in identification of BRONJ is heavily dependent on the use of contrast enhancing MR sequences and should be encountered as high considering the identification of all the

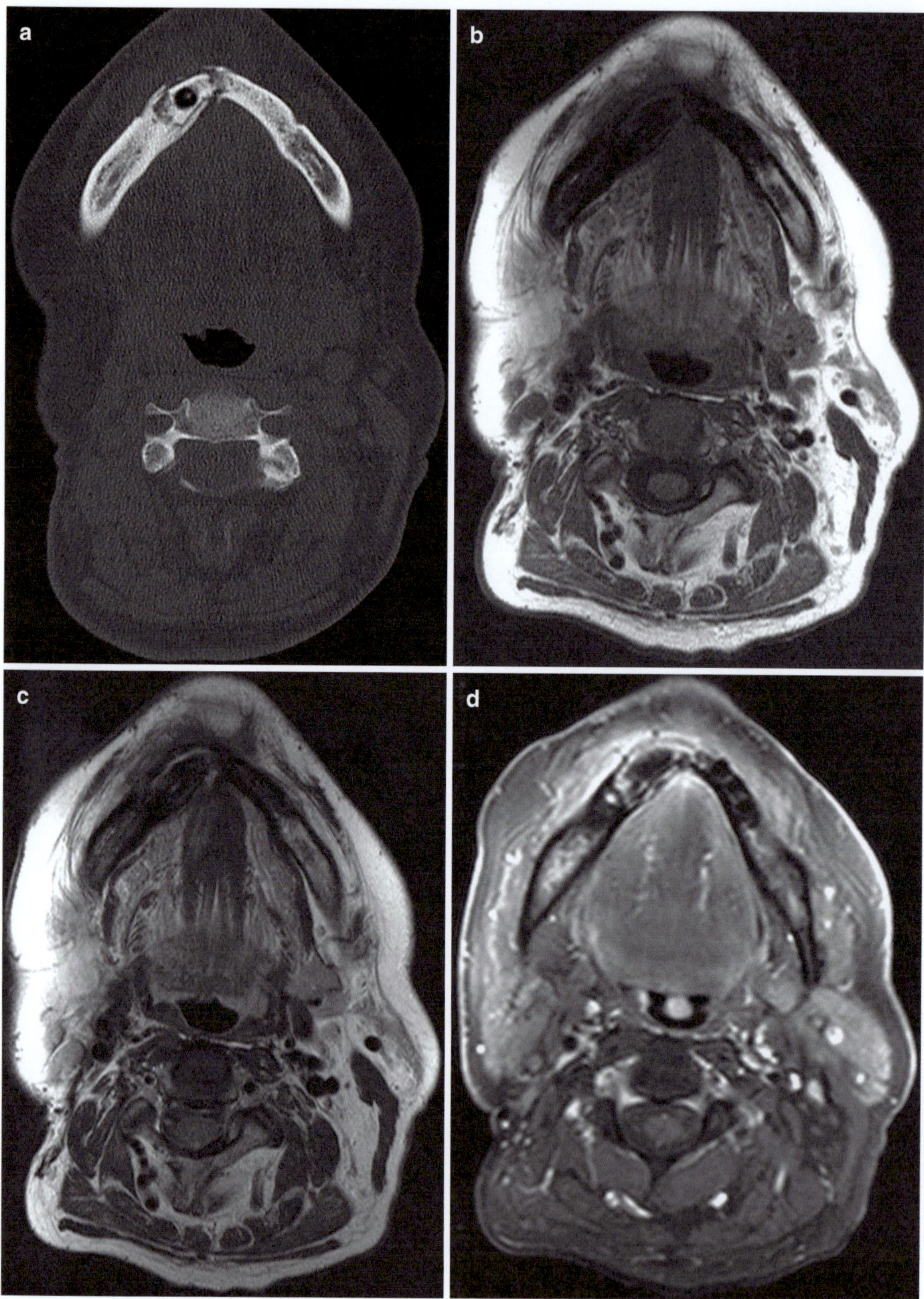

**Fig. 6.9** (**a–d**) A 60-year-old male with prostate cancer. Axial CT image (**a**) shows bony sequestrum in the right mandibular body as well as medullar and cortical sclerosis on both sides. The corresponding unenhanced T1-weighted image (**b**) demonstrates the sclerotic lesions as areas with low signal intensity, whereas the T2-weighted image (**c**) shows intermediate signal intensity. The MR images reveal also soft-tissue changes in the labial and lingual adjacent tissue. The soft-tissue inflammation presents with avid enhancement in the fat-saturated, post-contrast T1-weighted image (**d**)

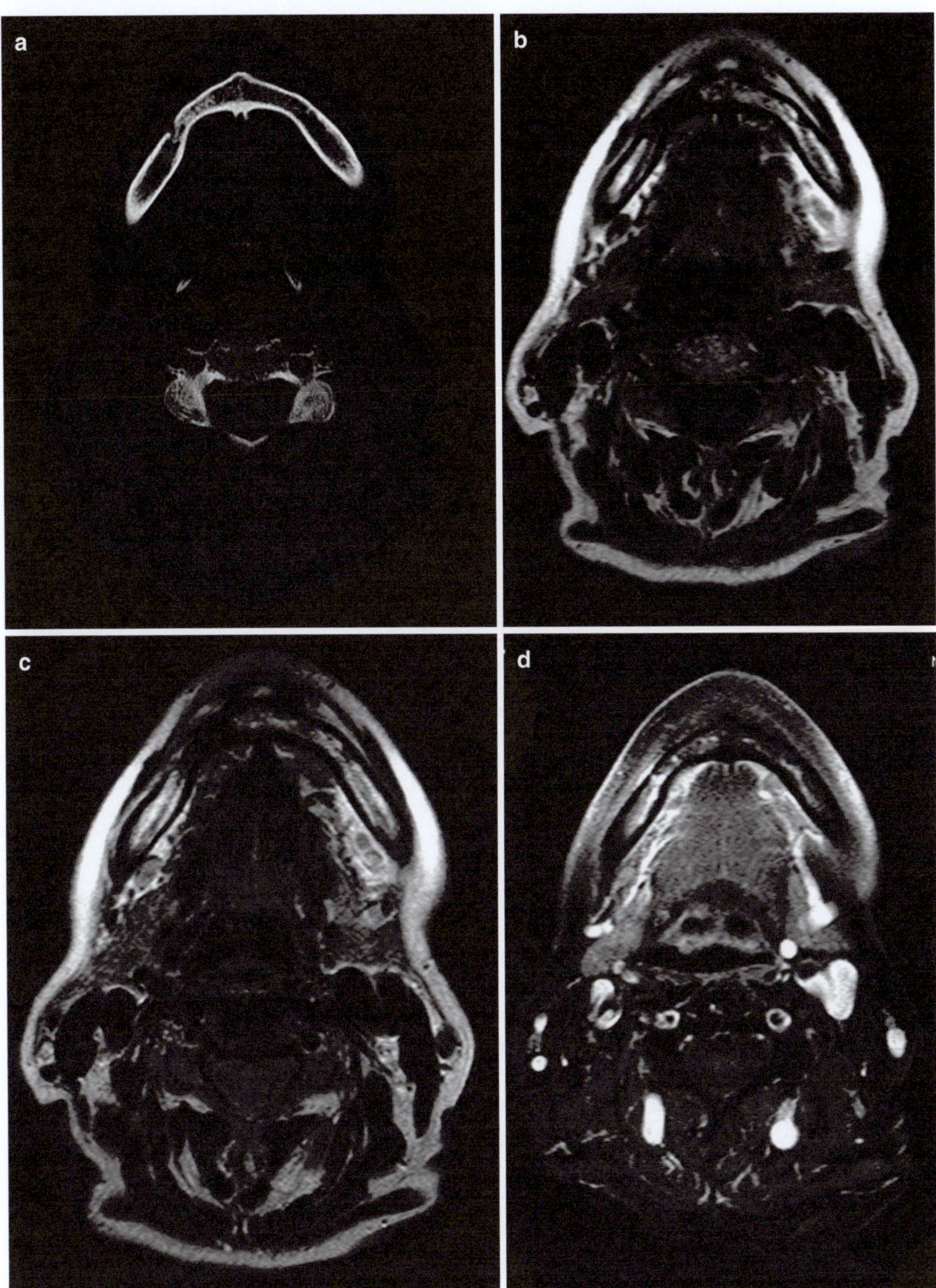

**Fig. 6.10** (**a–d**) A 54-year-old woman with breast cancer and intermittent pain on the right mandible. Axial CT image (**a**) shows subtle focal sclerosis on the right mandible next to the mental foramen. The suspected area appears with low signal intensity on unenhanced T1-weighted (**b**) and T2-weighted (**c**) images, whereas it shows remarkable gadolinium enhancement on fat-suppressed, post-contrast T1-weighted image (**d**) the contrast enhancement seems to follow the right inferior alveolar canal; focal inflammation of the gingival tissue is also present

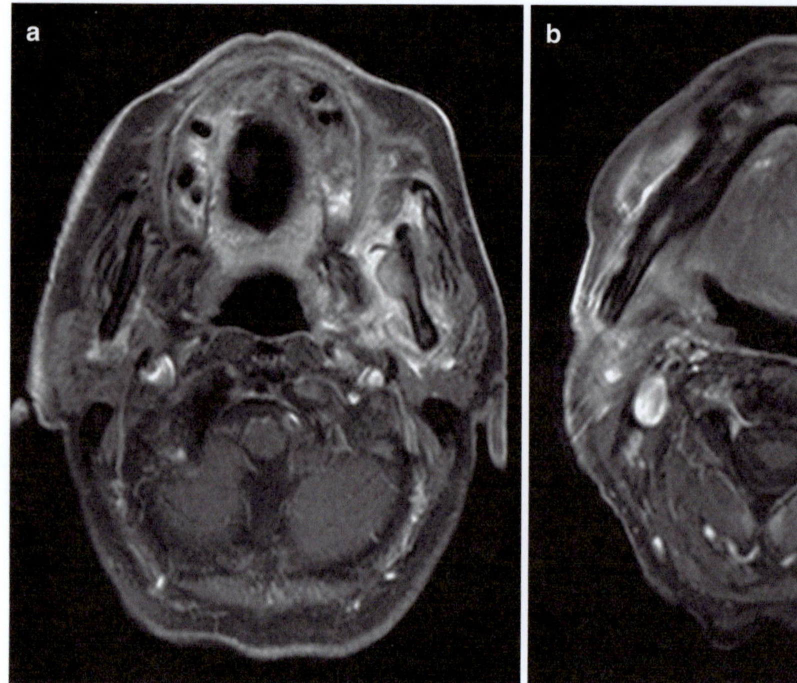

**Fig. 6.11** (**a–b**) Fat-suppressed, post-contrast, T1-weighted MR imaging of a 67-year-old woman with multiple myeloma and BRONJ lesions on the maxilla and mandible. Axial image (**a**) demonstrates increased gadolinium uptake in the maxilla and left mandible as well as prominent enhancement of the soft tissues adjacent to the left mandibular ramus. There is fluid collection on the buccal side of the maxilla and on the mandibular foramen. The adjacent axial section at the level of the mandible (**b**) reveals the extensive inflammatory changes in the buccal region as well as in the oropharyngeal space and the tonsillar region on the left side. The bony marrow shows increased gadolinium uptake and the left mandible is fragmented with sequestration

symptomatic lesions and additional lesions not appreciated at clinical examination [37, 43].

Taken together, MRI may be advantageous over other imaging modalities in helping to exclude other possible diseases, delimiting the area of the lesion with bone and soft-tissue involvement, and guiding the therapeutic approach (i.e., debridement in intractable cases not responding to conservative treatment).

## Nuclear Medicine Imaging Techniques

Functional imaging with bone scintigraphy, bone single-photon emission computed tomography (SPECT), positron emission tomography (PET), and combinations with computed tomography (SPECT/CT, PET/CT) finally complete the imaging spectrum of MRONJ imaging. While radiographs, CT, and MRI are able to display osteonecrotic pattern, they have low specificity for BRONJ lesions [8, 16, 44]. Reliable detection of early BRONJ lesions and assessment of the extent of a lesion are limited so far. Therefore, functional nuclear medicine techniques were investigated as well in the context of BRONJ imaging.

Bone scintigraphy was identified to present with alterations of radionuclide uptake in BRONJ lesions [6, 45, 46]. 99Tcm-MDP uptake is generally influenced by blood flow and osteoblastic metabolism. Chinadussi et al. reported decreased 99Tcm-MDP uptake in early stages when vascularization is lowered and increased uptake in later stages due to higher osteoblast activity in advanced disease [6]. SPECT confirmed the presence of increased uptake, and it was concluded that scintigraphy might be used as a screening test to detect subclinical osteonecrosis in patients receiving bisphosphonates [6]. A drawback of conventional bone scintigraphy and SPECT however is the low spatial resolution and a certain lack in anatomical information. Hybrid SPECT/CT can improve the accuracy of scintigraphy because SPECT/CT provides a functional–anatomical correlation. Accordingly, it was reported that SPECT/CT increased the accuracy of conventional imaging and differentiation between the necrosis and adjacent viable bone became possible [46].

A comparison between two functional imaging techniques, characterized, on the one hand, by a tracer showing oncotropic properties, such as Tc99m-sestamibi, and, on the other hand, a tracer taken up by inflammation such as FDG-PET, was reported to support differentiation between BRONJ lesions and myeloma osteolysis in a preliminary report [45, 47].

Further studies demonstrated focal enhancement on PET scans at sites of BRONJ lesions [43, 44, 48]. PET enhancement is related to vascularization and hypermetabolism. Therefore, uptake in BRONJ lesions may be due to hypermetabolism caused by superimposing infection or healing response and may not be caused by the necrosis itself [44]. In a present study based on 46 PET scans, it was shown that enhancement on a PET scan is not a reliable indicator of BRONJ and that a non-enhancing scan does not necessarily exclude the disease. In conclusion, the results did not support a routine use in the diagnostic of BRONJ [44]. However, Wilde et al. suggested that PET might serve as an option for visualizing the severity of BRONJ and could be valuable for evaluation of treatment effects. Combined PET/CT techniques may further improve the diagnosis of BRONJ by combining functional and anatomical information [48].

While scintigraphy, SPECT, and PET are not useful for metric analysis of BRONJ [9], combined PET/CT was assessed to detect more extensive involvement of BRONJ compared with panoramic views from CBCT and clinical examinations, although, comparable to contrast-enhanced MRI, the real dimension of a lesion may be overestimated [21].

## Conclusions

At present, panoramic radiographs can be considered as a primary modality for MRONJ imaging. In clinical routine, CT and CBCT are widely used to gain further three-dimensional information of the extent of osteonecrosis and to clarify if there are any further findings like pathological fractures or signs of sinusitis. So far, there is no final evidence that MRI is superior to CT in order to display the extent of the lesion or to detect early stages of BRONJ. Anyway, it seems like CT and MRI offer a wide spectrum of findings but those are often not very specific. Nuclear medicine tomographic imaging techniques may be useful in detecting early stages and monitoring the disease; however, they cannot be regarded as standard in MRONJ imaging at the moment.

# References


1. Ruggiero SL, Dodson TB, Assael LA, Landesberg R, Marx RE, Mehrotra B. American Association of Oral and Maxillofacial Surgeons position paper on bisphosphonate-related osteonecrosis of the jaws–2009 update. J Oral Maxillofac Surg. 2009;67(5 Suppl):2–12. PubMed PMID: 19371809. Epub 2009/04/25. eng.
2. Lo JC, O'Ryan FS, Gordon NP, Yang J, Hui RL, Martin D, et al. Predicting Risk of Osteonecrosis of the Jaw with Oral Bisphosphonate Exposure (PROBE) Investigators. Prevalence of osteonecrosis of the jaw in patients with oral bisphosphonate exposure. J Oral Maxillofac Surg. 2010;68(2):243–53. PubMed PMID: 19772941. Epub 2009/09/24. eng.
3. Hutchinson M, O'Ryan F, Chavez V, Lathon PV, Sanchez G, Hatcher DC, et al. Radiographic findings in bisphosphonate-treated patients with stage 0 disease in the absence of bone exposure. J Oral Maxillofac Surg. 2010;68(9):2232–40. PubMed PMID: 20728032. eng.
4. Rocha GC, Jaguar GC, Moreira CR, Neves EG, Fonseca FP, Pedreira EN. Radiographic evaluation of maxillofacial region in oncology patients treated with bisphosphonates. Oral Surg Oral Med Oral Pathol Oral Radiol. 2012;114(5 Suppl):S19–25. PubMed PMID: 23083951. Epub 2012/02/18. eng.
5. Arce K, Assael LA, Weissman JL, Markiewicz MR. Imaging findings in bisphosphonate-related osteonecrosis of jaws. J Oral Maxillofac Surg. 2009;67(5 Suppl):75–84. PubMed PMID: 19371818. eng.
6. Chiandussi S, Biasotto M, Cavalli F, Cova MA, Di Learda R. Clinical and diagnostic imaging of bisphosphonate-associated osteonecrosis of the jaws.

Dentomaxillofac Radiol. 2006;35:236–43. PubMed PMID: 16798918. eng.

7. Morag Y, Morag-Hezroni M, Jamadar DA, Ward BB, Jacobson JA, Zwetchkenbaum SR, et al. Bisphosphonate-related osteonecrosis of the jaw: a pictorial review. Radiographics. 2009;29(7):1971–84. PubMed PMID: 19926757. eng.

8. Popovic KS, Kocar M. Imaging findings in bisphosphonate-induced osteonecrosis of the jaws. Radiol Oncol. 2010;44(4):215–9. PubMed PMID: 22933918. Epub 2010/06/24. eng.

9. Stockmann P, Hinkmann FM, Lell MM, Fenner M, Vairaktaris E, Neukam FW, Nkenke E. Panoramic radiograph, computed tomography or magnetic resonance imaging. Which imaging technique should be preferred in bisphosphonate-associated osteonecrosis of the jaw? A prospective clinical study. Clin Oral Investig. 2010;14(3):311–7.

10. Wilde F, Heufelder M, Lorenz K, Liese S, Liese J, Helmrich J, et al. Prevalence of cone beam computed tomography imaging findings according to the clinical stage of bisphosphonate-related osteonecrosis of the jaw. Oral Surg Oral Med Oral Pathol Oral Radiol. 2012;114(6):804–11. PMID: 23159120. eng.

11. Phal PM, Myall RW, Assael LA, Weissman JL. Imaging findings of bisphosphonate-associated osteonecrosis of the jaws. AJNR Am J Neuroradiol. 2007;28(6):1139–45. PubMed PMID: 17569974. eng.

12. Torres SR, Chen CS, Leroux BG, Lee PP, Hollender LG, Santos EC, Drew SP, Hung KC, Schubert MM. Mandibular cortical bone evaluation on cone beam computed tomography images of patients with bisphosphonate-related osteonecrosis of the jaw. Oral Surg Oral Med Oral Pathol Oral Radiol. 2012;113(5):695–703. PubMed PMID: 22668629. Epub 2012/04/12. eng.

13. Groetz KA, Al-Nawas B. Persisting alveolar sockets— a radio- logic symptom of BP-ONJ? J Oral Maxillofac Surg. 2006;64:1571–2. PubMed PMID: 16982320. eng.

14. Durie BG, Katz M, Crowley J. Osteonecrosis of the jaw and bisphosphonates. N Engl J Med. 2005;353(1):99–102; discussion 99–102. PubMed PMID: 16000365. eng.

15. Hewitt C, Farah CS. Bisphosphonate-related osteonecrosis of the jaws: a comprehensive review. J Oral Pathol Med. 2007;36(6):319–28. PubMed PMID: 17559492. eng.

16. Bisdas S, Chambron Pinho N, Smolarz A, Sader R, Vogl TJ, Mack MG. Bisphosphonate-induced osteonecrosis of the jaws: CT and MRI spectrum of findings in 32 patients. Clin Radiol. 2008;63(1):71–7. PubMed PMID: 18068792. Epub 2007 Oct 22. eng.

17. Bianchi SD, Scoletta M, Cassione FB, Migliaretti G, Mozzati M. Computerized tomographic findings in bisphosphonate-associated osteonecrosis of the jaw in patients with cancer. Oral Surg Oral Med Oral Pathol Oral Radiol Endod. 2007;104(2):249–58. PMID: 17560140. Epub 2007/06/07.

18. Gill SB, Valencia MP, Sabino ML, Heideman GM, Michel MA. Bisphosphonate-related osteonecrosis of the mandible and maxilla: clinical and imaging features. J Comput Assist Tomogr. 2009;33(3):449–54. PubMed PMID: 19478642. eng.

19. Marx RE, Sawatari Y, Fortin M, Broumand V. Bisphosphonate-induced exposed bone (osteonecrosis/osteopetrosis) of the jaws: risk factors, recognition, prevention, and treatment. J Oral Maxillofac Surg. 2005;63(11):1567–75. PubMed PMID: 16243172. eng.

20. Bedogni A, Blandamura S, Lokmic Z, Palumbo C, Ragazzo M, Ferrari F, et al. Bisphosphonate-associated jawbone osteonecrosis: a correlation between imaging techniques and histopathology. Oral Surg Oral Med Oral Pathol Oral Radiol Endod. 2008;105(3):358–64. PubMed PMID: 18280968. eng.

21. Guggenberger R, Fischer DR, Metzler P, Andreisek G, Nanz D, Jacobsen C, et al. Bisphosphonate-induced osteonecrosis of the jaw: comparison of disease extent on contrast-enhanced MR imaging, [18F] fluoride PET/CT, and conebeam CT imaging. AJNR Am J Neuroradiol. 2013;34(6):1242–7. PMID: 23221951. Epub 2012/12/6. eng.

22. Assaf AT, Zrnc TA, Riecke B, Wikner J, Zustin J, Friedrich RE, et al. Intraoperative efficiency of fluorescence imaging by Visually Enhanced Lesion Scope (VELscope) in patients with bisphosphonate related osteonecrosis of the jaw (BRONJ). J Craniomaxillofac Surg. 2014;42(5):157–64. PubMed PMID: 24011463. eng.

23. Pautke C, Bauer F, Otto S, Tischer T, Steiner T, Weitz J, et al. Fluorescence-guided bone resection in bisphosphonate-related osteonecrosis of the jaws: first clinical results of a prospective pilot study. J Oral Maxillofac Surg. 2011;69(1):84–91. PubMed PMID: 20971542. Epub 2010/10/26. eng.

24. Elad S, Gomori MJ, Ben-Ami N, Friedlander-Barenboim S, Regev E, Lazarovici TS, Yarom N. Bisphosphonate-related osteonecrosis of the jaw: clinical correlations with computerized tomography presentation. Clin Oral Investig. 2010;14(1):43–50. PubMed PMID: 19603201. Epub 2009/07/15. eng.

25. Allen MR, Ruggiero SL. Higher bone matrix density exists in only a subset of patients with bisphosphonate-related osteonecrosis of the jaw. J Oral Maxillofac Surg. 2009;67(7):1373–7. PubMed PMID: 19531405. eng.

26. De Vos W, Casselman J, Swennen GR. Cone-beam computerized tomography (CBCT) imaging of the oral and maxillofacial region: a systematic review of the literature. Int J Oral Maxillofac Surg. 2009;38:609–25. PubMed PMID: 19464146. Epub 2009/05/21. eng.

27. Loubele M, Bogaerts R, Van Dijck E, et al. Comparison between effective radiation dose of CBCT and MSCT scanners for dentomaxillofacial applications. Eur J Radiol. 2009;71:461–8. PubMed PMID: 18639404. Epub 2008/07/18. eng.

28. Schulze D, Heiland M, Thurmann H, Adam G. Radiation exposure during midfacial imaging using 4- and 16-slice computed tomography, cone beam computed tomography systems and conventional radiography. Dentomaxillofac Radiol. 2004;33:83–6. PubMed PMID: 15313998. eng.

29. Barragan-Adjemian C, Lausten L, Ang DB, Johnson M, Katz J, Bonewald LF. Bisphosphonate-related osteonecrosis of the jaw: model and diagnosis with cone beam computerized tomography. Cells Tissues

Organs. 2009;189:284–8. Pubmed PMID: 18703870. Epub 2008/08/15. eng.

30. Fleisher KE, Doty S, Kottal S, Phelan J, Norman RG, Glickman RS. Tetracycline-guided debridement and cone beam computed tomography for the treatment of bisphosphonate-related osteonecrosis of the jaw: a technical note. J Oral Maxillofac Surg. 2008;66(12): 2646–53. PubMed PMID: 19022151. Epub 2008/11/22. eng.

31. Singer SR, Mupparapu M. Plain film and CBCT findings in a case of bisphosphonate-related osteonecrosis of the jaw. Quintessence Int. 2009;40:163–5. PubMed PMID: 19169448. eng.

32. Treister NS, Friedland B, Woo SB. Use of cone-beam computerized tomography for evaluation of bisphosphonate-associated osteonecrosis of the jaws. Oral Surg Oral Med Oral Pathol Oral Radiol Endod. 2010;109(5):753–64. PubMed PMID: 20303301. Epub 2010/05/29. eng.

33. Olutayo J, Olubanwo Agbaje J, Jacobs R, Verhaeghe V, Vande Velde F, Vinckier F. Bisphosphonate-related osteonecrosis of the jaw bone: radiological pattern and the potential role of CBCT in early diagnosis. J Oral Maxillofac Res. 2010;1:e3. Available at http://www.ejomr.org/JOMR/archives/2010/2/e3/e3ht.htm.

34. Kalender WA, Kyriakou Y. Flat-detector computed tomography (FD-CT). Eur Radiol. 2007;17:2767–79. PubMed PMID: 17587058. Epub 2007/06/23. eng.

35. Mast G, Otto S, Mucke T, Schreyer C, Bissinger O, Kolk A, et al. Incidence of maxillary sinusitis and oro-antral fistulae in bisphosphonate-related osteonecrosis of the jaw. J Craniomaxillofac Surg. 2012;40(7): 568–71. PubMed PMID: 22118926. Epub 2011/11/29. eng.

36. Maurer P, Sandulescu T, Kriwalsky MS, Rashad A, Hollstein S, Stricker I, et al. Bisphosphonate-related osteonecrosis of the maxilla and sinusitis maxillaris. Int J Oral Maxillofac Surg. 2011;40(3):285–91. PubMed PMID: 21163624. Epub 2010/12/15.

37. Garcia-Ferrer L, Bagan JV, Martinez-Sanjuan V, Hernandez-Bazan S, Garcia R, Jimenez-Soriano Y, et al. MRI of mandibular osteonecrosis secondary to bisphosphonates. AJR Am J Roentgenol. 2008; 190(4):949–55. PubMed PMID: 18356441. eng.

38. Takao M, Sugano N, Nishii T, Sakai T, Nakamura N, Yoshikawa H. Different magnetic resonance imaging features in two types of nontraumatic rabbit osteonecrosis models. Magnetic resonance imaging. Magn Reson Imaging. 2009;27(2):233–9.

39. Fatterpekar GM, Emmrich JV, Eloy JA, Aggarwal A. Bone-within-bone appearance: a red flag for biphosphonate-associated osteonecrosis of the jaw.

40. Khosla S, Burr D, Cauley J, Dempster DW, Ebeling PR, Felsenberg D, et al. Bisphosphonate-associated osteonecrosis of the jaw: report of a task force of the American Society for Bone and Mineral Research. J Bone Miner Res. 2007;22(10):1479–91. PubMed PMID: 17663640. eng.

41. Fox MG, Stephens T, Jarjour WN, Anderson MW, Kimpel DL. Contrast-enhanced magnetic resonance imaging positively impacts the management of some patients with rheumatoid arthritis or suspected RA. J Clin Rheumatol. 2012;18(1):15–22. PubMed PMID: 22157267. eng.

42. Wutzl A, Eisenmenger G, Hoffmann M, Czerny C, Moser D, Pietschmann P, et al. Osteonecrosis of the jaws and bisphosphonate treatment in cancer patients. Wien Klin Wochenschr. 2006;118(15–16):473–8. PubMed PMID: 16957978. eng.

43. Raje N, Woo SB, Hande K, Yap JT, Richardson PG, Vallet S, et al. Clinical, radiographic, and biochemical characterization of multiple myeloma patients with osteonecrosis of the jaw. Clin Cancer Res. 2008;14(8):2387–95. PubMed PMID: 18413829. eng.

44. Belcher R, Boyette J, Pierson T, Siegel E, Bartel TB, Aniasse E, et al. What is the role of positron emission tomography in osteonecrosis of the jaws? J Oral Maxillofac Surg. 2014;72(2):306–10. doi:10.1016/j.joms.2013.07.038. pii: S0278-2391(13)00950-6. PubMed PMID: 24075237. eng.

45. Catalano L, Del Vecchio S, Petruzziello F, Fonti R, Salvatore B, Martorelli C, et al. Sestamibi and FDG-PET scans to support diagnosis of jaw osteonecrosis. Ann Hematol. 2007;86(6):415–23. PubMed PMID: 17285274. Epub 2007 Feb 7. eng.

46. Dore F, Filippi L, Biasotto M, Chiandussi S, Cavalli F, Di Lenarda R. Bone scintigraphy and SPECT/CT of bisphosphonate-induced osteonecrosis of the jaw. J Nucl Med. 2009;50(1):30–5. PubMed PMID: 19091894. eng.

47. Fabbricini R, Catalano L, Pace L, Del Vecchio S, Fonti R, Salvatore M, Rotoli B. Bone scintigraphy and SPECT/CT in bisphosphonate-induced osteo-crosis of the jaw. J Nucl Med. 2009;50(8):1385; author reply 1385. Epub 2009/07/17. PubMed PMID: 19617329.

48. Wilde F, Steinhoff K, Frerich B, Schulz T, Winter K, Hemprich A, et al. Positron-emission tomography imaging in the diagnosis of bisphosphonate-related osteonecrosis of the jaw. Oral Surg Oral Med Oral Pathol Oral Radiol Endod. 2009;107(3):412–9. PubMed PMID: 19121962. Epub 2009/01/04. eng.

Christoph Pautke

**Abstract**

The medication-related osteonecrosis of the jaw (MRONJ) is considered a therapy-resistant osteonecrosis entity. Both conservative and surgical treatment regimens are recommended. Nevertheless, contradictory success rates of the different therapy strategies are reported. The more experience with MRONJ is gathered, the more the surgical therapy is recommended: the success rates are higher, the progression of the disease can be stopped, and the diagnosis of osteonecrosis can be proved histologically, while other causes for exposed bone can be excluded. Using surgical treatment protocols, success rates exceeding 90 % can be achieved. Novel techniques such as visualization of bone fluorescence can further help to delineate the extent of the osteonecrosis intraoperatively.

The bisphosphonate-related osteonecrosis of the jaw (BRONJ) was first described in 2003 as a new osteonecrosis entity [1–3]. Naturally, at this time no experiences with this disease existed, and there was a great uncertainty of how to treat the affected patients.

The first treatment recommendations were given by the bisphosphonate suppliers advising conservative therapy approaches including local and systemic antibiotic treatment, oral hygiene measures, local irrigations, pain control, protective covering of the exposed bone, and conservative

osteonecrosis removal [4, 5]. Due to the fact that a considerable number of BRONJ cases could be related to tooth extractions prior to the manifestation [1, 6, 7], surgical procedures were thought to worsen the situation and the BRONJ stage. It was postulated that "attempts to accomplish debridements, cover the exposed bone with flaps, or bone-contouring procedures have mostly been counterproductive and have led to further exposed bone, worsening of symptoms, and a greater risk for a pathologic fracture of the jaw" [7].

As a consequence, the first studies on the therapy of BRONJ used conservative treatment approaches – the results were disappointing if not devastating (see Fig. 7.1). In 2005, Marx and coworkers reported of the unsuccessful treatment of 119 (out of 119) cases applying conservative measures [7]. The success rates of Bamias et al.

C. Pautke, MD, DDS
Medizin & Aesthetik, Clinic for Oral
and Maxillofacial Surgery,
Lenbachplatz 2a, Munich D-80333, Germany
e-mail: christoph.pautke@gmx.net

S. Otto (ed.), *Medication-Related Osteonecrosis of the Jaws: Bisphosphonates, Denosumab, and New Agents*,
DOI 10.1007/978-3-662-43733-9_7, © Springer-Verlag Berlin Heidelberg 2015

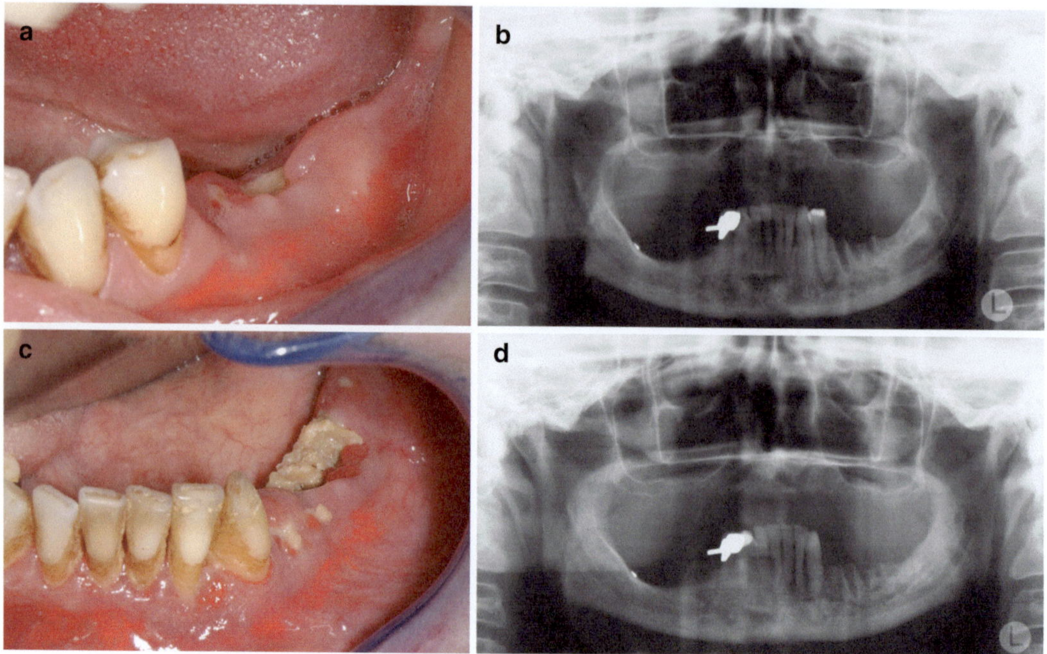

**Fig. 7.1** (**a**) A 68-year-old female patient suffering from multiple myeloma presented with a BRONJ stage I lesion in the left mandible. (**b**) The radiologic situation (orthopantograph) showed the typical signs of BRONJ, such as the absence of bone remodeling in the extraction sockets 7 months after tooth extraction. At that time, the patient refused surgical therapy, so the BRONJ was managed conservatively. (**c**) Clinical situation of the same patient 7 months later. Despite intensive conservative therapy, the disease progressed to a BRONJ stage II lesion with more exposed bone accompanied by a purulent and painful infection. (**d**) Displays the corresponding radiologic situation. All the remaining teeth in the left mandible were radiologically involved in the osteonecrosis (case published in 2011 [8] (Reprinted with kind permission of Elsevier))

as well as Migliorati et al. were similarly frustrating [5, 9].

Thus, after the first reports, BRONJ became the attribute of being very therapy refractory. Indeed, it was already recognized in 2004 by Ruggiero and coworkers that surgical therapy was necessary in most of the 63 cases of his study to improve or resolve BRONJ [10].

The treatment recommendations then changed with time: the more experience and knowledge with different BRONJ treatment strategies were gathered, the more the surgical therapy gained importance.

In 2006, it was suggested that the stages 1 and 2 should be treated conservatively, while extended cases (stage 3) should be treated surgically by debridement [11, 12].

In 2007 and 2009, the American Association of Oral and Maxillofacial Surgery (AAOMS) published stage-specific treatment recommendations

for BRONJ [13, 14] (Table 7.1) which are still up to date. Summarized, conservative treatment of BRONJ stages 0 and I, superficial debridement of stage II, and debridement stage III is recommended.

Although newer (from 2012), the guideline report for BRONJ of the German Dental and the German Oral and Maxillofacial Associations is less concrete abstaining therapy recommendations for certain stages of the disease [15]. The reason might be that there are significant drawbacks in current BRONJ staging as suggested by the AAOMS [14]. First, neither the extent of the exposed bone nor its localization is taken into account. Definitely, a large area of exposed bone is more difficult to treat than a small one. Second, combinations of different BRONJ symptoms (i.e., no exposed bone (stage 0) and sinusitis maxillaries (stage III)) cannot clearly be classified. Third, the general condition as

**Table 7.1** Staging and treatment strategies of bisphosphonate-related osteonecrosis of the jaw according to the position paper of the American Association of Oral and Maxillofacial Surgery 2009 [14] (Reprinted with kind permission of Elsevier)

| Stage | Description | Treatment strategies |
|---|---|---|
| 0 | No clinical evidence of necrotic bone, but nonspecific clinical findings and symptoms | Systemic management, including use of pain medication and antibiotics |
| I | Exposed and necrotic bone in asymptomatic patients without evidence of infection | Antibacterial mouth rinse<br>Clinical follow-up on quarterly basis<br>Patient education and review of indications for continued bisphosphonate therapy |
| II | Exposed and necrotic bone associated with infection as evidenced by pain and erythema in region of exposed bone with or without purulent drainage | Symptomatic treatment with oral antibiotics<br>Oral antibacterial mouth rinse<br>Pain control<br>Superficial debridement to relieve soft tissue irritation |
| III | Exposed and necrotic bone in patients with pain, infection, and one or more of the following: exposed and necrotic bone extending beyond the region of the alveolar bone (i.e., inferior border and ramus in the mandible, maxillary sinus, and zygoma in the maxilla), resulting in pathologic fracture, extraoral fistula, oroantral/oronasal communication, or osteolysis extending to the inferior border of the mandible or the sinus floor | Antibacterial mouth rinse<br>Antibiotic therapy and pain control<br>Surgical debridement/resection for longer-term palliation of infection and pain |

well as the patients' burden of suffering are not considered. In a stage I disease, a patient might not have pain, but symptoms such as halitosis might reduce the quality of the social life significantly. Indeed, it is of great importance whether a patient is treated because of osteoporosis without any comorbidity or because of bone metastasis in a final stage receiving additional chemotherapy and suffering from various comorbidities such as diabetes or peripheral artery disease.

With regard to the development of the treatment recommendations, the author (as Oral and Maxillofacial Surgeon) suggests further advances in the BRONJ therapy will be achieved if all BRONJ stages are treated surgically.

This is for several important good reasons:

(i) The diagnosis of an osteonecrosis should be confirmed by a histopathological investigation. Although until now the histopathological proof of an osteonecrosis is not a part of its definition, it can be excluded that other pathologic conditions such as jawbone metastasis [16] induce the clinical picture of the exposed bone. This is important as the therapy of a jawbone metastasis and BRONJ differs significantly.

(ii) Exposed bone is an entrance gate for bacterial colonization and infection such as for actinomyces bacteria [17, 18]. For this particular microbial strain, a possible role in the pathogenesis as well as an aggravating effect of an existing BRONJ is discussed. Therefore, the exposed bone always increases the risk of BRONJ progression. Due to the fact that conservative treatment approaches do commonly not resolve the exposed bone [7, 19], there is the risk of worsening of the BRONJ stage or secondary infection leading to abscess or pain, particularly in patients who are immunocompromised by chemotherapy (see Fig. 7.1).

(iii) The success rates of surgical approaches are significantly higher compared to conservative treatment regimens [20]. Given that a therapy success includes the removal of exposed bone and an intact mucosa, conservative management shows disappointing results of less than 20 % [7, 19, 21, 22]. In contrast, surgical approaches reveal success rates exceeding 85 % [8, 23–25]. A timely treatment has a positive effect on the outcome [10, 26], which is another reason to perform surgical therapy in the stages 0 and I.

(iv) The conservative therapy commonly takes months to years with weekly or twice a week consultations for conservative wound management [21, 22], which can be considered as additional burden for the affected patients. In contrast, the surgical treatment is usually completed 3–4 weeks after surgery [8]. It should be taken into account that effects similar to habituation of the microbial wound flora will take place after weeks or even months of antibiotic treatment [27]. Side effects such as microbial resistances or oral candidiasis might aggravate the treatment.

"Therapy literally means 'curing, healing' and is the attempted remediation of a health problem, usually following a diagnosis" [28].

BRONJ is currently diagnosed by the presence of exposed jawbone for a period that exceeds 8 weeks [13, 14, 29] (in combination with a positive drug history for bisphosphonates and no radiation of the head and neck region). Consequently, a therapy success is achieved when the exposed necrotic bone is removed and a mucosal integrity is restored. Therefore, the aim of the BRONJ therapy should resolve the leading symptom: the exposed bone.

Indeed, confusion is caused by studies applying conservative measures to treat BRONJ and reporting success rates exceeding 50 % [30, 31]. To understand this obvious discrepancy, it is important to take a closer look of how the success of a therapy is defined in these studies. The maintenance of the status quo, i.e., no worsening of the situation of the exposed bone [30, 31], can be considered as improvement of the patient's situation but not as therapy success with respect to the definition of the disease. Furthermore, studies on therapy success should not use retrospective but prospective study designs. In retrospective studies conducted with questionnaires without oral investigations, it is impossible to detect early stages with exposed bone that are not accompanied by infection or pain. Due to the fact that these "silent" BRONJ stages are a frequent finding, a significant number of BRONJ cases are not recorded in retrospective studies.

In spite of these considerations to treat all BRONJ stages surgically, the conservative therapy is useful and necessary to control the disease when the patient's general condition does not allow surgical intervention or when chemotherapy cannot be discontinued. Applying conservative measures, patients' condition improved or stay asymptomatic in up to 70 % of the cases [32].

Indeed, it is of crucial importance that the patient is thoroughly informed about the different treatment options, the duration and burden of each therapy way, as well as the success rates. In addition, the specific needs and discomforts of the patients should be considered for the choice of therapy.

Due to the fact that the necrotic and exposed bone will not be revitalized and turned into a vital bone again, BRONJ should be removed even if only small bone areas are affected. Thus, the aim of the surgical therapy is the complete removal of the osteonecrosis because even small residuals might lead to a recurrence or progression of BRONJ both by mechanical injury of the mucosa as well as by microbacteria remaining in the affected bone.

The therapy should be well planned beginning with the choice of the surgical approach. The mucosal incision should always be performed in consideration of a tension-free mucoperiosteal coverage of the area of the exposed bone. Mucosal dehiscences as well as fistulas should be included in the incision line. Subsequently, the marginal mucosa of these areas should be cut out, because the mucosa adjacent to BRONJ lesions is altered due to the chronic infection and less useful for reconstruction [33]. If teeth have to be removed, a marginal incision has to be performed in order to allow the wound closure with a mucoperiosteal flap. Unlike in osteoradionecrosis, the deperiostation of the bone has no unfavorable effect in the treatment of BRONJ. Indeed, a sufficient bone exposure helps to remove the osteonecrosis completely, to even sharp bone ridges, and to achieve a tension-free wound closure.

The exposed bone in BRONJ commonly shows a darker and yellowish color compared to the unaffected sites. The porosity is often increased, and the necrotic bone is often softer compared to the normal bone. Frequently, BRONJ is surrounded by sclerotic bone areas, which are harder and less vascularized pretending an avascular necrosis. The osteonecrosis including bone sequestra must be removed completely even if this causes large bone defects of the jawbones or broad oroantral fistulas.

If the osteonecrosis reaches or surrounds the teeth, the respective teeth have to be extracted in order to remove the osteonecrosis completely. After the surgical elimination of the osteonecrosis, it is of crucial importance to smooth sharp bone ridges such as the crestal bone of tooth extraction sockets in order to avoid failure. This is an important step in the treatment of BRONJ, because the bone turnover is reduced by the bisphosphonate administration and sharp bone sites will be remodeled very slowly. Spiky ridges can either hamper the mucosal healing or injure the mucosal coverage of the wound and increase the risk of recurrence of the exposed bone. There is an overlap of therapeutic and prophylactic measures. With respect to the conclusive pH-dependent BRONJ pathogenesis theory [34, 35], surgical procedures such as root resections or tooth extractions are recommended to eliminate chronic infections. Indeed, sharp bone ridges must also be removed following these procedures.

In most cases, buccal mucoperiosteal flaps are best suited to achieve a tension-free mucosal coverage. On the one hand, the mobilization of the buccal mucoperiosteum is easier compared to the palate mucosa in the maxilla or parts of floor of the mouth. On the other hand, the functional limitations are much less when using buccal mucoperiosteal flaps. Some surgeons suggest a two-layer coverage of the exposed bone to achieve safer wound closure. In the mandible, this can be achieved either by a muscle flap of the mylohyoid muscle [36] or a buccal fat flap. The latter is also suitable for a two-layer coverage in the maxilla in particular when oroantral fistulas are present after the BRONJ resection [37, 38] (see Fig. 7.2). The nasolabial flap is an additional option to reconstruct defects of both the mandible and the maxilla [39]. While a two-layer wound closure might be of use in broad oroantral fistulas, a monolayer coverage using a mucoperiosteal flap is usually sufficient when the osteonecrosis is completely removed. Although the mucosa in BRONJ patients can be of inferior quality and stability [33], soft tissue free flap reconstruction is only necessary in rare cases.

The demand for bony reconstruction arises more frequently, in particular when parts of the mandible have to be resected. The treatment options range from a resection without reconstruction [25], the stabilization of the jaw with osteosynthesis plates [25, 40, 41], to the bony jaw reconstruction using avascular [41] or microvascular bone flaps [42–44]. Although success rates of free flap bone reconstructions are good, the burden of the operation for the patients is not negligible. Indeed, the dental rehabilitation using dental implants is contraindicated in patients with intravenous bisphosphonate administration as well as a BRONJ in the medical history according to the recommendations of the AAOMS [14]. It should always be considered that the transplanted bone is also loaded with bisphosphonates. As a matter of fact, the transplanted bone can again be affected from BRONJ [45] not to mention failure of the transplant because of a higher operation risk due to the comorbidities. The limitations have to be considered especially the general condition of the patient suffering from bone metastasis as well as the prognosis and the stage of the underlying disease. Thus, a free flap bone reconstruction might be in option in the treatment of extended BRONJ cases, but it is not recommended as the first step in the therapy.

The exposed bone in BRONJ is always colonized with bacteria of the oral cavity such as actinomyces. Furthermore, the microbial adhesion to the bone appears to be altered under bisphosphonate therapy [46]. Thus, there is always a more or less active infection of the exposed bone [47]. Consequently, adjuvant measures that aim for disinfection of the bone are of use to support the surgical treatment such as ozone application [48], laser therapy [49], and in particular a prolonged antibiotic therapy [50]. Antibiotic prophylaxis had a significant impact on the incidence of BRONJ after dental procedures in patients under bisphosphonate medication. The administration of penicillin derivates is recommended. In case of allergy to penicillin, tetracycline derivates or clindamycin are an alternative treatment option. Due to the fact that tetracycline and its derivates bind to calcium, there might be a depot or long-term effect.

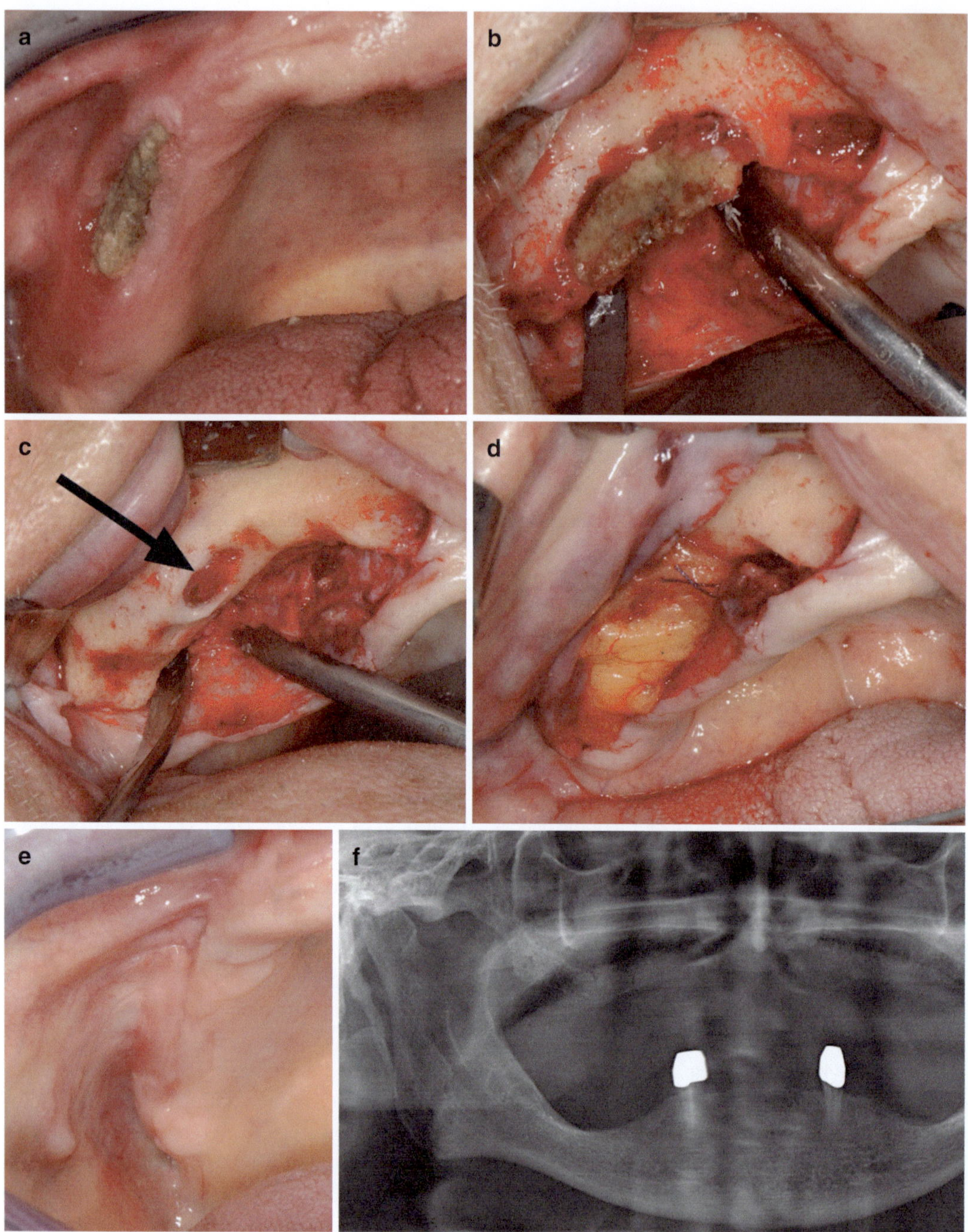

Fig. 7.2 (a) 79-year-old man suffering from prostate cancer presented (a) with a BRONJ stages I–II lesion in the right upper jaw. The patient was treated surgically. (b) Intraoperative presentation of the BRONJ. (c) Intraoperative situation after complete surgical resection of the osteonecrosis. Note the broad oroantral fistula (*arrow*). (d) Wound closure was performed in a two-layer technique using Bichat's buccal fat flap and muco-periosteum. (e) 4 weeks postoperatively, the patient was free of symptoms and showed complete mucosal healing. (f) The postoperative radiograph (case published in 2012 [34] (Reprinted with kind permission of Elsevier))

Additional measures such as the application of stem cells [51] and platelet-rich plasma [52], providing an alkaline environment [53], or the administration of parathyroid hormone [54, 55] are promising approaches; however, still on an experimental level.

The challenge as well as the limitations of the surgical therapy of BRONJ is that the margins of the osteonecrosis cannot be exactly determined; thus, a clear demarcation of the necrotic bone is difficult if not impossible [13, 29, 56]. However, the complete removal of the necrotic bone is of crucial importance as otherwise there is the risk of disease recurrence or progression [25, 57]. On the other hand, it must avoided to unintentionally and unnecessarily remove the healthy bone without signs of osteonecrosis in order neither to weaken the jawbone (danger of fracture) nor to make the situation for dental or prosthetic rehabilitation more difficult. The bone debridement cannot be standardized, as it is the surgeon who decides how much bone to be removed, because there is no modality, which is able to objectify the margins of the necrosis. Hence, the surgical therapy is dependent on the surgeon and neither comparable nor reproducible in another department.

There are numerous studies using various imaging modalities in attempts to objectify the extent of the osteonecrosis including panoramic radiography [58], CT, SPECT/CT [59], PET/CT, MRI, cone-beam CT imaging [37, 60], or bone scintigraphy [61]. However, none of these modalities is able to clearly depict the margins of the necrosis [15]. It could be demonstrated that the changes of the bone structure (depicted by x-ray techniques such as panoramic radiography, CT, or cone-beam imaging) are more helpful for operation planning compared to the depiction of the soft tissue reactions including the infection (e.g., by MRI, PET, or scintigraphy). Osteosclerosis around sites of inflammation (e.g., teeth with periodontitis), density confluence of cortical and cancellous bone, and prominence of the inferior alveolar nerve canal,

and a persisting alveolar socket can be early radiologic signs [58]. In later stages, bone sequestra, radiolucencies due to osteolysis, and cortical disruption as well as periosteal bone formation might be present [62]. However, these findings are not stage specific and cannot objectify the exact extent of the necrosis.

One of the most reliable parameters is the intraoperative impression of the surgeon [60]. The surgical debridement in BRONJ therapy is commonly performed until the bone appears to be "normal," i.e., the bone structure (porosity), color, and texture are similar to the non-affected bone sites. However, the personal feeling of a surgeon is neither reproducible nor transferable. As a consequence, the comparability of studies with different surgeons is limited. What is more, the bleeding of the bone is widely accepted to be a sign of a viable bone in the surgical therapy of osteonecrosis and in particular in BRONJ. However, it has been shown that bone bleeding does not correlate well with the histological findings of the vital bone. Thus, this finding is no appropriate parameter to determine the extent or the margins of an osteonecrosis [8, 40, 56].

A helpful technique to distinguish between viable and necrotic bone is the use of bone fluorescence [8, 40, 56, 63, 64]. In addition to the antibiotic effect of reducing inflammation and pain in patients suffering from BRONJ, tetracycline and its derivates possess fluorescence properties [65]. Under appropriate excitation light, tetracycline derivates show a greenish fluorescence at approximately 525–540 nm [66]. Due to its affinity to calcium, tetracycline is incorporated in the bone in particular in areas of bone remodeling and bone apposition [67]. Viable bone shows a green fluorescence that can be visualized intraoperatively by using a VELscope fluorescence lamp (LED Medical Diagnostics, British Columbia, Canada), a certified medical device approved by the American Dental Association for the detection of mucosal tissue abnormalities [8, 40, 56, 64, 68]. In contrast, the necrotic bone shows no or only pale fluorescence (see Figs. 7.3 and 7.4). Recent reports suggest that the VELscope system induces an autofluorescence of vital but not of necrotic bone leading to similar bone fluorescence findings without tetracycline bone labeling [69].

As a consequence, a viable and necrotic bone can be distinguished during the operation enabling to remove the osteonecrosis considerately but completely. The resection of the bone necrosis is performed until the complete bone is fluorescing under the VELscope light. Reddish fluorescence is considered as bacterial colonization of the bone. These areas should be further removed even if green bone fluorescence is present.

Due to the fact that this technique is easy to apply, is reproducible, and does not rely on the subjective impression of the surgeon, it is an important milestone towards a standardization of the surgical BRONJ therapy auguring an improvement of the treatment.

Recently, another osteonecrosis entity of the jaw has been reported which is due to the therapy with antibodies against receptor activator of nuclear factor kappaB ligand (RANKL) [70, 71]. The first treatment results suggested that this osteonecrosis entity might even be more refractory to conservative therapy compared to BRONJ [72]. Notably, in a recent report, it was demonstrated that the fluorescence-guided bone resection is a suitable and successful treatment modality for the RANKL-inhibitor or denosumab-related osteonecrosis of the jaw (DRONJ) [73]. Therefore, the author recommends to learn from the developments and pitfalls of the BRONJ therapy and not to hesitate too long with surgical procedures (In these patients, extensive dental surgery to treat MRONJ may exacerbate the condition) [74].

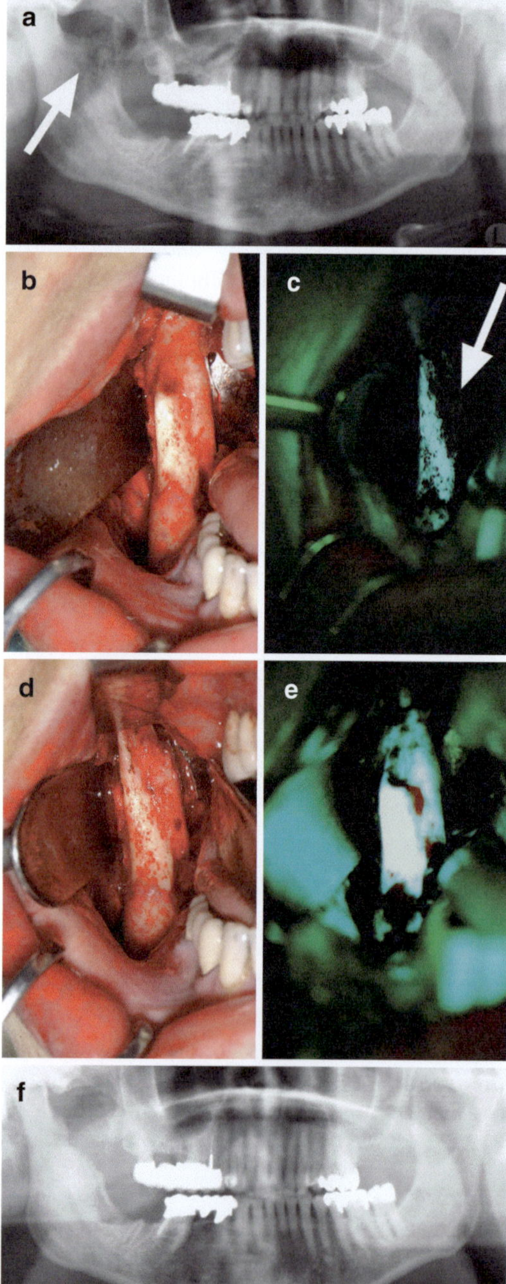

**Fig. 7.3** A 70-year-old female patient suffering from multiple myeloma which was treated with intravenous administrations of zoledronate presented with a pterygomandibular abscess on the right side (thus BRONJ stage II). (**a**) The radiograph showed an altered bone structure in the right muscular processus (*arrow*). (**b**) After surgical bone exposure, it was not possible to clearly delineate the osteonecrosis. (**c**) By the use of a fluorescence lamp (VELscope), a viable bone showed a greenish fluorescence, whereas the osteonecrosis revealed no or only very pale fluorescence (*arrow*). (**d**) Clinical picture after fluorescence-guided bone resection, which is performed until (**e**) the bone shows a homogeneous greenish fluorescence. (**f**) The postoperative radiograph. The patient is free of symptoms

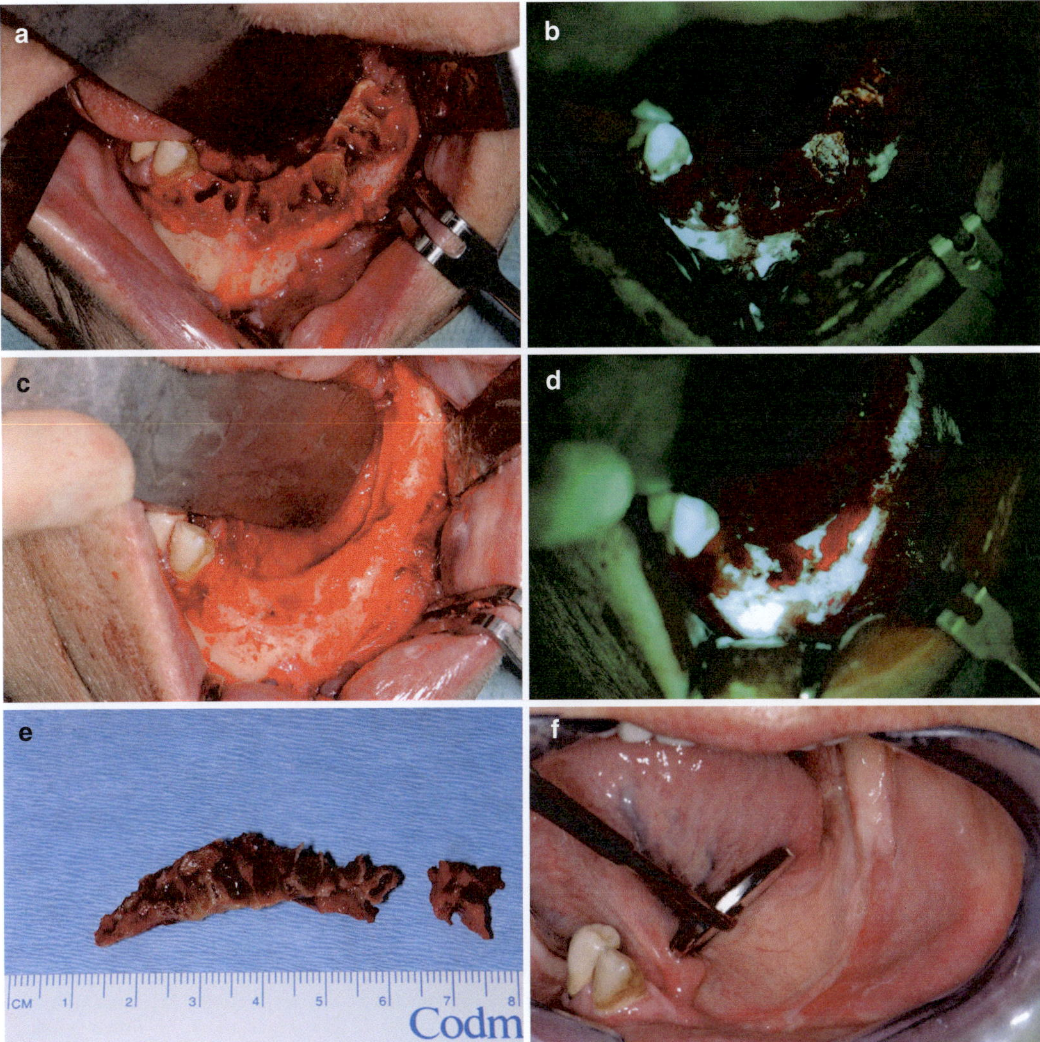

**Fig. 7.4** Surgical therapy of the same patient presented in Fig. 7.1. The surgical resection of the osteonecrosis was performed under fluorescence guidance. (**a**) Clinical picture after subperiosteal exploration. (**b**) The extent of the osteonecrosis became obvious using the fluorescence lamp. The reddish fluorescence is considered as bacterial infection. (**c**) After complete debridement, the bone showed a homogeneous greenish fluorescence indicating viable bone (**d**). (**e**) Resected necrotic bone. (**f**) Clinical situation with mucosal closure 4 weeks after the operation. The patient is free of symptoms (case published in 2011 [8] (Reprinted with kind permission of Elsevier))

Due to the fact that the antiresorptive effects of denosumab diminish with time, it is recommended that the therapy is discontinued preferably at least 3 months, if possible 6 months, before dentoalveolar surgeries. This is a crucial difference to the recommendations for BRONJ treatment. Bisphosphonates covalently bind to the bone, and bone parameters are altered for over 10 years. Currently, there is no evidence that the discontinuation of a bisphosphonate therapy leads either a lower BRONJ incidence after dental surgeries or to favorable treatment outcomes of BRONJ [15].

### Conclusion

Even though conservative treatment might be able to slow down disease progression and alleviate superinfection of the exposed bone, surgical treatment protocols have shown superior results with regard to complete mucosal healing. Surgical intervention should be considered in all MRONJ stages (also stages 0 and I) in terms of histological confirmation of the diagnosis MRONJ as well as preventing disease progression. The fluorescence-guided bone resection is an innovative and promising treatment modality for BRONJ which seems to be applicable for the treatment of denosumab-related osteonecrosis of the jaw (DRONJ) as well.

# References


1. Marx RE. Pamidronate (Aredia) and zoledronate (Zometa) induced avascular necrosis of the jaws: a growing epidemic. J Oral Maxillofac Surg. 2003;61(9):1115–7. PubMed PMID: 12966493. eng.
2. Migliorati CA. Bisphosphonates and oral cavity avascular bone necrosis. J Clin Oncol. 2003;21(22):4253–4. PubMed PMID: 14615459. Epub 2003/11/15. eng.
3. Wang J, Goodger NM, Pogrel MA. Osteonecrosis of the jaws associated with cancer chemotherapy. J Oral Maxillofac Surg. 2003;61(9):1104–7. PubMed PMID: 12966490. Epub 2003/09/11. eng.
4. Expert panel recommendations for the prevention, diagnosis, and treatment of osteonecrosis of the jaws. Professional education material. East Hanover, NJ, Novartis; 2004.
5. Migliorati CA, Schubert MM, Peterson DE, Seneda LM. Bisphosphonate-associated osteonecrosis of mandibular and maxillary bone: an emerging oral complication of supportive cancer therapy. Cancer. 2005;104(1):83–93. PubMed PMID: 15929121. Epub 2005/06/02. eng.
6. Badros A, Weikel D, Salama A, Goloubeva O, Schneider A, Rapoport A, et al. Osteonecrosis of the jaw in multiple myeloma patients: clinical features and risk factors. J Clin Oncol. 2006;24(6):945–52. PubMed PMID: 16484704. Epub 2006/02/18. eng.
7. Marx RE, Sawatari Y, Fortin M, Broumand V. Bisphosphonate-induced exposed bone (osteonecrosis/osteopetrosis) of the jaws: risk factors, recognition, prevention, and treatment. J Oral Maxillofac Surg. 2005;63(11):1567–75. PubMed PMID: 16243172. eng.
8. Pautke C, Bauer F, Otto S, Tischer T, Steiner T, Weitz J, et al. Fluorescence-guided bone resection in bisphosphonate-related osteonecrosis of the jaws: first clinical results of a prospective pilot study. J Oral Maxillofac Surg. 2011;69(1):84–91. PubMed PMID: 20971542. Epub 2010/10/26. eng.
9. Bamias A, Kastritis E, Bamia C, Moulopoulos LA, Melakopoulos I, Bozas G, et al. Osteonecrosis of the jaw in cancer after treatment with bisphosphonates: incidence and risk factors. J Clin Oncol. 2005;23(34):8580–7. PubMed PMID: 16314620. eng.
10. Ruggiero SL, Mehrotra B, Rosenberg TJ, Engroff SL. Osteonecrosis of the jaws associated with the use of bisphosphonates: a review of 63 cases. J Oral Maxillofac Surg. 2004;62(5):527–34. PubMed PMID: 15122554. eng.
11. Migliorati CA, Siegel MA, Elting LS. Bisphosphonate-associated osteonecrosis: a long-term complication of bisphosphonate treatment. Lancet Oncol. 2006;7(6):508–14. PubMed PMID: 16750501. Epub 2006/06/06. eng.
12. Ruggiero SL, Fantasia J, Carlson E. Bisphosphonate-related osteonecrosis of the jaw: background and guidelines for diagnosis, staging and management. Oral Surg Oral Med Oral Pathol Oral Radiol Endod. 2006;102(4):433–41. PubMed PMID: 16997108. Epub 2006/09/26. eng.
13. Advisory Task Force on Bisphosphonate-Related Ostenonecrosis of the Jaws, American Association of Oral and Maxillofacial Surgeons. J Oral Maxillofac Surg. 2007;65(3):369–76. PubMed PMID: 17307580. eng.
14. Ruggiero SL, Dodson TB, Assael LA, Landesberg R, Marx RE, Mehrotra B. American Association of Oral and Maxillofacial Surgeons position paper on bisphosphonate-related osteonecrosis of the jaws–2009 update. J Oral Maxillofac Surg. 2009;67(5 Suppl):2–12. PubMed PMID: 19371809. Epub 2009/04/25. eng.
15. Groetz KA, Piesold J-U, Al-Nawas B. Bisphosphonat-assoziierte Kiefernekrose (BP-ONJ) und andere Medikamenten-assoziierte Kiefernekrosen. AWMF online www.awmf.org. 2012.
16. Otto S, Schuler K, Ihrler S, Ehrenfeld M, Mast G. Osteonecrosis or metastases of the jaw or both? Case report and review of the literature. J Oral Maxillofac Surg. 2010;68(5):1185–8. PubMed PMID: 20144499. Epub 2010/02/11. eng.
17. Schipmann S, Metzler P, Rossle M, Zemann W, von Jackowski J, Obwegeser JA, et al. Osteopathology associated with bone resorption inhibitors – which role does Actinomyces play? A presentation of 51 cases with systematic review of the literature. J Oral Pathol Med. 2013;1. PubMed PMID: 23369166. Epub 2013/02/02. Eng.
18. Sedghizadeh PP, Kumar SK, Gorur A, Schaudinn C, Shuler CF, Costerton JW. Identification of microbial biofilms in osteonecrosis of the jaws secondary to bisphosphonate therapy. J Oral Maxillofac Surg. 2008;66(4):767–75. PubMed PMID: 18355603. Epub 2008/03/22. eng.
19. Montebugnoli L, Felicetti L, Gissi DB, Pizzigallo A, Pelliccioni GA, Marchetti C. Biphosphonate-associated osteonecrosis can be controlled by nonsurgical management. Oral Surg Oral Med Oral Pathol Oral Radiol Endod. 2007;104(4):473–7. PubMed PMID: 17482847. Epub 2007/05/08. eng.
20. Lesclous P, Grabar S, Abi Najm S, Carrel JP, Lombardi T, Saffar JL, et al. Relevance of surgical management of patients affected by bisphosphonate-associated osteonecrosis of the jaws. A prospective clinical and

radiological study. Clin Oral Investig. 2014;18(2):391–9. PubMed PMID: 23604698.

21. Hoff AO, Toth BB, Altundag K, Johnson MM, Warneke CL, Hu M, et al. Frequency and risk factors associated with osteonecrosis of the jaw in cancer patients treated with intravenous bisphosphonates. J Bone Miner Res. 2008;23(6):826–36. PubMed PMID: 18558816. Epub 2008/06/19. eng.

22. O'Ryan FS, Khoury S, Liao W, Han MM, Hui RL, Baer D, et al. Intravenous bisphosphonate-related osteonecrosis of the jaw: bone scintigraphy as an early indicator. J Oral Maxillofac Surg. 2009;67(7):1363–72. PubMed PMID: 19531404. Epub 2009/06/18. eng.

23. Stockmann P, Vairaktaris E, Wehrhan F, Seiss M, Schwarz S, Spriewald B, et al. Osteotomy and primary wound closure in bisphosphonate-associated osteonecrosis of the jaw: a prospective clinical study with 12 months follow-up. Support Care Cancer. 2010;18(4):449–60. PubMed PMID: 19609572. Epub 2009/07/18. eng.

24. Voss PJ, Joshi Oshero J, Kovalova-Muller A, Veigel Merino EA, Sauerbier S, Al-Jamali J, et al. Surgical treatment of bisphosphonate-associated osteonecrosis of the jaw: technical report and follow up of 21 patients. J Craniomaxillofac Surg. 2012;40(8):719–25. PubMed PMID: 22336489. Epub 2012/02/18. eng.

25. Carlson ER, Basile JD. The role of surgical resection in the management of bisphosphonate-related osteonecrosis of the jaws. J Oral Maxillofac Surg. 2009;67(5 Suppl):85–95. PubMed PMID: 19371819. Epub 2009/04/25. eng.

26. Otto S, Hafner S, Grotz KA. The role of inferior alveolar nerve involvement in bisphosphonate-related osteonecrosis of the jaw. J Oral Maxillofac Surg. 2009;67(3):589–92. PubMed PMID: 19231785. Epub 2009/02/24. eng.

27. Hoefert S, Eufinger H. Relevance of a prolonged preoperative antibiotic regime in the treatment of bisphosphonate-related osteonecrosis of the jaw. J Oral Maxillofac Surg. 2011;69(2):362–80. PubMed PMID: 21122968. Epub 2010/12/03. eng.

28. Definition of "therapy" according to wikipedia. http://en.wikipedia.org/wiki/Therapy.

29. Khosla S, Burr D, Cauley J, Dempster DW, Ebeling PR, Felsenberg D, et al. Bisphosphonate-associated osteonecrosis of the jaw: report of a task force of the American Society for Bone and Mineral Research. J Bone Miner Res. 2007;22(10):1479–91. PubMed PMID: 17663640. eng.

30. Badros A, Terpos E, Katodritou E, Goloubeva O, Kastritis E, Verrou E, et al. Natural history of osteonecrosis of the jaw in patients with multiple myeloma. J Clin Oncol. 2008;26(36):5904–9. PubMed PMID: 19018084. Epub 2008/11/20. eng.

31. Van den Wyngaert T, Claeys T, Huizing MT, Vermorken JB, Fossion E. Initial experience with conservative treatment in cancer patients with osteonecrosis of the jaw (ONJ) and predictors of outcome. Ann Oncol. 2009;20(2):331–6. PubMed PMID: 18953067. Epub 2008/10/28. eng.

32. Lerman MA, Xie W, Treister NS, Richardson PG, Weller EA, Woo SB. Conservative management of bisphosphonate-related osteonecrosis of the jaws: staging and treatment outcomes. Oral Oncol. 2013;3. PubMed PMID: 23830962.

33. Lorenzo SD, Trapassi A, Corradino B, Cordova A. Histology of the oral mucosa in patients with BRONJ at III Stage: a microscopic study proves the unsuitability of local mucosal flaps. J Clin Med Res. 2013;5(1):22–5. PubMed PMID: 23390472. Pubmed Central PMCID: 3564564.

34. Otto S, Schreyer C, Hafner S, Mast G, Ehrenfeld M, Sturzenbaum S, et al. Bisphosphonate-related osteonecrosis of the jaws – characteristics, risk factors, clinical features, localization and impact on oncological treatment. J Craniomaxillofac Surg. 2012;40(4):303–9. PubMed PMID: 21676622. Epub 2011/06/17. eng.

35. Otto S, Hafner S, Mast G, Tischer T, Volkmer E, Schieker M, et al. Bisphosphonate-related osteonecrosis of the jaw: is pH the missing part in the pathogenesis puzzle? J Oral Maxillofac Surg. 2010;68(5):1158–61. PubMed PMID: 20138420. Epub 2010/02/09. eng.

36. Lemound J, Eckardt A, Kokemuller H, von See C, Voss PJ, Tavassol F, et al. Bisphosphonate-associated osteonecrosis of the mandible: reliable soft tissue reconstruction using a local myofascial flap. Clin Oral Investig. 2012;16(4):1143–52. PubMed PMID: 21818568.

37. Mast G, Otto S, Mucke T, Schreyer C, Bissinger O, Kolk A, et al. Incidence of maxillary sinusitis and oroantral fistulae in bisphosphonate-related osteonecrosis of the jaw. J Craniomaxillofac Surg. 2012;40(7):568–71. PubMed PMID: 22118926. Epub 2011/11/29. eng.

38. Gallego L, Junquera L, Pelaz A, Hernando J, Megias J. The use of pedicled buccal fat pad combined with sequestrectomy in bisphosphonate-related osteonecrosis of the maxilla. Med Oral Patol Oral Cir Bucal. 2012;17(2):e236–41. PubMed PMID: 22143692. Pubmed Central PMCID: 3448310.

39. Eckardt AM, Kokemuller H, Tavassol F, Gellrich NC. Reconstruction of oral mucosal defects using the nasolabial flap: clinical experience with 22 patients. Head Neck Oncol. 2011;3:28. PubMed PMID: 21605443. Pubmed Central PMCID: 3121716.

40. Pautke C, Bauer F, Bissinger O, Tischer T, Kreutzer K, Steiner T, et al. Tetracycline bone fluorescence: a valuable marker for osteonecrosis characterization and therapy. J Oral Maxillofac Surg. 2010;68(1):125–9. PubMed PMID: 20006166. Epub 2009/12/17. eng.

41. Marx RE. Reconstruction of defects caused by bisphosphonate-induced osteonecrosis of the jaws. J Oral Maxillofac Surg. 2009;67(5 Suppl):107–19. PubMed PMID: 19371821. Epub 2009/04/25. eng.

42. Ferrari S, Bianchi B, Savi A, Poli T, Multinu A, Balestreri A, et al. Fibula free flap with endosseous implants for reconstructing a resected mandible in bisphosphonate osteonecrosis. J Oral Maxillofac Surg. 2008;66(5):999–1003. PubMed PMID: 18423292. Epub 2008/04/22. eng.

43. Mücke T, Haarmann S, Wolff KD, Holzle F. Bisphosphonate related osteonecrosis of the jaws treated by surgical resection and immediate osseous microvascular reconstruction. J Craniomaxillofac Surg. 2009;37(5):291–7. PubMed PMID: 19179088. Epub 2009/01/31. eng.

44. Engroff SL, Kim DD. Treating bisphosphonate osteone- crosis of the jaws: is there a role for resection and vascu- larized reconstruction? J Oral Maxillofac Surg. 2007;65(11):2374–85. PubMed PMID: 17954344. eng.

45. Pautke C, Otto S, Reu S, Kolk A, Ehrenfeld M, Sturzenbaum S, et al. Bisphosphonate related osteo- necrosis of the jaw–manifestation in a microvascular iliac bone flap. Oral Oncol. 2011;47(5):425–9. PubMed PMID: 21478047. Epub 2011/04/12. eng.

46. Kos M, Junka A, Smutnicka D, Bartoszewicz M, Kurzynowski T, Gluza K. Pamidronate enhances bac- terial adhesion to bone hydroxyapatite. Another puz- zle in the pathology of bisphosphonate-related osteonecrosis of the jaw? J Oral Maxillofac Surg. 2013;71(6):1010–6.

47. Lesclous P, Abi Najm S, Carrel JP, Baroukh B, Lombardi T, Willi JP, et al. Bisphosphonate-associated osteonecrosis of the jaw: a key role of inflammation? Bone. 2009;45(5):843–52. PubMed PMID: 19631301. Epub 2009/07/28. eng.

48. Agrillo A, Filiaci F, Ramieri V, Riccardi E, Quarato D, Rinna C, et al. Bisphosphonate-related osteonecro- sis of the jaw (BRONJ): 5 year experience in the treat- ment of 131 cases with ozone therapy. Eur Rev Med Pharmacol Sci. 2012;16(12):1741–7. PubMed PMID: 23161050.

49. Vescovi P, Manfredi M, Merigo E, Guidotti R, Meleti M, Pedrazzi G, et al. Early surgical laser-assisted man- agement of bisphosphonate-related osteonecrosis of the jaws (BRONJ): a retrospective analysis of 101 treated sites with long-term follow-up. Photomed Laser Surg. 2012;30(1):5–13. PubMed PMID: 22054203.

50. Montefusco V, Gay F, Spina F, Miceli R, Maniezzo M, Teresa Ambrosini M, et al. Antibiotic prophylaxis before dental procedures may reduce the incidence of osteonecrosis of the jaw in patients with multiple myeloma treated with bisphosphonates. Leuk Lymphoma. 2008;49(11):2156–62. PubMed PMID: 19021059.

51. Cella L, Oppici A, Arbasi M, Moretto M, Piepoli M, Vallisa D, et al. Autologous bone marrow stem cell intralesional transplantation repairing bisphosphonate related osteonecrosis of the jaw. Head Face Med. 2011;7:16. PubMed PMID: 21849044. Pubmed Central PMCID: 3175443.

52. Curi MM, Cossolin GS, Koga DH, Zardetto C, Christianini S, Feher O, et al. Bisphosphonate-related osteonecrosis of the jaws–an initial case series report of treatment combining partial bone resection and autolo- gous platelet-rich plasma. J Oral Maxillofac Surg. 2011;69(9):2465–72. PubMed PMID: 21763050.

53. Dayisoylu EH, Ungor C, Tosun E, Ersoz S, Duman MK, Taskesen F, et al. Does an alkaline environment prevent the development of bisphosphonate-related osteonecrosis of the jaw? An experimental study in rats. Oral Surg Oral Med Oral Pathol Oral Radiol. 2014;117(3):329–34. PubMed PMID: 24368141.

54. Cheung A, Seeman E. Teriparatide therapy for alendronate-associated osteonecrosis of the jaw. N Engl J Med. 2010;363(25):2473–4. PubMed PMID: 20950167.

55. Dayisoylu EH, Senel FC, Ungor C, Tosun E, Cankaya M, Ersoz S, et al. The effects of adjunctive parathy- roid hormone injection on bisphosphonate-related osteonecrosis of the jaws: an animal study. Int J Oral Maxillofac Surg. 2013;42(11):1475–80. PubMed PMID: 23746422.

56. Pautke C, Bauer F, Tischer T, Kreutzer K, Weitz J, Kesting M, et al. Fluorescence-guided bone resection in bisphosphonate-associated osteonecrosis of the jaws. J Oral Maxillofac Surg. 2009;67(3):471–6. PubMed PMID: 19231768. Epub 2009/02/24. eng.

57. Mücke T, Koschinski J, Deppe H, Wagenpfeil S, Pautke C, Mitchell DA, et al. Outcome of treatment and parameters influencing recurrence in patients with bisphosphonate-related osteonecrosis of the jaws. J Cancer Res Clin Oncol. 2011;137(5):907–13. PubMed PMID: 20927569. Epub 2010/10/12. eng.

58. Hutchinson M, O'Ryan F, Chavez V, Lathon PV, Sanchez G, Hatcher DC, et al. Radiographic findings in bisphosphonate-treated patients with stage 0 disease in the absence of bone exposure. J Oral Maxillofac Surg. 2010;68(9):2232–40. PubMed PMID: 20728032. Epub 2010/08/24. eng.

59. Dore F, Filippi L, Biasotto M, Chiandussi S, Cavalli F, Di Lenarda R. Bone scintigraphy and SPECT/CT of bisphosphonate-induced osteonecrosis of the jaw. J Nucl Med. 2009;50(1):30–5. PubMed PMID: 19091894.

60. Guggenberger R, Fischer DR, Metzler P, Andreisek G, Nanz D, Jacobsen C, et al. Bisphosphonate-induced osteonecrosis of the jaw: comparison of disease extent on contrast-enhanced MR imaging, [18F] fluoride PET/CT, and conebeam CT imaging. AJNR Am J Neuroradiol. 2013;34(6):1242–7. PubMed PMID: 23221951.

61. Van den Wyngaert T, Huizing MT, Fossion E, Vermorken JB. Prognostic value of bone scintigraphy in cancer patients with osteonecrosis of the jaw. Clin Nucl Med. 2011;36(1):17–20. PubMed PMID: 21157201.

62. Wilde F, Heufelder M, Lorenz K, Liese S, Liese J, Helmrich J, et al. Prevalence of cone beam computed tomography imaging findings according to the clini- cal stage of bisphosphonate-related osteonecrosis of the jaw. Oral Surg Oral Med Oral Pathol Oral Radiol. 2012;114(6):804–11. PubMed PMID: 23159120. Epub 2012/11/20. eng.

63. Pautke C, Tischer T, Neff A, Horch HH, Kolk A. In vivo tetracycline labeling of bone: an intraoperative aid in the surgical therapy of osteoradionecrosis of the mandible. Oral Surg Oral Med Oral Pathol Oral Radiol Endod. 2006;102(6):e10–3. PubMed PMID: 17138157. eng.

64. Fleisher KE, Doty S, Kottal S, Phelan J, Norman RG, Glickman RS. Tetracycline-guided debridement and cone beam computed tomography for the treatment of

bisphosphonate-related osteonecrosis of the jaw: a technical note. J Oral Maxillofac Surg. 2008;66(12):2646–53. PubMed PMID: 19022151. Epub 2008/11/22. eng.

65. Harris WH. A microscopic method of determining rates of bone growth. Nature. 1960;188:1039–9. PubMed PMID: 13711801. eng.

66. Pautke C, Vogt S, Kreutzer K, Haczek C, Wexel G, Kolk A, et al. Characterization of eight different tetracyclines: advances in fluorescence bone labeling. J Anat. 2010;217(1):76–82. PubMed PMID: 20456523. Pubmed Central PMCID: 2913014.

67. Rauch F, Travers R, Glorieux FH. Intracortical remodeling during human bone development–a histomorphometric study. Bone. 2007;40(2):274–80. PubMed PMID: 17049943. eng.

68. Assaf AT, Zrnc TA, Riecke B, Wikner J, Zustin J, Friedrich RE, et al. Intraoperative efficiency of fluorescence imaging by Visually Enhanced Lesion Scope (VELscope) in patients with bisphosphonate related osteonecrosis of the jaw (BRONJ). J Craniomaxillofac Surg. 2013;4. PubMed PMID: 24011463.

69. Ristow O, Pautke C. Auto-fluorescence of the bone and its use for delineation of bone necrosis – a technical note. Int J Oral Maxillofac Surg (2014), in press, http://dx.doi.org/10.1016/j.ijom.2014.07.017.

70. Taylor KH, Middlefell LS, Mizen KD. Osteonecrosis of the jaws induced by anti-RANK ligand therapy. Br J Oral Maxillofac Surg. 2010;48(3):221–3. PubMed PMID: 19836866. Epub 2009/10/20. eng.

71. Aghaloo TL, Felsenfeld AL, Tetradis S. Osteonecrosis of the jaw in a patient on Denosumab. J Oral Maxillofac Surg. 2010;68(5):959–63. PubMed PMID: 20149510. Epub 2010/02/13. eng.

72. Saad F, Brown JE, Van Poznak C, Ibrahim T, Stemmer SM, Stopeck AT, et al. Incidence, risk factors, and outcomes of osteonecrosis of the jaw: integrated analysis from three blinded active-controlled phase III trials in cancer patients with bone metastases. Ann Oncol. 2012;23(5):1341–7. PubMed PMID: 21986094. Epub 2011/10/12. eng.

73. Otto S, Baumann S, Ehrenfeld M, Pautke C. Successful surgical management of osteonecrosis of the jaw due to RANK-ligand inhibitor treatment using fluorescence guided bone resection. J Craniomaxillofac Surg. 2013;41(7):694–8. PubMed PMID: 23830772.

74. Important Safety Information: www.xgeva.com.

Thomas Mücke and David A. Mitchell

**Abstract**

Medication-and especially Bisphosphonate-related osteonecrosis of the jaw (MRONJ/BRONJ, also known as bisphosphonate-induced osteonecrosis and antiresorptive drug-induced osteonecrosis) is considered a therapy-resistant form of osteonecrosis. Despite this conservative and surgical treatment, regimens have been attempted and recommended in the years since it was first identified.

The key points after surgical debridement of the exposed bone sites are to close the wounds in a watertight manner to avoid exposure to the oral milieu and reinfection of the bone surface that has been rendered almost impossible to respond to challenges that require remodeling – essentially the purpose of the bisphosphonate and related drugs. While there are techniques described in the literature capable of achieving this aim, the relevance of patients' comorbidities and prognosis plays a very substantial part in planning logical individualized treatment. Many of these patients, often those worst affected, are suffering from malignant diseases with limited prognosis. Therefore, the choice of defect closure technique should also consider the individual situation of each patient; was the drug used for prophylaxis in osteoporosis or for advanced metastatic malignancy?

Therapeutic planning and treatment for MRONJ and BRONJ should be considered in two different ways. On the one hand, there is the need for removal of the exposed and necrotic bone, as described in the treatment chapter by Pautke [1]. On the other hand, there is a need for a watertight defect closure to minimize the risk of microbial contamination of the bone and ensure good healing of the bone. It is essential to realize this bone undergoes a different type of healing process due to the pathophysiology and the metabolism of the bisphosphonates (or other antiresorptives) [2, 3]. Additionally, these patients

T. Mücke, MD, DDS, PhD (✉)
Department of Oral and Maxillofacial Surgery, Klinikum Rechts der Isar der Technischen Universität München, Ismaninger Str. 22, 81675 München, Germany
e-mail: th.mucke@gmx.de

D.A. Mitchell, MBBS, BDS, FDS, FRCS
Bradford Teaching Hospitals NHS Foundation Trust, Oral and Facial Specialties Department Duckworth Ln, West Yorkshire BD9 6RJ, Bradford, UK
e-mail: david@davidamitchell.me.uk

S. Otto (ed.), *Medication-Related Osteonecrosis of the Jaws: Bisphosphonates, Denosumab, and New Agents*, 93
DOI 10.1007/978-3-662-43733-9_8, © Springer-Verlag Berlin Heidelberg 2015

may be immunosuppressed or have carcinomatosis which also contributes to a prolonged and complicated healing of all wound defects. This is demonstrated by a very high relapse rate of patients after completion of therapy of MRONJ and BRONJ [4]. The relapse rate varies between 11 and 50 % in these patients observed mostly over a 2-year period. There are only a few studies with a close follow-up period [1, 4–12]. The impact of MRONJ and BRONJ for these patients in their daily quality of life is well known [13]. The need for further effective treatment which is acceptable in conjunction with their oncological treatments and does not further damage their remaining quality of life is challenging [13].

In view of this, there are several options for defect closure dependent on several factors which should be considered in the choice of treatment [7, 12, 14, 15]. If the bone can be completely debrided and there are enough soft tissues available, a simple technique should be favored [4]. Local tissue techniques in conjunction with a standardized routine conservative treatment (antibiotics, mouth rinse, omit dentures, soft diet, or in extended cases nasogastric tube) are of value [16, 17]. Large areas of exposed bone are more difficult to treat than small ones for self-evident reasons [4]. Patients with multiple relapses of BRONJ and exposed bone also require more extensive surgery, since the soft tissues around the damaged bone have been shown to undergo damaging change which reduces the effectiveness of local tissue for surgical wound closure [4, 10, 18]. The more recurrences are observed, the more likely the need for more extensive surgery due to the loss of surrounding healthy soft tissue [4, 10].

Early proactive treatment has a positive effect on the outcome [19, 20] and maximizes the chance to prevent further complications such as mandibular fractures, pain, extension of MRONJ and BRONJ, and the development of fistulas. This, in turn, reduces the demand for more extensive surgical procedures [4, 10, 20]. The primary concept is to remove all necrotic bone, retain vascularized apparently healthy bone, restore mucosal integrity to cover the underlying bone, prevent abnormal movement, and seal any abnormal communications. To achieve this, bearing in mind the extent of hard and soft tissue destruction and the comorbidity and prognosis of the patient, all approaches even microvascular free flaps should be considered

if necessary [14, 15, 21]. Patients with reasonable life expectancy with regard to their malignant disease who are having significant life-altering symptoms should be considered for reconstruction by any appropriate means up to and including microvascular tissue transfer after aggressive resection of the affected region [14, 15, 21]. Only a very limited number of patients are likely to be in this category and are not sufficient to clarify a new standard treatment modality [14, 15, 21] but just as metastasectomy and hip replacement can improve quality of life in palliative oncology patients so can radical resection and reconstruction of painful, malodorous, or dysfunctional MRONJ and BRONJ. Individualized therapy seems to be appropriate for the patient in accordance to the stage of the oncological disease, the extension of MRONJ and BRONJ as well as the motivation and life expectancy of each individual [13].

Beyond the conservative treatment options, there are a broad variety of surgical options. As the bone is debrided, several versions of wound closure are available dependent on the area of exposure, presence or absence of intact healthy bone as well as the available soft tissue. We outline some of the more suitable and common techniques.

## Local Flaps

## Mucosal Flap

The mucosal flap is a local flap providing tissue close to the area of the exposed bone. The incision should be minimal and aim for tensionless defect coverage and a broad supply of the minimally mobilized mucosa. The rationale for minimizing the flaps is that subperiosteal dissection will also require osteoclast activation – the essential underlying defect in MRONJ and BRONJ. For this reason, the ideal socket closure is achieved by reducing the intrasocket alveolar bone by bur and allowing the surrounding mucosa to "collapse" over the socket and sutured to create a watertight seal. Larger local mucosal flaps are necessary for mucosal dehiscences, and fistulas should be included in the surgical planning of the incision line. The surrounding mucosal parts of the exposed bone should be excised since they are chronically inflamed and unlikely to heal [18]. The mucosal flap should be inserted into

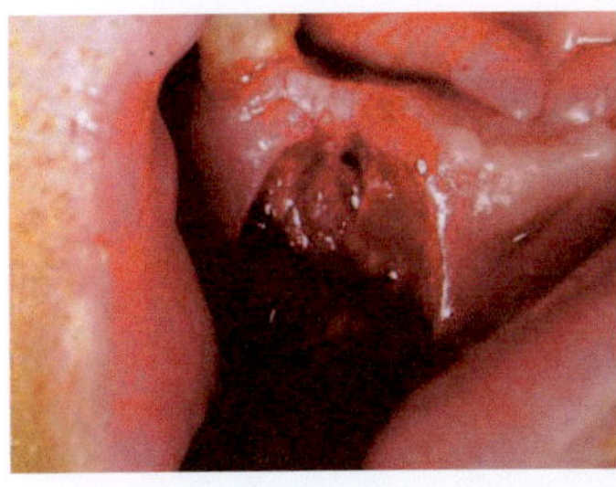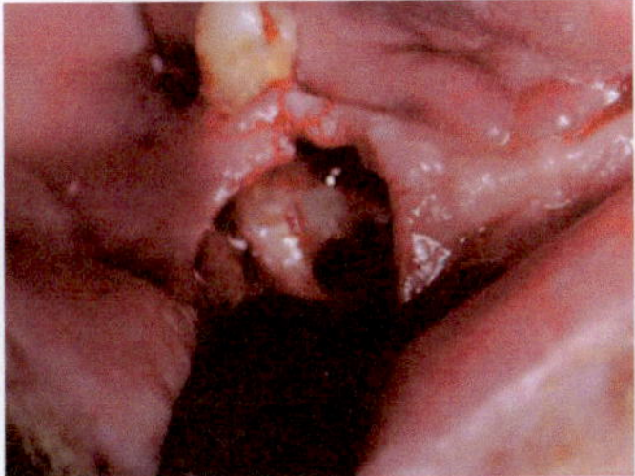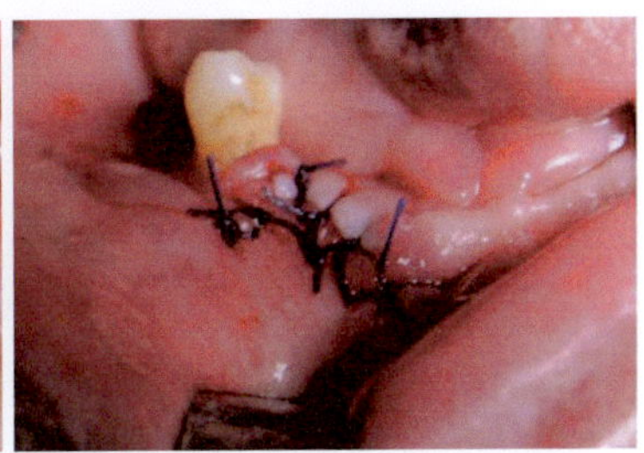

**Fig. 8.1** Example of a BRONJ defect in the lower right jaw with a persistent exposed alveolus (*left*). The mucosal flap is designed in a trapezoid manner, and the decortica-tion and debridement are performed (*middle*). After peri-osteal incision, the mucosal flap is sutured into the defect (*right*)

the defect area in a watertight manner by circular suturing. With the help of marionette sutures and circular careful mobilization of the mucosa, a water-tight wound closure can be achieved (Fig. 8.1).

## Buccal Mucosal Flap

The buccal mucosal flap is also a very versatile axial- or random-pattern flap with a much greater and better flexibility than the palatal flap [22–24]. Palatal bone is exposed in the palatal flap tech-nique which is counterproductive in a patient with MRONJ and BRONJ. Therefore, the palatal flap is not indicated, but the buccal mucosal flap can be useful in small defects [24].

This flap can be based on the anterior or pos-terior part of the buccal mucosa, incorporating the buccal branch of the facial artery with some parts of the buccinator muscle if necessary [22–24]. The mucosa is incised including underlying glandular tissue, but the parotid duct should be preserved [22]. As mentioned above, parts of the buccinator muscle can be integrated as an axial-pattern flap if necessary [22, 23]. We prefer ante-riorly based buccal mucosal flaps for defects in the incisional area of the alveolar crest and pos-teriorly based flaps for defects in the premolar or molar area.

## Buccal Fat Pad Flap

The buccal fat pad flap is one of the most reliable flaps in the management of BRONJ in the upper jaw, as this flap offers additional tissue to cover mucosal defects [25, 26]. The exposed fat rapidly mucosalizes by epithelial seeding. The buccal fat pad is located in the cheek and surrounded by a thin capsule [27, 28]. The fat pad consists of four parts in the buccal, temporal, pterygoidal, and pterygo-palatine area. The central and buccal parts are the most reliable and can easily be used for additional coverage especially in the upper but also in the lower jaw if necessary [27, 28]. The vascular sup-ply of this flap is provided by small branches aris-ing from the maxillary, facial, and superficial temporal artery [27, 28] entering the deep surface of the fat pad. This flap can be exposed and mobi-lized easily by incising the periosteum underlying a buccal mucoperiosteal flap [27, 28]. This flap can be combined with a standard mucosal flap (Fig. 8.2).

## Mylohyoid Flap

The mylohyoid flap can be used if the lingual part of the mandible is affected. In such cases mucosal flaps are not best suited due to the ten-sion of the floor of the mouth as well as the alveolar crest and the vestibular mucosa [29]. Especially in cases of relapsing BRONJ at this site, the mylohyoid muscle flap can be used for defect coverage in the same manner as the buccal fat pad flap for additional coverage of the bone [4]. The mylohyoid flap is a myofas-cial flap which is accessible at the lingual bor-der of the mandible, inserting at the mylohyoid line. The muscle is detached from here, mobi-lized and placed over the decorticated mandible with interrupted and tensionless sutures [29]. A mucosal flap should also be used, but is not essential due to the capacity of intraoral exposed muscle flaps to rapidly mucosalize albeit with fibrosis and scarring [30] (Fig. 8.3).

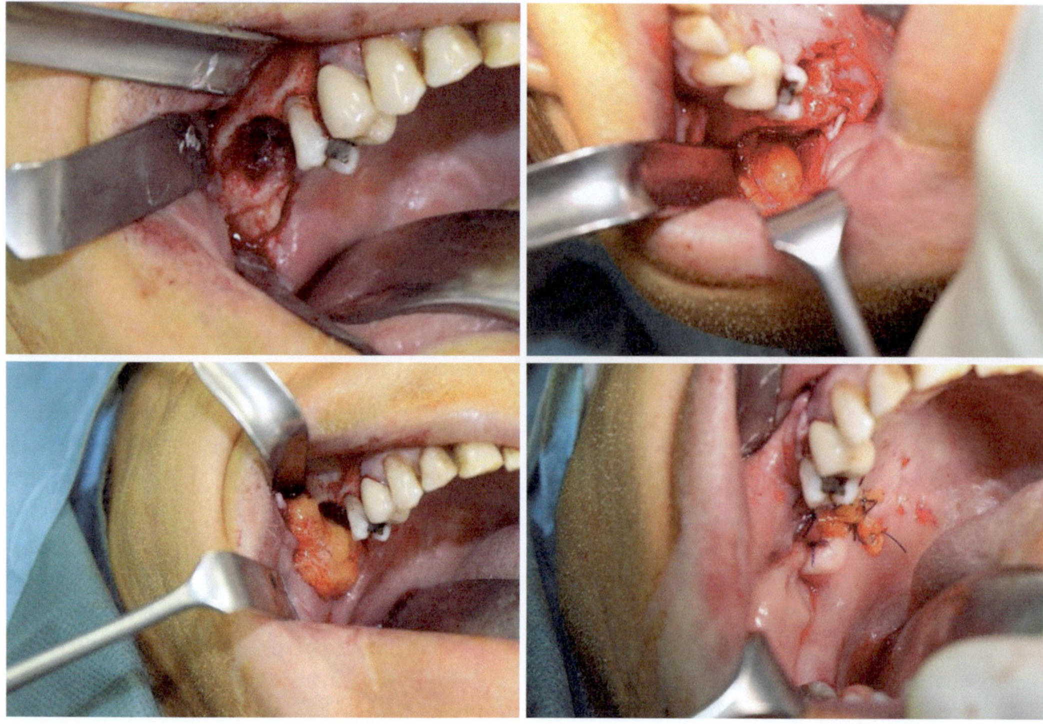

**Fig. 8.2** Example of a BRONJ defect in the upper right jaw with exposure of the maxillary sinus (*upper left*). The buccal fat pad flap can be exposed at the pterygopalatine line (*upper right*). After careful mobilization (*lower left*), the buccal fat pad flap is sutured into the defect and covered by an additional mucosal flap (*lower right*)

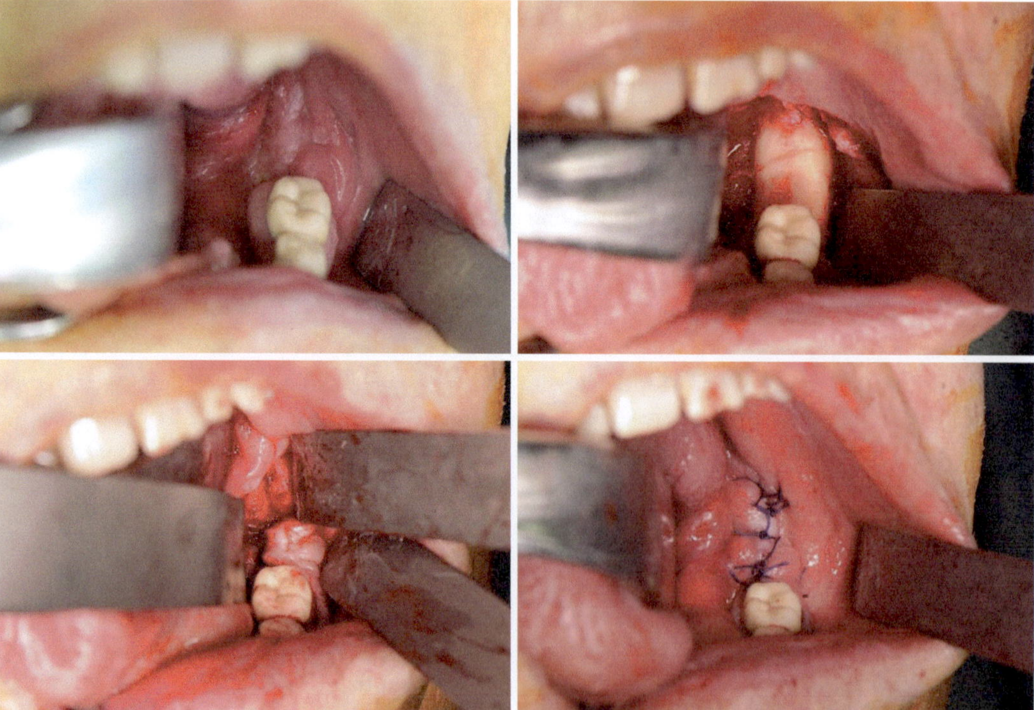

**Fig. 8.3** Example of a BRONJ defect in the lower left jaw with exposure of the lingual part of the mandible (*upper left*). The mylohyoid muscle flap can be exposed at the mylohyoid line and mobilized (*upper right*). After careful fixation over the debrided mandible (*lower left*), this flap is covered by an additional mucosal flap (*lower right*)

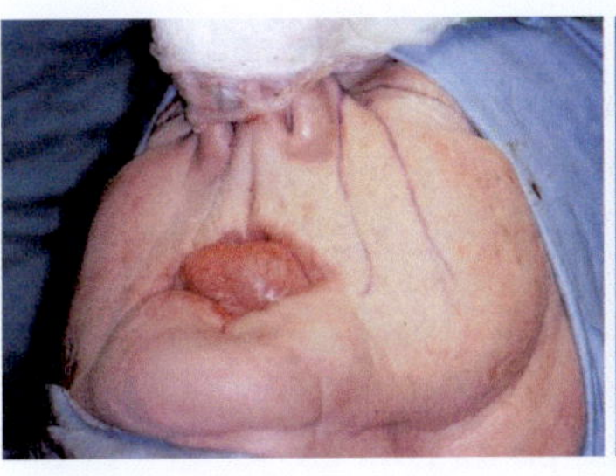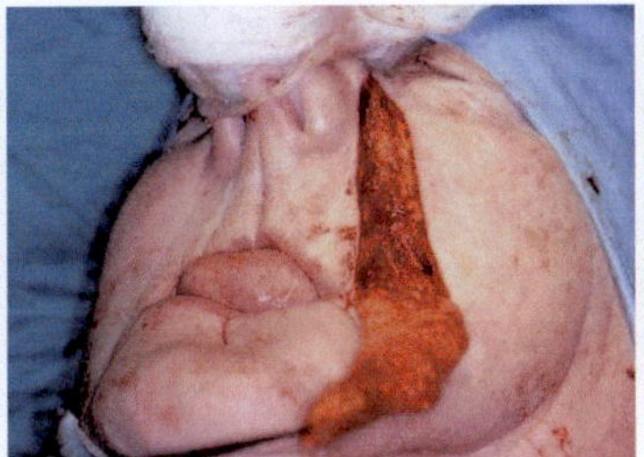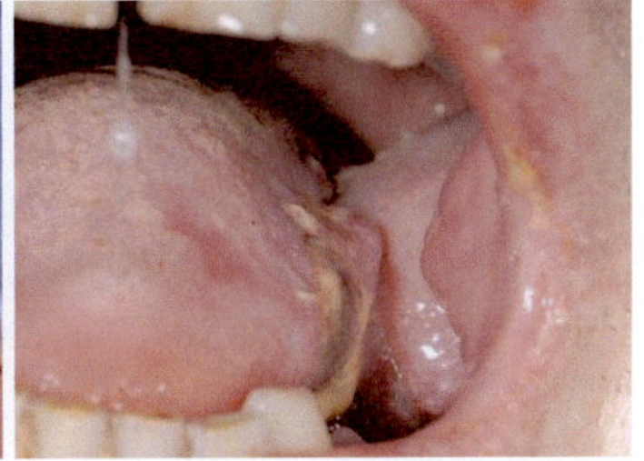

**Fig. 8.4** Example of a nasolabial flap after planning (*left*). The flap is prepared (*middle*). After intraoral transposition, the flap is sutured into the defect (*right*)

## Nasolabial Flap

The nasolabial flap is a random-pattern flap relying on the subdermal plexus of vessels arising from small branches of the facial artery and accompanying veins. While it can be raised on the facial vessels, this by definition disrupts the muscles of facial expression and is entirely unnecessary. This flap can be based on a cranial or caudal pedicle, although the caudally based type of this flap is more valuable for intraoral reconstruction [31]. The incision is outlined in the nasolabial fold and as far lateral as needed. The incision is through skin and subcutaneous fat [31, 32]. The distal part of the flap includes thin lower eyelid skin and the proximal thicker subcutaneous flap. The facial vessels are often seen in the deeper fat of the face and are not included in the flap itself. A tunnel is created just above this point through into the mouth. This is widened by blunt dissection and the distal end of the flap passed into the mouth for inset. Parrafin gauze is wrapped around the base of the pedicle to prevent it healing into the tunnel [31, 32]. The flap is limited by its axis of rotation and is not a good choice in the dentate patient. The donor site defect in the nasolabial fold is surprisingly easily closed directly in two layers [31, 32]. The singular disadvantage to this technique is the need to divide and inset the pedicle at 3 weeks necessitating a second operation, although the second stage can be performed under local anesthesia. With this type of flap, both defects of the upper and lower jaw can be covered [32, 33] (Fig. 8.4).

## Microvascular Free Flaps

### Radial Forearm Flap

This reliable, common flap provides thin, pliable, and reliable skin from the forearm. The skin is hair bearing in many men. The flap design was first described in 1981 [34]. Before this flap can be raised, an Allen test should be performed to ensure the perfusion of the hand [35]. The flap raising is straightforward, but the microvascular anastomoses of the accompanying venae comitans might be more challenging in some patients due to their small diameter. Flap harvesting normally starts at the ulnar site of the forearm, raising a fasciocutaneous portion of the forearm being careful to leave the paratenon which creates a donor site of muscle and paratenon which readily accepts a split- or full-thickness skin graft. The radial artery and accompanying venae are identified at the most distal point of the flap, usually 2 cm proximal to the flexor crease (minimizing the tension on the repairing skin graft). These vessels should be ligated and then dissected after identifying the superficial branch of the radial nerve, which should be preserved. The flap can be raised with the cephalic vein and the lateral antebrachial cutaneous nerve of the forearm [34]. Neither is essential for success of the flap. The vascular pedicle lies between the flexor carpi radialis muscle and the brachioradialis muscle. The vascular bundle should be dissected from the deep septum (which carries perforating vessels to the radius in 40 % of which can be included creating an osteocutaneous flap) followed by ligation or even bipolar coagulation of the muscular perforators arising from the radial artery and its concomitant veins. The pedicle length can be dissected to the length dictated by the site of reconstruction and microvascular anastomosis. If necessary, the microanastomoses can also be performed at the contralateral neck of reconstruction if needed. The donor site should be closed by a full-thickness skin graft or a split-thickness skin graft [36].

## Osteocutaneous Fibular Flap

Reconstruction with the fibular bone flap was first described by Taylor et al. in 1975 [37] and was modified by Chen and coworkers with an integrated skin paddle [38]. The skin paddle allows good defect coverage of the affected mucosa and makes this type of flap suitable in patients with extensive MRONJ. This flap is especially beneficial in cases with pathological fractures of the mandible requiring continuity resections and additional mucosal reconstruction [14, 15, 21].

The vessels of the lower leg should be assessed by magnetic resonance imaging or computed tomography combined with an angiographic visualization [39]. While it is extremely unlikely that the fibula will be a site of metastases of the primary disease, this should be excluded. It may be helpful to assess the perforator inserted into the skin paddle by a Doppler examination. The dissection starts with an incision along the fibular bone on the peroneus longus muscle 2 cm anterior to the intermuscular lateral septum. In the area of the anticipated perforator, the incision should be curved anterior to the line of the fibula. The subcutaneous tissue is dissected down to the muscular fascia and intermuscular septum to the peroneal muscles. The perforator vessels become visible in most cases. The lateral part of the fibular bone should be dissected, and the flexor hallucis muscle is dissected from the soleus muscle. The peroneal artery can be palpated behind the fibular bone and is carefully dissected. The distal osteotomy of the fibular bone should be performed 6–8 cm above the lateral malleolus. The proximal osteotomy should preserve a similar amount of fibular bone below the fibular head. The fibular bone is then mobilized by dissection of the intermuscular fascia and interosseous membrane. The guide to this part of the preparation is the tibialis posterior muscle with its v-shaped muscle bundles. The pedicle should be cut after ligation at the most distal part of the fibular bone. The skin paddle is then incised, but the intermuscular septum should be left intact as the perforators are located in this area. The pedicle is further dissected and the flap raised completely, then either detached and shaped on a side table or osteotomized to a preformed template on the leg while still perfused to allow reconstruction of the mandible and the soft tissue defect. The anastomosis can be performed to the standard vessels of the neck as they are of good diameter and the pedicle length is long.

The shaping of the fibula is one of the advantages described in the literature but also prolongs overall operation time [40, 41]. The flexibility of the skin paddle is another advantage of the fibular free flap but also is time consuming due to the handling of the skin paddles containing small perforators [42]. The cutaneous component of the flap provides additional soft tissue for reconstruction of resected fistulas as in the presented cases and helps to establish tension-free wounds in the oral cavity as well [14].

The fibula flap is associated with significantly fewer complications such as infections at the recipient site and free flap loss compared to the iliac crest flap [41]. Debate continues as to whether the ileum or the fibula leave the more significant donor site defect although a majority would agree the ileum is more morbid. The DCIA composite flap has an unreliable skin component although the bulky internal oblique muscle can be used as a well-vascularized space filler which subsequently scars down into fibrous neomucosa.

Although bisphosphonates are also integrated into the transferred fibular flap, as they are systemic and present in all bones, the evidence to date is that this kind of bone with a direct blood supply and minimal demand on osteoclasts in integrating into the neomandible by internal fixation and prevention of contamination by a watertight mucosal seal has little risk of developing osteonecrosis related to bisphosphonates [14, 15, 21]. This is a high-risk strategy as

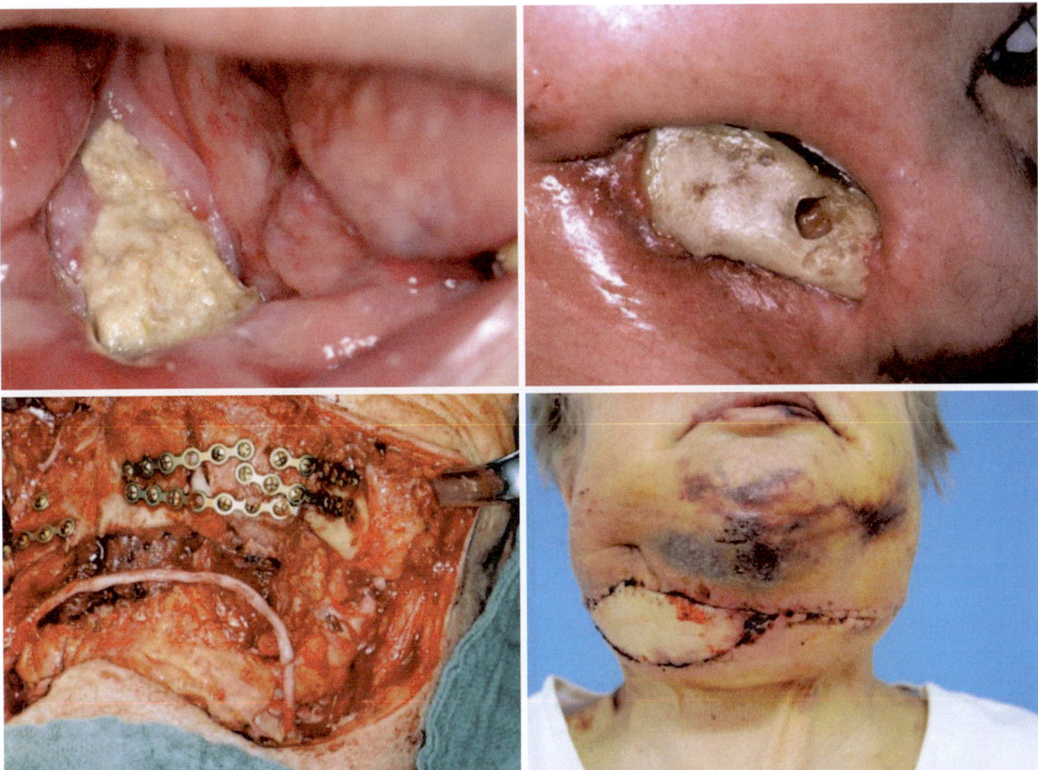

**Fig. 8.5** Example of a patient with an extensive BRONJ at the intra- and extraoral part of the mandible (*upper row*). After continuity resection, the fibular osteocutaneous free flap was inserted (*lower left*) containing a skin paddle for the extraoral defect site (*lower right*)

if the fibula flap is not well perfused, the risk of flap failure and total necrosis of the transferred flap and surrounding bone would be increased [14, 15, 21]. The risk of occurrence of BRONJ within the flap should be critically observed, although just one report can be found in the literature [43]. While this may be due to technical failure, management of this risk should be kept in focus if a microvascular free flap is considered. The surgeon's objective should always be to "do no net harm."

Therapeutic options for treating established MRONJ range from comparatively simple to the much more complex and require intensive communication between the patient, contributing professionals, and an experienced surgeon. An interdisciplinary approach should be favored to provide best possible outcome for the patient. The limitations of each therapeutic concept have to be considered in accordance with the general condition of the patient, their needs, wants and aspirations, life expectancy, or other significant prognosis due to the stage and nature of the underlying disease. Thus, a microvascular free flap reconstruction containing bone might be an option in the treatment of extended MRONJ cases, but it is not recommended as the first step in the therapy. It should, however, be critically appraised for special cases (Fig. 8.5).

---

### Conclusion

Several conservative and surgical options are available to treat patients with established MRONJ. Prevention will always be better than cure. Each patient's demands require an individualized therapy approach integrating an interdisciplinary decision making process including all of the available treatment options. Depending on the prognosis of the underlying disease, the patients' symptoms, and their individual needs and wants, a cautious therapeutic plan is recommended. Extensive surgery should only be applied in special cases respecting the surgeons´ experience and extent of MRONJ of the patient.

## References


1. Pautke C, Bauer F, Tischer T, Kreutzer K, Weitz J, Kesting M, et al. Fluorescence-guided bone resection in bisphosphonate-associated osteonecrosis of the jaws. J Oral Maxillofac Surg. 2009;67(3):471–6.
2. Otto S, Pautke C, Opelz C, Westphal I, Drosse I, Schwager J, et al. Osteonecrosis of the jaw: effect of bisphosphonate type, local concentration, and acidic milieu on the pathomechanism. J Oral Maxillofac Surg. 2010;68(11):2837–45.
3. Chuah C, Barnes DJ, Kwok M, Corbin A, Deininger MW, Druker BJ, et al. Zoledronate inhibits proliferation and induces apoptosis of imatinib-resistant chronic myeloid leukaemia cells. Leukemia. 2005;19(11):1896–904.
4. Mücke T, Koschinski J, Deppe H, Wagenpfeil S, Pautke C, Mitchell DA, et al. Outcome of treatment and parameters influencing recurrence in patients with bisphosphonate-related osteonecrosis of the jaws. J Cancer Res Clin Oncol. 2011;137(5):907–13.
5. Abu-Id MH, Acil Y, Gottschalk J, Kreusch T. Bisphosphonate-associated osteonecrosis of the jaw. Mund Kiefer Gesichtschir. 2006;10(2):73–81.
6. Boonyapakorn T, Schirmer I, Reichart PA, Sturm I, Massenkeil G. Bisphosphonate-induced osteonecrosis of the jaws: prospective study of 80 patients with multiple myeloma and other malignancies. Oral Oncol. 2008;44(9):857–69.
7. Stockmann P, Vairaktaris E, Wehrhan F, Seiss M, Schwarz S, Spriewald B, et al. Osteotomy and primary wound closure in bisphosphonate-associated osteonecrosis of the jaw: a prospective clinical study with 12 months follow-up. Support Care Cancer. 2010;18(4):449–60.
8. Vescovi P, Merigo E, Meleti M, Manfredi M. Bisphosphonate-associated osteonecrosis (BON) of the jaws: a possible treatment? J Oral Maxillofac Surg. 2006;64(9):1460–2.
9. Wutzl A, Eisenmenger G, Hoffmann M, Czerny C, Moser D, Pietschmann P, et al. Osteonecrosis of the jaws and bisphosphonate treatment in cancer patients. Wien Klin Wochenschr. 2006;118(15–16):473–8.
10. Carlson ER, Basile JD. The role of surgical resection in the management of bisphosphonate-related osteonecrosis of the jaws. J Oral Maxillofac Surg. 2009;67(5 Suppl):85–95.
11. Pautke C, Bauer F, Otto S, Tischer T, Steiner T, Weitz J, et al. Fluorescence-guided bone resection in bisphosphonate-related osteonecrosis of the jaws: first clinical results of a prospective pilot study. J Oral Maxillofac Surg. 2011;69(1):84–91.
12. Voss PJ, Joshi Oshero J, Kovalova-Muller A, Veigel Merino EA, Sauerbier S, Al-Jamali J, et al. Surgical treatment of bisphosphonate-associated osteonecrosis of the jaw: technical report and follow up of 21 patients. J Craniomaxillofac Surg. 2012;40(8):719–25.
13. Miksad RA, Lai KC, Dodson TB, Woo SB, Treister NS, Akinyemi O, et al. Quality of life implications of bisphosphonate-associated osteonecrosis of the jaw. Oncologist. 2011;16(1):121–32.
14. Mücke T, Haarmann S, Wolff KD, Hölzle F. Bisphosphonate related osteonecrosis of the jaws treated by surgical resection and immediate osseous microvascular reconstruction. J Craniomaxillofac Surg. 2009;37(5):291–7.
15. Nocini PF, Saia G, Bettini G, Ragazzo M, Blandamura S, Chiarini L, et al. Vascularized fibula flap reconstruction of the mandible in bisphosphonate-related osteonecrosis. Eur J Surg Oncol. 2009;35(4):373–9.
16. American Association of Oral and Maxillofacial Surgeons position paper on bisphosphonate-related osteonecrosis of the jaws. J Oral Maxillofac Surg. 2007;65(3):369–76.
17. Ruggiero SL, Dodson TB, Assael LA, Landesberg R, Marx RE, Mehrotra B. American Association of Oral and Maxillofacial Surgeons position paper on bisphosphonate-related osteonecrosis of the jaws–2009 update. J Oral Maxillofac Surg. 2009;67(5 Suppl):2–12.
18. Lorenzo SD, Trapassi A, Corradino B, Cordova A. Histology of the oral mucosa in patients with BRONJ at III Stage: a microscopic study proves the unsuitability of local mucosal flaps. J Clin Med Res. 2013;5(1):22–5.
19. Otto S, Hafner S, Grotz KA. The role of inferior alveolar nerve involvement in bisphosphonate-related osteonecrosis of the jaw. J Oral Maxillofac Surg. 2009;67(3):589–92.
20. Ruggiero SL, Mehrotra B, Rosenberg TJ, Engroff SL. Osteonecrosis of the jaws associated with the use of bisphosphonates: a review of 63 cases. J Oral Maxillofac Surg. 2004;62(5):527–34.
21. Engroff SL, Kim DD. Treating bisphosphonate osteonecrosis of the jaws: is there a role for resection and vascularized reconstruction? J Oral Maxillofac Surg. 2007;65(11):2374–85.
22. Pribaz J, Stephens W, Crespo L, Gifford G. A new intraoral flap: facial artery musculomucosal (FAMM) flap. Plast Reconstr Surg. 1992;90(3):421–9.
23. Stofman GM. Facial artery musculomucosal flap. Plast Reconstr Surg. 1993;91(6):1170–1.
24. Axausen G. Über den plastischen Verschluss von Antrum-Mundhöhlen-Verbindungen. Dtsch Monatsschr Zahnheilk. 1930;3:193.

25. Mast G, Otto S, Mucke T, Schreyer C, Bissinger O, Kolk A, et al. Incidence of maxillary sinusitis and oroantral fistulae in bisphosphonate-related osteonecrosis of the jaw. J Craniomaxillofac Surg. 2012;40(7): 568–71.

26. Gallego L, Junquera L, Pelaz A, Hernando J, Megias J. The use of pedicled buccal fat pad combined with sequestrectomy in bisphosphonate-related osteonecrosis of the maxilla. Med Oral Patol Oral Cir Bucal. 2012;17(2):e236–41.

27. Dean A, Alamillos F, Garcia-Lopez A, Sanchez J, Penalba M. The buccal fat pad flap in oral reconstruction. Head Neck. 2001;23(5):383–8.

28. Nabil S, Ramli R. The use of buccal fat pad flap in the treatment of osteoradionecrosis. Int J Oral Maxillofac Surg. 2013;42(4):548–9.

29. Lemound J, Eckardt A, Kokemuller H, von See C, Voss PJ, Tavassol F, et al. Bisphosphonate-associated osteonecrosis of the mandible: reliable soft tissue reconstruction using a local myofascial flap. Clin Oral Investig. 2012;16(4):1143–52.

30. Wolff KD, Metelmann HR. Applications of the lateral vastus muscle flap. Int J Oral Maxillofac Surg. 1992;21(4):215–8.

31. Lazaridis N, Zouloumis L, Venetis G, Karakasis D. The inferiorly and superiorly based nasolabial flap for the reconstruction of moderate-sized oronasal defects. J Oral Maxillofac Surg. 1998;56(11):1255–9; discussion 60.

32. Lazaridis N. Unilateral subcutaneous pedicled nasolabial island flap for anterior mouth floor reconstruction. J Oral Maxillofac Surg. 2003;61(2):182–90.

33. Eckardt AM, Kokemuller H, Tavassol F, Gellrich NC. Reconstruction of oral mucosal defects using the nasolabial flap: clinical experience with 22 patients. Head Neck Oncol. 2011;3:28.

34. Yang GF, Chen PJ, Gao YZ, Liu XY, Li J, Jiang SX, et al. Forearm free skin flap transplantation: a report of 56 cases. 1981. Br J Plast Surg. 1997;50(3):162–5.

35. Cable DG, Mullany CJ, Schaff HV. The Allen test. Ann Thorac Surg. 1999;67(3):876–7.

36. Loeffelbein DJ, Al-Benna S, Steinstrasser L, Satanovskij RM, Rohleder NH, Mücke T, et al. Reduction of donor site morbidity of free radial forearm flaps: what level of evidence is available? Eplasty. 2012;12:e9.

37. Taylor GI, Miller GD, Ham FJ. The free vascularized bone graft. A clinical extension of microvascular techniques. Plast Reconstr Surg. 1975;55(5):533–44.

38. Chen ZW, Yan W. The study and clinical application of the osteocutaneous flap of fibula. Microsurgery. 1983;4(1):11–6.

39. Hölzle F, Ristow O, Rau A, Mücke T, Loeffelbein DJ, Mitchell DA, et al. Evaluation of the vessels of the lower leg before microsurgical fibular transfer. Part II: magnetic resonance angiography for standard preoperative assessment. Br J Oral Maxillofac Surg. 2011;49(4):275–80.

40. Shen Y, Sun J, Li J, Shi J, Ow A. Long-term results of partial double-barrel vascularized fibula graft in symphysis for extensive mandibular reconstruction. J Oral Maxillofac Surg. 2012;70(4):983–91.

41. Mücke T, Loeffelbein DJ, Kolk A, Wagenpfeil S, Kanatas A, Wolff KD, et al. Comparison of outcome of microvascular bony head and neck reconstructions using the fibular free flap and the iliac crest flap. Br J Oral Maxillofac Surg. 2013;51(6): 514–9.

42. Loeffelbein DJ, Holzle F, Wolff KD. Double-skin paddle perforator flap from the lateral lower leg for reconstruction of through-and-through cheek defect – a report of two cases. Int J Oral Maxillofac Surg. 2006;35(11):1016–20.

43. Pautke C, Otto S, Reu S, Kolk A, Ehrenfeld M, Sturzenbaum S, et al. Bisphosphonate related osteonecrosis of the jaw–manifestation in a microvascular iliac bone flap. Oral Oncol. 2011;47(5): 425–9.

# Adjuvant Treatment Options in the Management of Medication-Related Osteonecrosis of the Jaw

**9**

Paolo Vescovi, Maddalena Manfredi, and Elisabetta Merigo


**Abstract**

MRONJ therapy is currently controversially discussed and remains a dilemma: there are no evidence-based guidelines on the management of this disorder [1]. The first objective of MRONJ treatment is to alleviate pain, reduce infection and stabilise the progression of disease with the closure of bone exposure. Several authors reported in literature two opposite approaches: surgical and non-surgical treatment [2]. Non-invasive treatment options include medical therapy, hyperbaric oxygen therapy, ozone therapy and the use of laser. The main problem of medical therapy (local or systemic) is the temporary clinical successful result with abscess, pain and swelling improvement but followed, after a mean of 3 weeks, by a relapse of infection and symptoms [3]. Moreover, it is important not to forget that these patients undergo chemotherapy, are debilitated by their malignancy and are thus not always able to bear the side effects of prolonged therapeutic antibiotic schedules. The risk of opportunistic infections is high as well as the possible side effects to the respiratory tract with a high mortality rate in old and immune-compromised patients. The adjuvant treatments, such as hyperbaric oxygen therapy, low-level laser applications and laser surgery, can help to reduce the antibiotic cycles and improve clinical results [4].


## Hyperbaric Oxygen Therapy

The usefulness of hyperbaric oxygen (HBO) is well reported in literature when normal wound healing is impaired such as in the osteoradionecrosis or osteomyelitis of the jaws. Impaired vascularisation has been indicated among the etiopathogenetic factors of MRONJ. HBO possesses significant angiogenic potential and therefore may contribute to


P. Vescovi, DDS, MSc (✉) • M. Manfredi, DDS, PhD
E. Merigo, DDS
Polo Clinico di Odontostomatologia – Unità di Odontostomatologia, Dipartimento di Scienze Biomediche, Biotecnologiche e Traslazionali, Università di Parma, Via Gramsci 14, Parma 43100, Italy
e-mail: paolo.vescovi@unipr.it; maddalena.manfredi@unipr.it; elisabetta.merigo@unipr.it



S. Otto (ed.), *Medication-Related Osteonecrosis of the Jaws: Bisphosphonates, Denosumab, and New Agents*, DOI 10.1007/978-3-662-43733-9_9, © Springer-Verlag Berlin Heidelberg 2015

the hypervascularisation of the osteomyelitic part of the jawbones. The benefits of this treatment have been attributed to the improvement of vascular flow in both hard and soft tissue due to its antibacterial activity by the oxygen gradients. Recent studies have revealed that HBO mediates the increase of reactive oxygen species (ROS) and reactive nitrogen species (RNS) production associated with different types of tissue wound healing [5, 6].

Furthermore, other studies showed that HBO is effective for the treatment of MRONJ counteracting a BP-induced suppression of osteoclasts. ROS stimulates the expression of RANKL changing the RANKL/osteoprotegerin ratio and favouring osteoclasts differentiation. In addition, bisphosphonate-induced apoptosis can be suppressed by oxygen-sensitive osteoclastogenic cytokines (tumour necrosis factor-$\alpha$, macrophage colony-stimulating factor, RANKL and interleukin-6$\alpha$). HBO may be also useful in MRONJ treatment due to its bactericidal activity against anaerobic species with an improvement of necrotising infections and hypoxic wounds, oedema, reduction of inflammation, stem cell mobilisation, angiogenesis and cell proliferation [7].

However, the main limit of HBO is its contraindication in oncological patients due to the presence of malignancy and metastatic bone disease and in patients affected by claustrophobia and/or ear or lung diseases. In addition, HBO is always recommended in combination with medical or surgical therapy and not alone: it is difficult to evaluate if the clinical results obtained are completely due to HBO or to the other conventional treatments [4].

## Ozone Therapy

Ozone has positive effects on hard and soft tissues by stimulation of endogenous antioxidant systems and by blocking the xanthine/xanthine oxidase pathway for ROS generation with an improvement of blood flow. Moreover, ozone increases red blood cell concentration and haemoglobin rate and stimulates diapedesis and phagocytosis of reticulo-histiocytes system [8]. Authors proposed the use of ozone combined with surgical therapy in the management of MRONJ or to improve healing of alveolar sockets after dental extractions in patients receiving bisphosphonates [9]. Stimulating effects of ozone represent a possible help for patients affected by avascular necrosis, thanks to ozone antibacterial and analgesic properties. The protocol consisted of local minor surgical curettage and pre-, intra- and post-operative ozone therapy. Ozone was applied during follow-up twice a week for 5 min for 20 days until wound healing [10]. A preliminary open label, prospective phase I–II study in patients treated with bisphosphonate was planned to evaluate the treatment effect and tolerability of medical ozone (O(3)) delivered in an oil suspension on MRONJ lesions $\leq 2.5$ cm. Ten consecutive patients with MRONJ lesions, who were not responsive to conservative treatment, were pretreated for 10 days with antibiotics to reduce purulent secretions on the gum. The exposed bone and osteomucosal edges were cleaned using an ultrasonic scaler. MRONJ lesions were then treated with 10 local applications of medical O(3) delivered in an oil suspension for 10 min. In all patients, mucosal lesions resolved with complete reconstitution of oral and jaw tissue, with 3–10 applications. No toxicity was reported. Unexpectedly, total sequestration of the necrotic bone, with spontaneous expulsion in 8 patients and new bone formation around the necrotic area in two patients, was observed. No patient required surgical intervention. In two patients with pre- and post-treatment X-rays, no residual bone lesions were observed after treatment [11]. Other authors presented their protocol based upon medical treatment, antibiotic and antimycotic agents, together with minimally invasive surgery and ozone therapy as regenerating factor for tissues. In 90 % of the cases, the results confirmed the procedure with successful outcomes [12]. These preliminary results show the efficacy and tolerability of O(3) applied directly to MRONJ lesions without side effects and contraindications with a safe and easy technique.

## Laser Therapy

### Low-Level Laser Therapy (LLLT)

Several studies have shown the positive effect of laser applications at low intensity (low-level laser therapy [LLLT]) on the repair process of human tissues. The effects of LLLT on the trophism of skin and mucosa and stimulation of blood capillaries have been reported by several authors and these observations could, to some extent, give support for a possible usefulness of laser bio-stimulation in the treatment of MRONJ [13]. LLLT improves reparative process, increases inorganic matrix of bone and mitotic osteoblastic index and stimulates lymphatic and blood capillary growth. Most of the studies published regarding LLLT and mucosal wound healing have examined the effects of laser beam on fibroblast cell growth and locomotion and production of collagen [14]. LLLT improves bone healing in traumatised sites and increases mineralisation during the regenerative bone process after dental implant placement [15, 16]. Different wavelengths have been used for LLLT such as He-Neon, Er:YAG, diode, CO2 and Nd:YAG. Laser beam produces some changes in cellular metabolism: the light is absorbed by the primary photoacceptors and this event triggers the usual machinery of the existing cell regulation mechanism. The universality of the LLLT effects and the possibility of using different wavelengths for irradiation are accounted by the fact that the primary photoacceptors of monochromatic visible light are the respiratory chain components. The intensity of the effects depends on the physiological state of the cell at the moment of irradiation and on the wavelength. LLLT has probably a photochemical mechanism with energy firstly absorbed by intracellular mitochondrial chromophores and thus converted to metabolic one involving the respiratory cytochrome chain [17]. Laser light increases the singlet oxygen, which acts as free radical that influences the production of ATP and the formation of transmembrane electrochemical proton gradients in mitochondria. The irradiation seems to increase the release of PGE2 and this reaction contributes to the process of bone and mucosal healing [18]. A two-step mechanism is involved in the interaction of the laser irradiation and the bone repair process: the first is probably related to the activation of osteoblasts to produce bone matrix. In a subsequent stage, an inhibitory photobiological mechanism would decrease the osteoblasts activity and LLLT would stimulate osteoclasts activity to promote bone resorption and remodelling [19].

In a study, out of 14 MRONJ patients treated with LLLT using Nd:YAG laser (1.25 W and 15 Hz) and antibiotic therapy (2 g of amoxicillin and 1.5 g of metronidazole a day for 2 weeks), 9 had had complete mucosal healing and 3 improved their symptomatology. The clinical success was maintained in 12 patients (85.7 %) during 6 months of follow-up [20]. Other studies reported clinical success with LLLT performed with a pulsed diode laser. In the majority of patients after 4 weeks of treatment, the authors observed a significant reduction of pain, oedema, size of bone exposure, pus, fistulas and halitosis [21, 22].

Trauma during dental surgery is a predisposing factor for MRONJ. However, about 40 % of cases of MRONJ are not related to dental invasive procedures, being probably associated to endodontic or periodontal infections. Extraction of non-treatable teeth is considered a reliable choice, to improve symptoms and to reduce the risk of MRONJ. In our experience, antibiotic treatment (administered 3 days before and 2 weeks after tooth extractions) associated with intra-operative LLLT and during 4 weeks after surgical procedure using Nd:YAG laser (1064 nm, power 1.25 W, frequency 15 Hz, fibre diameter 320 μm, 5 application of 1 min each) has proved to be a good protocol to prevent the onset of MRONJ [23].

LLLT appears a good option to prevent and treat MRONJ: it represents a safe and non-invasive procedure, well tolerated by patients and without side effects. It is recommended for both cancer and noncancer patients and it could be important for cases of MRONJ that require a nonsurgical management.

                                                                                                    

## Mini-invasive Laser Surgery

In MRONJ patients, laser can be also used for conservative surgery. A clinical example is given in Fig. 9.1a–e. In particular, necrotic bone may be vaporised until healthy bone is reached. The surgical technique involves Er:YAG (2,940 nm), a solid-state laser where the active medium is a crystal of yttrium-aluminium-garnet doped with erbium. The erbium laser penetrates only very slightly (0.1 mm), providing safety guarantees and allowing for precision, minimally invasive treatment, inducing a much lower increase in temperature in bone than conventional rotary

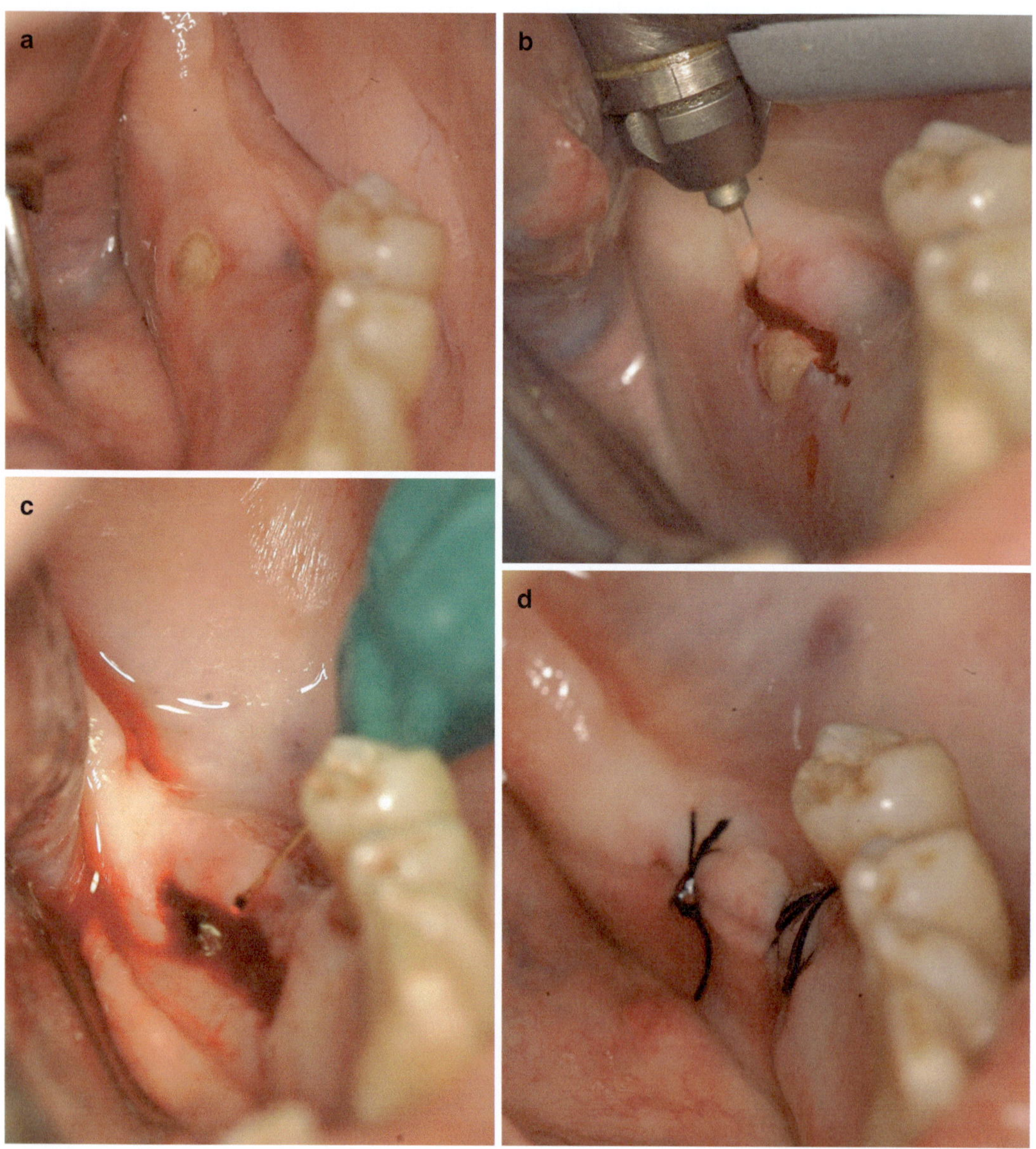

**Fig. 9.1** (**a**) MRONJ stage 1: spontaneous bone exposure without inflammation or pus discharge in a patient with prostatic cancer and bone metastasis treated with intravenous zoledronic acid for 15 months. (**b**) Minimally invasive bone evaporation with erbium laser (Er:YAG 2,940 nm). (**c**) Intra-operative laser bio-stimulation (Nd:YAG 1064 nm). (**d**) Wound closure using two resorbable stitches. (**e**) Complete mucosal healing after 1-year follow-up (Reprinted with kind permission of Springer Science + Business Media)

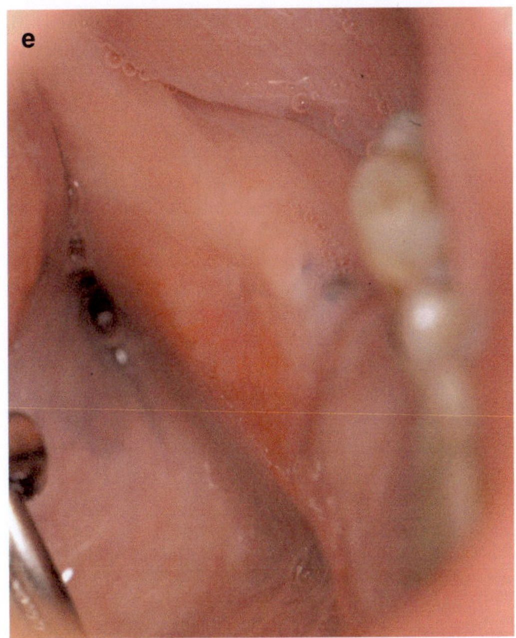


**Fig. 9.1** (continued)

tools (cold ablation) [24]. One undoubted advantage of this technique is the bactericidal and bio-stimulatory action of the laser beam, as it is frequently reported in literature on periodontal bacteria [25]. The Er:YAG laser can help versus the *Actinomyces* and anaerobes species in MRONJ treatment [26].

Pourzarandian et al. reported quicker healing of bone and of coating tissues following surgery with the erbium laser [27]. The histological examination 14 days after surgery performed with Er:YAG laser showed an improvement in the bone repair compared to the other side treated with conventional instruments [28].

The use of erbium laser allows bone resection of the upper and lower jaw affected by MRONJ even under local anaesthesia. Surgical debridement can also be performed, evaporating gradually the portion of the necrotic bone at increasing depths close to the healthy bone [29]. This mini-invasive technique of bone evaporation allows to obtain bone surfaces cut on regular basis and can be used to create micro-perforations at the base for renewed vascularisation.

In our experience, early treatment of MRONJ lesions (also in stage 1) allows better results and it is possible to perform minimally invasive interventions [30]. Laser device can be used in noncontact or near-contact way on three different surgery techniques: sequestrectomy and debridement, sequestrectomy and corticotomy and vaporisation [31–33].

Surgical approach allows better results in comparison to medical treatment alone in the management of MRONJ and laser surgery represents a valid therapeutic option, allowing a minimally invasive treatment of early stages of the disease [34, 35].

### Conclusions

MRONJ therapy remains a controversial issue and there are no evidence-based guidelines. The principal treatment goal for patients affected by jaw osteonecrosis is to provide relief from signs and symptoms (sometimes difficult to control with drugs) caused by lesions that, when present, often determine a worsening of their quality of life status, already influenced by their pathology. Medical treatment (antiseptics and/or antibiotics prolonged for 2–3 months) induces a temporary relief often followed by a rapid worsening of signs and symptoms. However, the associations of antibiotics with adjuvant treatments in comparison to medical therapy alone may determine a greater improvement of the lesions for a longer period of time. Applications of HBO, ozone or laser (always associated with medical therapy) may offer an aid in the treatment of MRONJ lesions, especially for patients that for different reasons (e.g. bleeding problems, immune depression, age, co-morbidities) cannot be treated with conventional surgery. These additional techniques represent a non-invasive treatment to manage symptoms of MRONJ, but, in the long term, the results regarding complete mucosal healing are improved when combined with a surgical approach.

The erbium laser allows surgical debridement of jaw bone under local anaesthesia through a minimal invasive intervention and with a bactericidal and bio-stimulatory action and a better post-operative recovery.

For these reasons, in our experience, the laser applications (LLLT and laser surgery) appear to be a promising modality of MRONJ treatment.

# References


1. Vescovi P. Bisphosphonates and osteonecrosis: an open matter. Clin Cases Miner Bone Metab. 2012;9(3):142–4.
2. Ruggiero SL, Dodson TB, Assael LA, Landesberg R, Marx RE, Mehrotra B. AAOMS (American Association of Oral and Maxillofacial Surgeons): position paper on bisphosphonate-related osteonecrosis of the Jaws – 2009 update. J Oral Maxillofac Surg. 2009;67:2–12.
3. Montebugnoli L, Felicetti L, Bartolomeo Gissi D, Pizzigallo A, Pelliccioni GA, Marchetti C. Bisphosphonate associated osteonecrosis can be controlled by nonsurgical management. Oral Surg Oral Med Oral Pathol Oral Radiol Endod. 2007;104(4):473–7.
4. Vescovi P, Nammour S. Bisphosphonate-Related Osteonecrosis of the Jaw (BRONJ) therapy. A critical review. Minerva Stomatol. 2010;59(4):181–213.
5. Boykin Jr JV, Baylis C. Hyperbaric Oxygen Therapy mediates increased nitric oxide production associated with wound healing: a preliminary study. Adv Skin Wound Care. 2007;20(7):382–8.
6. Asano T, Kaneko E, Shinozaki S, Imai Y, Shibayama M, Chiba T, Ai M, Kawakami A, Asaoka H, Nakayama T, Mano Y, Shimokado K. Hyperbaric oxygen induces basic fibroblast growth factor and hepatocyte growth factor expression and enhances blood perfusion and muscle regeneration in mouse ischemic and limbs. Circ J. 2007;71(3):405–11.
7. Freiberger JJ, Padilla-Burgos R, Chhoeu AH, Kraft KH, Boneta O, Moon RE, Piantadosi CA. Hyperbaric Oxygen Treatment and bisphosphonate-induced osteonecrosis of the jaw: a case series. J Oral Maxillofac Surg. 2007;65(7):1321–7.
8. Agrillo A, Petrucci MT, Tedaldi M, Mustazza MC, Marino SMF, Gallucci C, Iannetti G. New therapeutic protocol in the treatment of avascular necrosis of the jaws. J Craniofac Surg. 2006;17(6):1080–3.
9. Agrillo A, Sassano P, Rinna C, Priore P, Iannetti G. Ozone therapy in extractive surgery on patients treated with bisphosphonates. J Craniofac Surg. 2007;18(5):1068–70.
10. Ripamonti CI, Maniezzo M, Canpa T, Fagnoni E, Brunelli C, Saibene G, Bareggi C, Ascani L, Cislaghi E. Decreased occurrence of osteonecrosis of the jaw after implementation of dental preventive measures in solid tumor patients with bone metastases treated with bisphosphonates. The experience of the National Cancer Institute of Milan. Ann Oncol. 2009;20(1):137–45.
11. Ripamonti CI, Cislaghi E, Mariani L, Maniezzo M. Efficacy and safety of medical ozone (O(3)) delivered in oil suspension applications for the treatment of osteonecrosis of the jaw in patients with bone metastases treated with bisphosphonates: preliminary results of a phase I-II study. Oral Oncol. 2011;47(3):185–90.
12. Agrillo A, Filiaci F, Ramieri V, Riccardi E, Quarato D, Rinna C, Gennaro P, Cascino F, Mitro V, Ungari C. Bisphosphonate-related osteonecrosis of the jaw (BRONJ): 5 year experience in the treatment of 131 cases with ozone therapy. Eur Rev Med Pharmacol Sci. 2012;16(12):1741–7.
13. Vescovi P, Manfredi M, Meleti M, Merigo E. Bisphosphonate-associated osteonecrosis (BON) of the jaws: a possible treatment? J Oral Maxillofac Surg. 2006;64(9):1460–2.
14. Posten W, Wrone DA, Dover JS, Arndt KA, Silapunt S, Alam M. Low-Level Laser Therapy for wound healing: mechanism and efficacy. Dermatol Surg. 2005;31(3):334–40.
15. Guzzardella GA, Fini M, Torricelli P, Giavaresi G, Giardino R. Laser stimulation on bone defect healing: an in vitro study. Lasers Med Sci. 2002;17(3):216–20.
16. Khandra M, Ronold HJ, Lyngstaddas SP, Ellingsen JE, Haanaes HR. Low-level laser therapy stimulates bone implant interaction: an experimental study in rabbits. Clin Oral Implants Res. 2004;15:325–32.
17. Khadra M, Kasem N, Haanaes HR, Ellingsen JE, Lyngstadaas SP. Enhancement of bone formation in rat calvarial bone defects using low-level laser therapy. Oral Surg Oral Med Oral Pathol Oral Radiol Endod. 2004;97(6):693–700.
18. Medrado AR, Pugliese LS, Reis SR, Andrade ZA. Influence of low level laser therapy on wound healing and its biological action upon myofibroblasts. Lasers Surg Med. 2003;32(3):239–44.
19. Garavello-Freitas I, Baranauskas V, Joazeiro PP, Padovani CR, Dal Pai-Silva M, da Cruz-Höfling MA. Low-power laser irradiation improves histomorphometrical parameters and bone matrix organization during tibia wound healing in rats. J Photochem Photobiol B. 2003;70(2):81–9.
20. Vescovi P, Merigo E, Manfredi M, Meleti M, Fornaini M, Bonanini M, Rocca JP, Nammour S. Nd:YAG laser biostimulation in the treatment of bisphosphonate-associated necrosis of the jaw: clinical experience in 28 cases. Photomed Laser Surg. 2008;26(1):37–46.
21. Scoletta M, Arduino PG, Reggio L, Delmasso P, Mozzati M. Effect of Low- Level Laser Irradiation on bisphosphonate-induced osteonecrosis of the jaws: preliminary results of prospective study. Photomed Laser Surg. 2010;110(1):46–53.
22. Romeo U, Galanakis A, Marias G, Del Vecchio A, Tenore G, Palaia G, Vescovi P, Polimeni A. Observation of pain control in patients with bisphosphonate-induced osteonecrosis using low level laser therapy: preliminary results. Photomed Laser Surg. 2011;29(7):447–52.

23. Vescovi P, Meleti M, Merigo E, Manfredi M, Fornaini C, Guidotti R, Nammour S. Case series of 589 tooth extractions in patients under bisphosphonates therapy. Proposal of a clinical protocol supported by Nd:YAG low-level laser therapy. Med Oral Patol Oral Cir Bucal. 2013;18(4):e680–5.

24. Curti M, Rocca JP, Bertrand MF, Nammour S. Morpho structural aspect of Er:YAG prepared class V cavities. J Clin Laser Med Surg. 2004;22(2):119–24.

25. Akado I, Aoki A, Watanabe H, Hishikawa I. Bactericidal effect of Erbium YAG laser on periodontopathic bacteria. Laser Surg Med. 1996;19:190–200.

26. Vescovi P, Conti S, Merigo E, Ciociola T, Polonelli L, Manfredi M, Meleti M, Fornaini C, Rocca JP, Nammour S. In vitro bactericidal effect of Nd:YAG laser on Actinomyces israelii. Lasers Med Sci. 2013;28(4):1131–5.

27. Pourzarandian A, Watanabe H, Aoki A, Ichinose S, Sasaki KM, Nitta H, Ishikawa I. Histological and TEM examination of early stages of bone healing after Er:YAG laser irradiation. Photomed Laser Surg. 2004;22(4):343–50.

28. de Mello ED, Pagnoncelli RM, Munin E, Filho MS. Comparative histological analysis of bone healing of standardized bone defects performed with the Er:YAG laser and steel burs. Lasers Med Sci. 2008;23(3):253–60.

29. Vescovi P, Manfredi M, Merigo E, Meleti M, Fornaini C, Rocca JP, Nammour S. Surgical approach with Er:YAG laser on osteonecrosis of the jaws (ONJ) in patients under bisphosphonate therapy (BPT). Lasers Med Sci. 2010;25(1):101–13.

30. Angiero F, Sannino C, Borloni R, Crippa R, Benedicenti S, Romanos GE. Osteonecrosis of the jaws caused by bisphosphonates: evaluation of a new therapeutic approach using the Er:YAG laser. Laser Med Sci. 2009;24:849–56.

31. Vescovi P, Merigo E, Meleti M, Manfredi M. Early surgical approach preferable to medical therapy for bisphosphonates related osteonecrosis of the jaw. J Oral Maxillofac Surg. 2008;66:931–3.

32. Vescovi P, Romeo U, Merigo E, Del Vecchio A, Meleti M, Palaia G, Nammour S. Use of laser therapy in the treatment of jaw bone diseases. Dent Cadmos. 2011;79(3):133–48.

33. Vescovi P, Merigo E, Meleti M, Manfredi M, Guidotti R, Nammour S. Bisphosphonates-related osteonecrosis of the jaws: a concise review of the literature and a report of a single-centre experience with 151 patients. J Oral Pathol Med. 2012;41(3):214–21.

34. Graziani F, Vescovi P, Campisi G, Favia G, Gabriele M, Gaeta GM, Gennai S, Gioia F, Miccoli M, Peluso F, Scoletta M, Solazzo L, Colella G. Resective surgical approach shows a high performance in the management of advanced cases of bisphosphonate-related osteonecrosis of the Jaws: a retrospective survey of 347 Cases. J Oral Maxillofac Surg. 2012;70(11):2501–7.

35. Campisi G, Bedogni A, Di Fede O, Vescovi P, Fusco V, Lo Muzio L. Osteonecrosis of the jaw related to bisphosphonates, denosumab and anti-angiogenics in cancer and osteoporotic patients: diagnosis and management. Dent Cadmos. 2013;9:566–89.

# New and Innovative Treatment Strategies for Medication-Related Osteonecrosis of the Jaw

Riham M. Fliefel and Pit J. Voss


**Abstract**

A large variety of treatment options have been proposed for the management of medication-related osteonecrosis of the jaw in particular for osteonecrosis of the jaw due to bisphosphonate intake. More recently, regenerative concepts using stem cells from different sources and growth factors have been introduced for the treatment of medication-related osteonecrosis of the jaws. These new and innovative concepts seem to be promising future options in the management of osteonecrosis of the jaws.


## Introduction

In the current literature, treatment options for patients with established medication-related osteonecrosis of the jaw differ. While the first guidelines focused on preserving the patient's quality of life by controlling pain and secondary infection, nowadays there is a trend to a more surgical approach with the aim of complete mucosal healing of the lesions [1, 2].

As described in the previous chapters, a large variety of treatment modalities have been reported including conservative medical management, various types of surgery, hyperbaric oxygen, and ozone and laser therapy [3–5]. In large lesions with pathological fractures, reconstruction with vascularized or nonvascularized bone has been described, but remains problematic due to poor bone healing and an obligatory graft resorption phase, donor site morbidity, and infection of foreign material. Because bisphosphonates are often administered in patients with generalized bone pathologies and the molecules not only bind to the jaws, it is not unlikely that the transferred bone will either be affected by bony metastases or also develop osteonecrosis of the jaws [6, 7].

In osteonecrotic lesions, among others, the lack of osteogenic precursors and a shortage of endothelial progenitor cells (EPCs) cause an insufficient vascular support, so that safe


R.M. Fliefel, MSc
Faculty of Dentistry, Oral and Maxillofacial Surgery,
Alexandria University, Am Bergsteig 9.,
Munich 81541, Bayern, Germany
e-mail: riham.fliefel@med.uni-muenchen.de

P.J. Voss, MD, DDS (✉)
Department of Oral and Maxillofacial Surgery,
Regional Plastic Surgery, Albert-Ludwigs-
University Freiburg, University Hospital Freiburg,
Hugstetter St. 55, 79106 Freiburg, Germany
e-mail: pit.voss@uniklinik-freiburg.de



S. Otto (ed.), *Medication-Related Osteonecrosis of the Jaws: Bisphosphonates, Denosumab, and New Agents*, 111
DOI 10.1007/978-3-662-43733-9_10, © Springer-Verlag Berlin Heidelberg 2015

alternative therapies are needed to enhance the osteogenesis and vasculogenesis [8, 9].

While tissue engineering is the branch that brings biology, bioengineering, clinical sciences, and biotechnology together for the purpose of generating new tissues and organs and the development of biologic substitutes that can restore and maintain normal function, a variety of approaches are utilized that combine the use of morphogens, growth factors, and cytokines, with scaffolds and carriers and cells [10–12].

During the last years, the increased interest on stem cells allowed the evolution of new horizons in treatment perspectives. Stem cells are immature, undifferentiated cells that can divide and multiply for an extended period of time, differentiating into specific types of cells and tissues. They are defined as cells that self-replicate and are able to differentiate into at least two different cell types, and both criteria must be present for a cell to be called a "stem cell" [13, 14]. Embryonic stem cells (ESCs), adult stem cells (ASCs), and induced pluripotent stem cells (iPSCs) represent the three different major types of stem cells [15].

During embryonic development, embryonic stem cells are derived from cells of the inner cell mass of the blastocysts. They are pluripotent and give rise to all derivatives of the three primary germ layers. The most important and potential use of ESCs is clinically in transplantation medicine, where they can be used to develop cell replacement therapies [13, 14, 16, 17]. In contrast, iPSCs refer to adult or somatic stem cells that have been genetically reprogrammed to behave like ESC [18].

ASCs are multipotent because their potential is normally limited to one or more lineages of specialized cells [16]. In addition to bone marrow, various tissues have been found to harbor mesenchymal stem cell (MSC)-like populations including adipose tissues, muscles, tendons, dental pulps, periodontal ligaments, umbilical cord blood, placenta, periosteum, liver, cartilage, synovium, synovial fluid, spleen, and thymus [19–25]. In vitro expanded bone marrow stem cells (BMMSCs) may be a rich source of osteogenic progenitor cells that are capable of promoting the repair or regeneration of skeletal defects when cultured in the presence of dexamethasone,

inorganic phosphate, and vitamin C. BMMSCs can be induced to become osteoblast-like cells in vitro and form calcified nodules [26, 27].

## Cell-Based Therapy in Craniofacial Tissue Engineering

The bone is the second most frequently transplanted tissue with increasing frequency. Reconstruction of craniofacial components is one of the most important and intricate objectives in stem cell-mediated regenerative medicine [28–30]. The craniofacial bone has an essential role in supporting the adjacent soft tissue, providing anchoring for dental structures and providing a stable although flexible framework for craniofacial cartilage structures. Embryologically, most craniofacial bones are derived from mesenchymal tissue through membranous ossification [31].

Facial development, including that of the teeth and oral cavity, is a classic act of interactions by stem cells of the epithelium, craniofacial mesoderm, and neural crest-derived mesenchyme [32, 33]. Cranial neural crest cells (CNC) play an important role in development of the teeth, alveolar crest, and jaw bone [34]. Thus, the biologically unique features of cranial neural crest cell-derived bone should be considered in the etiopathology of antiresorptive drug-induced osteonecrosis of the jaw.

Stem cell-based strategies are currently a promising approach in craniofacial bone tissue engineering as they supply sufficient numbers of cells that can not only form bone and associated tissues but also maintain bone as it undergoes turnover throughout life [12, 35]. Regenerative medicine for bone healing has reached the patient in the form of cell therapy approaches to treat localized bone defects or systemic diseases of the skeleton [36].

Mesenchymal stem cells (MSCs) have been isolated from a variety of mesenchymal tissues, and they can differentiate into a wide array of cell types, including osteoblasts, chondrocytes, and adipocytes. They participate in regeneration of injured tissues in different ways. On one hand, they directly differentiate into tissue-specific cells and thus substitute damaged or lost cells. On the other hand, they indirectly influence tissue regeneration by secretion of soluble factors. Thirdly, they are able to modulate the inflammatory response. Thus, they can promote vascularization, cell proliferation, and differentiation and modulate inflammatory processes [37].

As a result of their slower growth rate and the absence of telomerase activity in vitro, mesenchymal stem cells (MSCs) are presumed to have a lower risk for tumor formation compared with embryonic stem cells (ESCs) [38]. This suggests that mesenchymal stem cells may have broader therapeutic applications compared to other adult stem cells.

Bone marrow-derived mesenchymal stem cells (BMMSCs) can be concentrated from bone marrow aspirate with different techniques. The FICOLL method (synthetic polysaccharide) and the BMAC method (bone marrow aspirate concentrate) are established methods for mononuclear cell concentration from iliac crest aspirate [28]. Percutaneous or intraoperative local administration of cell suspensions delivers progenitor or lineage-committed cells directly to the wound site.

Mesenchymal stem cells functional properties have been proved by several experimental and clinical studies using autologous BMMSC implants for healing, cell architecture repair, and recovery of local blood flow on injured and ischemic tissues for alveolar ridge augmentation and long bone defects [39–41].

Autologous bone marrow or autologous mesenchymal stem cells were successfully implanted in a number of patients to enhance fracture and osteotomy healing; fill bone defects; treat pseudarthrosis, bone cysts, and osteonecroses; or enhance spinal fusion [37]. In a randomized controlled trial, it has been shown that the new bone formation in sinus lift procedures using autologous mesenchymal stem cells in combination with bovine bone mineral is equivalent to autologous bone and bovine bone mineral [42].

## Experimental and Clinical Cell-Based Therapy in Medication-Related Osteonecrosis of the Jaw

Several authors have focused on the treatment of osteonecrosis of the jaw with mesenchymal stem cells. With the ability to induce ectopic bone formation and angiogenesis, MSCs might become a promising treatment option for antiresorptive drug-induced osteonecrosis of the jaws [43].

In a mouse model, a mesenchymal stem cell-based approach to treat osteonecrosis of the jaw was tested. At 2 weeks after tooth extraction, ONJ-like wild-type mice receiving intravenous infusions with mesenchymal stem cells healed with complete soft tissue and bone regeneration at the extracted alveolar socket suggesting that cell-based immunotherapy using T regulatory cells (Tregs) or mesenchymal stem cells are promising therapeutic strategies to prevent and treat ONJ-like lesions in wild-type mice. It is discussed that cell-based therapy using systemic mesenchymal stem cell infusions can prevent or cure antiresorptive drug-induced osteonecrosis of the jaws via reestablishment of the immune balance between inhibition of T-helper-producing interleukin 17 cells (th17) and increase in Tregs [44].

In a swine model, Li et al. reported the treatment of ONJ lesions with allogenic mesenchymal stem cells and concluded to have discovered that allogenic mesenchymal stem cell-based infusions provide a safe and effective therapeutic modality for treating ONJ lesions, which sheds light on potential clinical applications for treating patients suffering from medication-related osteonecrosis of the jaws [45].

In a case report, Cella et al. published to have cured a patient with refractory osteonecrosis of the jaw, with autologous mesenchymal stem cells that were aspirated from the iliac crest and transplanted intralesionally on a gelatin sponge carrier after concentration with the FICOLL method. This procedure allowed a clinical improvement of symptoms and induced novel ossification with complete remission from a stage 3 bisphosphonate-induced osteonecrosis of the jaw [46]. In another case report, Elad et al. presented a patient with bisphosphonate-induced osteonecrosis of the jaw, where bone marrow cells were resuspended in saline and injected along the mucosal margins of two areas of exposed bone. No complications were observed with considerable reduction in the size of the alveolar bone exposures following the local infiltration of the hematopoietic stem cells. Complete healing of the lesion was achieved within a few months of the procedure showing the great potential of hematopoietic stem cells to treat osteonecrosis of the jaws [8, 47].

In our own experience, a case series of 8 patients with refractory bisphosphonate-induced osteonecrosis of the jaws, the lesions was managed with surgical resection of necrotic bone followed by mesenchymal stem cell grafting (Fig. 10.1a–j). Marrow-derived cells were aspirated from the iliac crest and concentrated using a chair-side bone marrow concentration procedure (BMAC) to obtain mesenchymal stem cells. These MSCs were then grafted into the defect with autologous thrombin and a BioGide membrane. In all cases bony edges were rounded, and the wound was closed using a three-layer

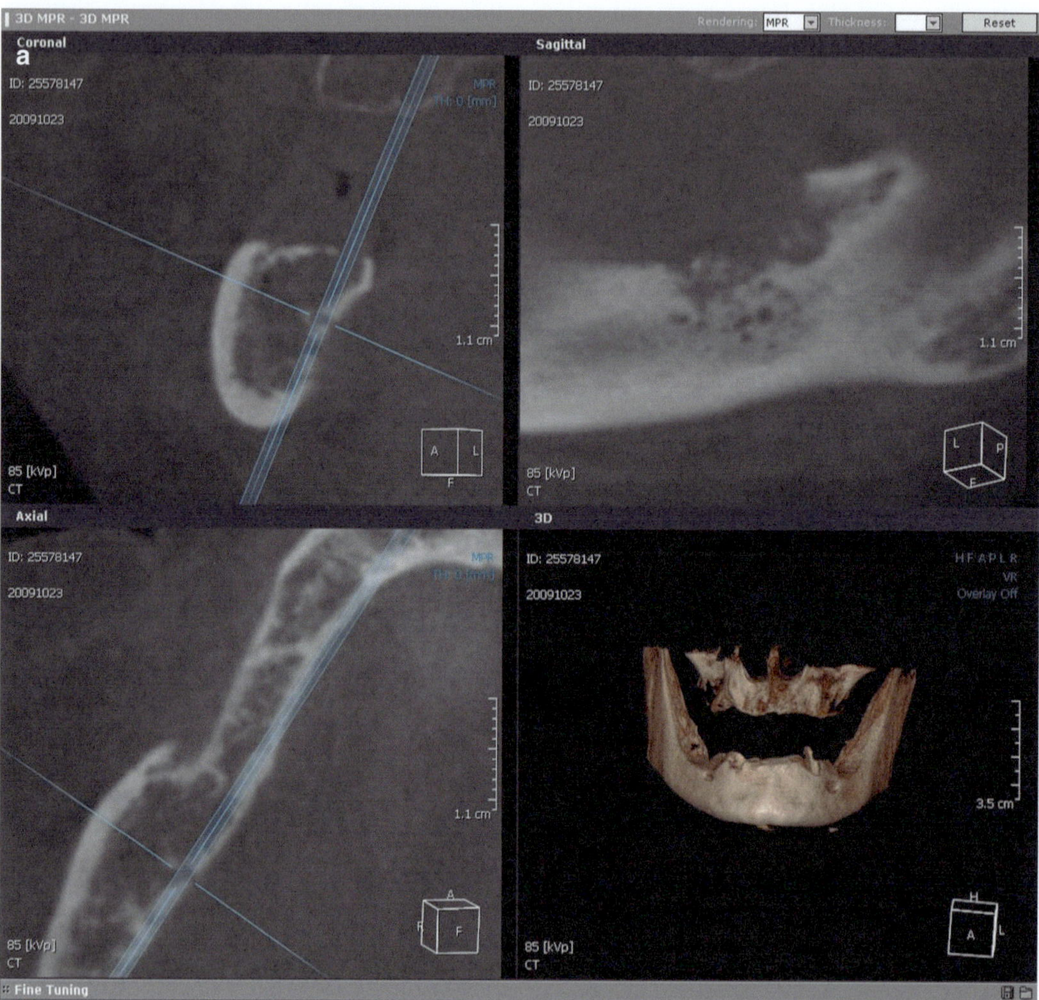

**Fig. 10.1** (**a**) Preoperative cone beam CT of a 57-year-old female patient suffering from bisphosphonate-induced osteonecrosis of the jaw in the right mandible after oral bisphosphonate treatment for osteoporosis due to rheumatoid arthritis and glucocorticoid treatment. (**b**) Intraoperative exposure of the osteonecrotic lesion in the right mandible. (**c**) Exposure of the inferior alveolar nerve after complete removal of the affected bone. (**d**) Puncture of the posterior iliac crest for sampling of 50 ml bone marrow aspirate. (**e**) Transfer of the bone marrow aspirate into the SmartPReP2 centrifuge. (**f**) The suspension is centrifuged for 14 min. (**g**) Close-up of the smaller of the two chambers of the BMAC™ kit. The white line is composed of mononuclear cells including progenitor cells and mesenchymal stem cells. (**h**) BMAC is mixed with autologous thrombin and inserted under a collagen membrane. (**i**) The defect is covered with a multiple layer technique. After slitting of the vestibular periosteum, the mobile part is quilted under the lingual mucoperiosteal flap. (**j**) The wound is closed with backstitches and a running suture

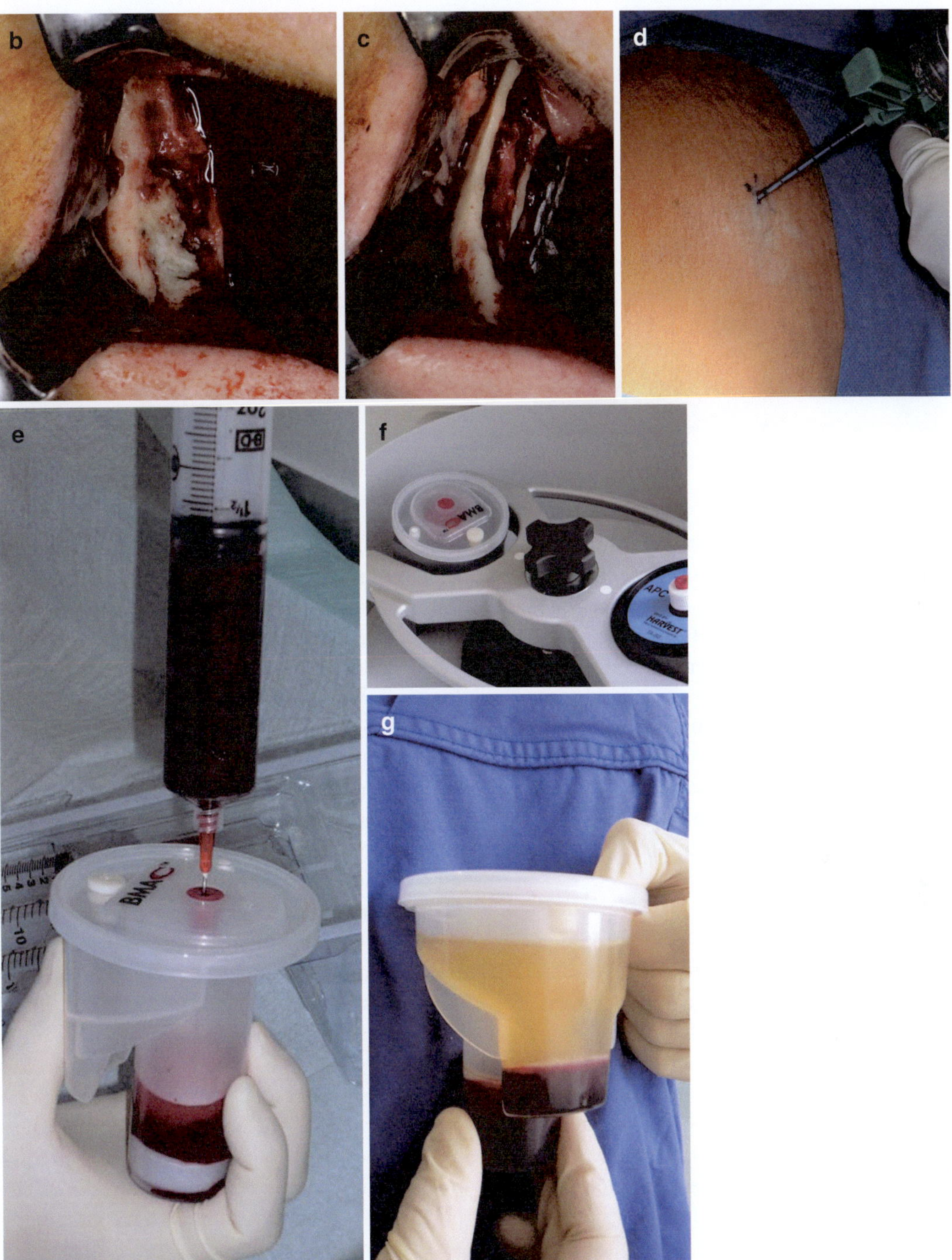

**Fig. 10.1**  (continued)

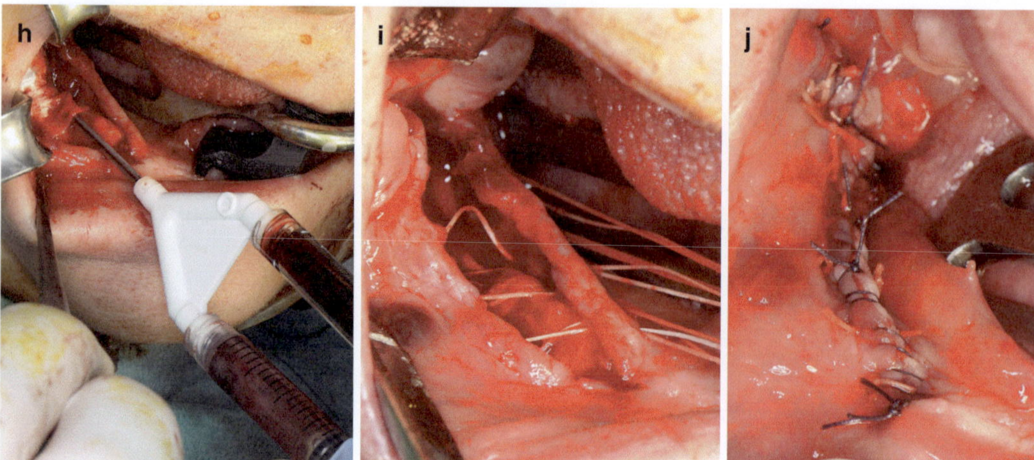

**Fig. 10.1** (continued)

technique. At 12–15 months follow-up, all patients showed satisfactory healing with no signs of wound infection, dehiscence, or recurrence of osteonecrosis of the jaw. Only one patient developed significant complications, that of sepsis of unknown origin, 2 months postoperatively (unpublished own data).

## Growth Factors in Treatment of Medication-Related Osteonecrosis of the Jaw

Growth factors are soluble-secreted signaling polypeptides capable of instructing specific cellular responses in a biological environment [48]. The specific cellular response triggered by growth factor signaling can result in a very wide range of cell actions, including cell survival, control over migration, differentiation, or proliferation of a specific subset of cells [49]. A variety of growth factors produced by osteogenic cells, platelets, and inflammatory cells—including bone morphogenetic proteins (BMPs), insulin-like growth factors 1 and 2, transforming growth factor-β1 (TGF-β1), platelet-derived growth factor, and fibroblast growth factor 2—are functionally involved in bone healing. The bone matrix serves as a reservoir for these growth factors [50–52].

Growth factor application to patients suffering osteonecrosis of the jaws can be considered a challenge because of improving the soft and hard tissues healing. Acting like chemotactic agents, they stimulate angiogenesis, migration, proliferation, and differentiation of stem cells from the surrounding mesenchymal tissues into bone-forming cells in an area of injury [53, 54].

The discovery of bone morphogenic proteins (BMPs) as osteoinductive factors and the subsequent development of commercially available recombinant forms of BMPs have offered the potential to replace traditional grafting techniques with de novo bone formation [55, 56]. Bone morphogenetic protein type 2 (BMP-2) application substituting the necrotic bone removal could be considered a therapeutic option for reconstruction of localized bone defects of medication-related osteonecrosis of the jaws. rhBMP-2 was applied using an absorbable collagen sponge carrier to 20 patients who underwent surgical removal of necrotic bone related to bisphosphonate therapy. The collagen was fixed to the soft tissue by an absorbable suture. The postoperative controls showed an increase in the soft tissue healing and new bone formation of the treated sites [57].

Some researchers have proposed also the use of platelet-rich plasma (PRP) in ONJ surgery based on surgical debridement and reconstruction combined with the use of platelet-rich plasma produced from the patient's autologous blood [58–68]. The rationale for the employment of PRP in patients affected by osteonecrosis of the jaws is based on the thesis that the presence of growth factors constitutes stimulations for bone healing, which is similar to physiological healing. The growth factors in platelet-rich plasma might accelerate epithelial wound healing, decrease tissue inflammation after surgery, improve the regeneration of bone and soft tissues, and promote tissue vascularization. The additional advantages related to the use of this product are its biocompatibility and safety as an autologous product [69, 70].

In a prospective study, Scoletta et al. reported of only one wound dehiscence after extraction of 202 teeth in 63 patients under intravenous bisphosphonate treatment. After extraction, the sockets were filled with scaffold-like autologous PRP [71]. In a case series of 25 patients with osteonecrotic lesions due to bisphosphonate intake, treatment of ONJ with a combination of bone resection and platelet-rich plasma was found to be an effective therapy that should be considered an alternative treatment modality for the management of advanced ONJ cases [72].

Lee et al. also described the successful management of complications of dental implant surgery of 2 patients taking the oral form of bisphosphonates, including platelet-rich plasma and hyperbaric oxygen [60]. Several other studies reported of enhanced mucosal healing of patients with ONJ due to bisphosphonate intake treated with surgical removal of the exposed bone, platelet-rich plasma, and primary closure under antibiotic coverage [61–63, 65].

Nitrogen-containing bisphosphonates are able to inhibit pyrophosphate synthase in the mevalonate pathway. The consequently decreased synthesis of the metabolite geranylgeraniol is believed to largely account for the development of bisphosphonate-induced osteonecrosis of the jaws. In an in vitro study, Ziebart et al. demonstrated that geranylgeraniol can rescue the negative effect of bisphosphonates in human umbilical cord vein endothelial cells, fibroblasts, and osteogenic cells [73]. Geranylgeraniol could lead to new treatment strategies for bisphosphonate-induced osteonecrosis of the jaws that have to be proven in animal studies.

**Conclusion**

The implementation of stem cell-based concepts and the use of growth factors are promising future treatment modalities for patients suffering from medication-related osteonecrosis of the jaw.

# References


1. Ruggiero SL, Drew SJ. Osteonecrosis of the jaws and bisphosphonate therapy. J Dent Res. 2007;86:1013–21.
2. Grötz KA, Piesold JU, Al-Nawas B. Bisphosphonat-assoziierte Kiefernekrose (BP-ONJ) und andere Medikamenten-assoziierte Kiefernekrosen. S3-Leitlinie AWMF-Register-Nr. 007/091, 15.04.2012. http://www.awmf.org/uploads/tx_szleitlinien/007-0911_S3_Bisphosphonat-assoziierte_Kiefernekrose_2012-04.pdf.
3. Freiberger JJ, Padilla-Burgos R, Chhoeu AH, Kraft KH, Boneta O, Moon RE, et al. Hyperbaric oxygen treatment and Bisphosphonates induced osteonecrosis of the jaw: a case series. J Oral Maxillofac Surg. 2007;65:1321–7.
4. Erkan M, Bilgi O, Mutluoglu M, Uzun G. Bisphosphonates-related osteonecrosis of the jaw in cancer patients and hyperbaric oxygen therapy. JOP. 2009;10:579–80.
5. Ficarra G, Beninati F. Bisphosphonate-related osteonecrosis of the jaws: an update on clinical, pathological and management aspects. Head Neck Pathol. 2007;1:132–40.
6. Mulliken JB, Glowacki J. Induced osteogenesis for repair and construction in the craniofacial region. Plast Reconstr Surg. 1980;65:553–60.
7. Bostrom R, Mikos A. Synthetic biodegradable polymer scaffolds. In: Atala A, Mooney DJ, Vacanti JP, Langer R, editors. Tissue engineering of bone. Boston: Birkhauser; 1997. p. 215–34.
8. Gonzálvez-García M, Rodríguez-Lozano FJ, Villanueva V, Segarra-Fenoll D, Rodríguez-González MA, Oñate-Sánchez R, et al. Mesenchymal stem cells and bisphosphonate-related osteonecrosis of the jaw: the future? Oral Dis. 2012;18:823–4.
9. Fournier P, Boissier S, Filleur S, Guglielmi J, Cabon F, Colombel M, et al. Bisphosphonates inhibit angiogenesis in vitro and testosterone-stimulated vascular regrowth in the ventral prostate in castrated rats. Cancer Res. 2002;62:6538–44.
10. Langer R, Vacanti JP. Tissue engineering. Science. 1993;260:920–6.
11. Koh CJ, Atala A. Tissue engineering, stem cells, and cloning: opportunities for regenerative medicine. J Am Soc Nephrol. 2004;15:1113–25.
12. Robey PG. Cell sources for bone regeneration: the good, the bad, and the ugly (but promising). Tissue Eng Part B Rev. 2011;17:423–30.

13. Mao JJ, Collins FM. Stem cells: sources, therapies and the dental professional. http://www.ineedce.com/courses/1486/PDF/StemCells.pdf.

14. Mao JJ. Stem cell and future of dental care. N Y State Dent J. 2008;74:20–4.

15. Leventhal A, Chen G, Negro A, Boehm M. The benefits and risks of stem cell technology. Oral Dis. 2012;18:217–22.

16. Reznick JB. Stem cells: emerging medical and dental therapies for the dental professional. http://www.stemsave.com/Docs/News/Dentaltown%20StemCell%20CE.pdf.2008.

17. Nedel F, André Dde A, de Oliveira IO, Cordeiro MM, Casagrande L, Tarquinio SB, et al. Stem cells: therapeutic potential in dentistry. J Contemp Dent Pract. 2009;10:90–6.

18. Yu J, Vodyanik MA, Smuga-Otto K, Antosiewicz-Bourget J, Frane JL, Tian S, Thomson JA, et al. Induced pluripotent stem cell lines derived from human somatic cells. Science. 2007;318:1917–20.

19. Nakahara H, Bruder SP, Haynesworth SE, Holecek JJ, Baber MA, Goldberg VM, et al. Bone and cartilage formation in diffusion chambers by subcultured cells derived from the periosteum. Bone. 1990;11:181–8.

20. Gronthos S, Mankani M, Brahim J, Robey PG, Shi S. Postnatal human dental pulp stem cells (DPSCs) in vitro and in vivo. Proc Natl Acad Sci U S A. 2000;97:13625–30.

21. Romanov YA, Svintsitskaya VA, Smirnov VN. Searching for alternative sources of postnatal human mesenchymal stem cells: candidate MSC-like cells from umbilical cord. Stem Cells. 2003;21:105–10.

22. Seo BM, Miura M, Gronthos S, Bartold PM, Batouli S, Brahim J, et al. Investigation of multipotent postnatal stem cells from human periodontal ligament. Lancet. 2004;364:149–55.

23. Pountos I, Giannoudis PV. Biology of mesenchymal stem cells. Injury. 2005;36:S8–12.

24. Bi Y, Ehirchiou D, Kilts TM, Inkson CA, Embree MC, Sonoyama W, et al. Identification of tendon stem/progenitor cells and the role of the extracellular matrix in their niche. Nat Med. 2007;13:1219–27.

25. Zannettino AC, Paton S, Arthur A, Khor F, Itescu S, Gimble JM, et al. Multipotential human adipose-derived stromal stem cells exhibit a perivascular phenotype in vitro and in vivo. J Cell Physiol. 2008;214:413–21.

26. Krebsbach PH, Robey PG. Dental and skeletal stem cells: potential cellular therapeutics for craniofacial regeneration. J Dent Educ. 2002;66:766–73.

27. Gronthos S, Graves SE, Ohta S, Simmons PJ. The STRO-1+ fraction of adult human bone marrow contains the osteogenic precursors. Blood. 1994;84:4164–73.

28. Warren SM, Fong KD, Chen CM, Loboa EG, Cowan CM, Lorenz HP, et al. Tools and techniques for craniofacial tissue engineering. Tissue Eng. 2003;9:187–200.

29. Cowan CM, Shi YY, Aalami OO, Chou YF, Mari C, Thomas R, et al. Adipose-derived adult stromal cells heal critical-size mouse calvarial defects. Nat Biotechnol. 2004;22:560–7.

30. Warnke PH, Springer IN, Wiltfang J, Acil Y, Eufinger H, Wehmöller M, et al. Growth and transplantation of a custom vascularised bone graft in a man. Lancet. 2004;364:766–70.

31. Schantz JT, Machens HG, Schilling AF, Teoh SH. Regenerative medicine: implications for craniofacial surgery. J Craniofac Surg. 2012;23:530–6.

32. Thesleff I. The genetic basis of tooth development and dental defects. Am J Med Genet A. 2006;140:2530–5.

33. Cordero DR, Brugmann S, Chu Y, Bajpai R, Jame M, Helms JA. Cranial neural crest cells on the move: their roles in craniofacial development. Am J Med Genet A. 2011;155A:270–9.

34. Chung IH, Yamaza T, Zhao H, Choung PH, Shi S, Chai Y. Stem cell property of postmigratory cranial neural crest cells and their utility in alveolar bone regeneration and tooth development. Stem Cells. 2009;27:866–77.

35. Sanchez-Lara PA, Warburton D. Impact of stem cells in craniofacial regenerative medicine. Front Physiol. 2012;3:188–96.

36. Horwitz EM, Gordon PL, Koo WK, Marx JC, Neel MD, McNall RY, et al. Isolated allogeneic bone marrow-derived mesenchymal cells engraft and stimulate growth in children with osteogenesis imperfecta: implications for cell therapy of bone. Proc Natl Acad Sci U S A. 2002;99:8932–7.

37. Schmitt A, van Griensven M, Imhoff AB, Buchmann S. Application of stem cells in orthopedics. Stem Cells Int. 2012;2012:394962.

38. Rosenthal N. Prometheus's vulture and the stem-cell promise. N Engl J Med. 2003;349:267–74.

39. Sun Y, Feng Y, Zhang C. The effect of bone marrow mononuclear cells on vascularization and bone regeneration in steroid-induced osteonecrosis of the femoral head. Joint Bone Spine. 2009;76:685–90.

40. Iohara K, Nakashima M, Ito M, Ishikawa M, Nakasima A, Akamine A. Dentin regeneration by dental pulp stem cell therapy with recombinant human bone morphogenetic protein 2. J Dent Res. 2004;83:590–5.

41. Ueda M, Yamada Y, Ozawa R, Okazaki Y. Clinical case reports of injectable tissue-engineered bone for alveolar augmentation with simultaneous implant placement. Int J Periodontics Restorative Dent. 2005;25:129–37.

42. Sauerbier S, Rickert D, Gutwald R, Nagursky H, Oshima T, Xavier SP, Christmann J, Kurz P, Menne D, Vissink A, Raghoebar G, Schmelzeisen R, Wagner W, Koch FP. Bone marrow concentrate and bovine bone mineral for sinus floor augmentation: a controlled, randomized, single-blinded clinical and histological trial–per-protocol analysis. Tissue Eng Part A. 2011;17(17–18):2187–97.

43. Handschel J, Meyer U. Infection, vascularization, remodelling – are stem cell the answers for bone disease of the jaw? Head Face Med. 2011;7:5.

44. Kikuiri T, Kin I, Yamaza T, Akiyama K, Zhang Q, Li Y, et al. Cell-based immunotherapy with mesenchymal stem cells cures bisphosphonate-related osteonecrosis of the jaw – like disease in mice. J Bone Miner Res. 2010;25:1668–79.

45. Li Y, Xu J, Mao L, Liu Y, Gao R, Zheng Z, et al. Allogeneic mesenchymal stem cell therapy for bisphosphonate-related jaw osteonecrosis in Swine. Stem Cells Dev. 2013;22:2047–56.

46. Cella L, Oppici A, Arbasi M, Moretto M, Piepoli M, Vallisa D, et al. Autologous bone marrow stem cell intralesional transplantation repairing bisphosphonate related osteonecrosis of the jaw. Head Face Med. 2011;7:16–21.

47. Elad S, Czerninski R, Avgil M, Or R. Hematopoietic stem cells local transplantation for the treatment of osteonecrosis of the jaws. Support Care Cancer. 2005;13:455 (abstract).

48. Cross M, Dexter TM. Growth factors in development, transformation, and tumorigenesis. Cell. 1991; 64:271–80.

49. Lee K, Silva EA, Mooney DJ. Growth factor delivery-based tissue engineering: general approaches and a review of recent developments. J R Soc Interface. 2011;8:153–70.

50. Reddi AH. Cartilage morphogenetic proteins: role in joint development, homoeostasis, and regeneration. Ann Rheum Dis. 2003;62:73–8.

51. Tsumaki N, Tanaka K, Arikawa-Hirasawa E, Nakase T, Kimura T, Thomas JT, et al. Role of CDMP-1 in skeletal morphogenesis: promotion of mesenchymal cell recruitment and chondrocyte differentiation. J Cell Biol. 1999;144:161–73.

52. Gruber R, Mayer C, Schulz W, Graninger W, Peterlik M, Watzek G, et al. Stimulatory effects of cartilage-derived morphogenetic proteins 1 and 2 on osteogenic differentiation of bone marrow stromal cells. Cytokine. 2000;12:1630–8.

53. Nase JB, Suzuki JB. Osteonecrosis of the jaw and oral bisphosphonate treatment. J Am Dent Assoc. 2006;137:1115–9.

54. Badros A, Weikel D, Salama A, Goloubeva O, Schneider A, Rapoport A, et al. Osteonecrosis of the jaw in multiple myeloma patients: clinical features and risk factors. J Clin Oncol. 2006;20:945–52.

55. Wozney J. The bone morphogenetic protein family and osteogenesis. Mol Reprod Dev. 1992;32:160–7.

56. Boyne PJ. Application of bone morphogenetic proteins in the treatment of clinical oral and maxillofacial osseous defects. J Bone Joint Surg. 2001;83A:146–50.

57. Cicciù M, Herford AS, Juodžbalys G, Stoffella E. Recombinant human bone morphogenetic protein type 2 application for a possible treatment of bisphosphonates-related osteonecrosis of the jaw. J Craniofac Surg. 2012;23:784–8.

58. Cetiner S, Sucak GT, Kahraman SA, Aki SZ, Kocakahyaoglu B, Gultekin SE, et al. Osteonecrosis of the jaw in patients with multiple myeloma treated with zoledronic acid. J Bone Miner Metab. 2009;27:435–43.

59. Curi MM, Cossolin GS, Koga DH, Araújo SR, Feher O, dos Santos MO, et al. Treatment of avascular osteonecrosis of the jaw in cancer patients with a history of bisphosphonate therapy by combining bone resection and autologous platelet-rich plasma: report of 3 cases. J Oral Maxillofac Surg. 2007;65:349–55.

60. Lee CY, David T, Nishime M. Use of platelet-rich plasma in the management of oral bisphosphonate-associated osteonecrosis of the jaw: a report of 2 cases. J Oral Implantol. 2007;33:371–82.

61. Bocanegra-Perez S, Vicente-Barrero M, Knezevic M, Castellano-Navarro JM, Rodriguez-Bocanegra E, Rodrıguez-Millares J, et al. Use of platelet-rich plasma in the treatment of bisphosphonate-related osteonecrosis of the jaw. Int J Oral Maxillofac Surg. 2012;41:1410–5.

62. Adornato MC, Morcos I, Rozanski J. The treatment of bisphosphonate associated osteonecrosis of the jaws with bone resection and autologous platelet-derived growth factors. J Am Dent Assoc. 2007;138: 971–7.

63. Mozzati M, Gallesio G, Arata V, Pol R, Scoletta M. Platelet-rich therapies in the treatment of intra-venous bisphosphonate-related osteonecrosis of the jaw: a report of 32 cases. Oral Oncol. 2012; 48:469–74.

64. Coviello V, Peluso F, Dehkhargani SZ, Verdugo F, Raffaelli L, Manicone PF, et al. Platelet-rich plasma improves wound healing in multiple myeloma bisphosphonate-associated osteonecrosis of the jaw patients. J Biol Regul Homeost Agents. 2012; 26:151–5.

65. Dohan Ehrenfest DM, Rasmusson L, Albrektsson T. Classification of platelet concentrates: from pure platelet-rich plasma (PPRP) to leukocyte- and platelet-rich fibrin (L-PRF). Trends Biotechnol. 2009;27:158–67.

66. Marx RE. Platelet-rich plasma: evidence to support its use. J Oral Maxillofac Surg. 2004;62:489–96.

67. Oliver R. Bisphosphonates and oral surgery. Oral Surg. 2009;2:56–63.

68. Tischler M. Platelet rich plasma. The use of autologous growth factors to enhance bone and soft tissue grafts. N Y State Dent J. 2002;68:22–4.

69. Carlson NE, Roach RB. Platelet-rich plasma: clinical applications in dentistry. J Am Dent Assoc. 2002;133:1383–6.

70. Nikolidakis D, Jansen JA. The biology of platelet-rich plasma and its application in oral surgery: literature review. Tissue Eng Part B Rev. 2008;14:249–58.

71. Scoletta M, Arata V, Arduino PG, Lerda E, Chiecchio A, Gallesio G, Scully C, Mozzati M. Tooth extractions in intravenous bisphosphonate-treated patients: a refined protocol. J Oral Maxillofac Surg. 2013;71(6):994–9. doi:10.1016/j.joms.2013.01.006. Epub 2013 Feb 21.

72. Curi MM, Cossolin GS, Koga DH, Zardetto C, Christianini S, Feher O, et al. Bisphosphonate-related osteonecrosis of the jaws–an initial case series report of treatment combining partial bone resection and autologous platelet-rich plasma. J Oral Maxillofac Surg. 2011;69:2465–72.

73. Ziebart T, Koch F, Klein MO, Guth J, Adler J, Pabst A, Al-Nawas B, Walter C. Geranylgeraniol – a new potential therapeutic approach to bisphosphonate associated osteonecrosis of the jaw. Oral Oncol. 2011;47(3):195–201.

# Microbiology and Antibiotics in the Context of Medication-Related Osteonecrosis of the Jaw

**11**

Sebastian Hoefert

**Abstract**

Microbial infections play a crucial role in the etiology of antiresorptive drug-induced osteonecrosis of the jaw. Numerous reasons are discussed to explain why the bone affected by osteonecrosis of the jaw lacks sufficient healing. Therefore, antibiotics are essential in the treatment of medication-related osteonecrosis of the jaw (MRONJ). Although antibiotic treatment as a singular therapy was able to heal MRONJ only in limited number of cases, it can support disease control. Ideally, antibiotic treatment should be adapted to an antibiogram. Without antibiogram, the antibiotic regime should cover the oral microbial bacteria and the bacteria expected in odontogenic infections. Additional factors have been discussed supporting the idea that bisphosphonates themselves attract bacteria at the bone as certain phyla and species could be found more frequently in osteonecrotic bone when compared to other infections.

## Bacterial Infection and MRONJ

Resistance to infection by microbes involves a series of interactions between cells of the immune system, in which activated macrophages, neutrophils, lymphocytes are essential. The immune system responds to bacterial infection with the secretion of a variety of cytokines that control key events in the initiation, resolution, and repair process of inflammation; mediate phagocytosis; and coordinate the destruction of infectious pathogens [1].

Oral infection is considered to play a leading role in the pathogenesis of antiresorptive drug-induced osteonecrosis of the jaw, i.e., more concrete, the microbial infection of the "affected" bone is one of the main causes for MRONJ. Consequently, antibiotic therapy has become a mainstay of MRONJ therapy [2, 3]. One of the convincing ideas of MRONJ in case of bisphosphonate medication is a promoted oral infection caused by a immunosuppression (see pathogenesis chapter). This idea includes compromised monocytes/macrophages, neutrophils, and T cells, especially γδ T-cell function [1, 2, 4–9].

S. Hoefert, DDS, MD
Department of Oral and Maxillofacial Surgery,
University Hospital Tuebingen,
Osianderstrasse 2-8, Tuebingen, BW, Germany
e-mail: sebastian.hoefert@med.uni-tuebingen.de

S. Otto (ed.), *Medication-Related Osteonecrosis of the Jaws: Bisphosphonates, Denosumab, and New Agents*,
DOI 10.1007/978-3-662-43733-9_11, © Springer-Verlag Berlin Heidelberg 2015

The oral cavities inhabit up to 750 different species, all of which could invade the bone [2, 10]. Although it is not clear whether it is the invasion in consequence of bone exposure, bacterial contamination (and infection) is regularly observed [5]. Bone exposition during surgery or during tooth extraction opens a "wide door" for bacterial invasion [3].

The American Association of Oral and Maxillofacial surgeons (AAOMS) classifies patients into stage 1 "with no clinical infectious symptoms but with clinical manifestations of the exposed bone" and stages 2 and 3 having signs of infection. Infection is one of the defined characteristics of MRONJ (see clinical presentation chapter) [9].

Assuming a local immunosuppression, a bacterial invasion and following subsequent infection are of utmost importance.

Studies suggest that periodontitis may predispose patients to develop MRONJ. Dental plaque contains another $1.0 \times 10^{11}$ pathogenic microorganisms per milligram [11]. Thumbigere-Math et al. demonstrated that MRONJ patients had a higher number of missing teeth, a higher average of clinical attachment level, a lower average of bone height, and a larger number of teeth with less than half of tooth length [12].

The exposed jaw bone (stage 1) leads to the colonization often followed by infection of the affected bone by oral microbes. The formation of complex biofilms has also been described in connection with MRONJ bone [5] and may have a direct MRONJ onset [8].

Interestingly, studies analyzing the risk of MRONJ in the jaw and long bone in an animal model showed that MRONJ is not limited to the jaw bone, if bacteria (*Aggregatibacter actinomycetemcomitans*) are injected into the jaw and non-jaw sites [13], supporting also the idea of the key role of infection and local immunosuppression due to bisphosphonates.

Microbial contamination and in consequence infection is one of the dominant clinical signs of MRONJ in stages.

Tsurushima et al. demonstrated in Wistar rats that bone exposed to zoledronate developed wider MRONJ regions when exposed to *Aggregatibacter actinomycetemcomitans*. Interestingly, the mandible and the femur were affected similarly [13].

The authors concluded that the infectious stimulus is all important because MRONJ was not limited to the jaw bone [11].

Infected bone is described to get secondarily avascular, which forms the necrotic bone. Homeostasis problems caused by the infection of the bone (marrow) might be the reason for the disruption of the blood supply resulting finally in avascular necrosis [7]. Furthermore, tissue destruction by bacterial enzymes like collagenases and subsequent tissue invasion may allow bacteria to evade the host's immune response and gain access to more anaerobic regions deep inside the bone [8].

Specimens of osteonecrotic bone regularly show bacterial contamination and biofilms (Figs. 11.1 and 11.2). Biofilms may play a key role in the pathogenesis of MRONJ. Several of the predominant species (both Gram-positive and Gram-negative) like *Prevotella, Bacteroides, Fusobacterium,* and *Peptostreptococcus* support the adaptation of other microbial species and the formation of certain biofilm structures that compromise antimicrobial treatment [10].

Biofilms are usually defined as surface-associated microbial communities, surrounded by an extracellular matrix of polymeric substances. Biofilm bacteria demonstrate coordinated behavior such as the formation of complex three-dimensional structures and functionally heterogeneous bacterial communities. The biofilm formation itself is an important microbial survival strategy [8, 14]. The bacterial size in biofilms ranges from 0.5 to 10 μm [8]. They are able to persist in a stationary phase-like dormancy within the biofilm, which may be responsible for their general resistance to antibiotics. Even if the matrix may not inhibit the penetration of antibiotics into the biofilm completely, it may reduce the rate of penetration enough to induce the expression of genes within the biofilm to mediate resistance. The (electrostatic) charge of polymers and the antibiotic-degrading enzymes in the matrix may lead to reduced binding and deactivation. Even dead cells may dilute antibiotics. Another mechanism of tolerance is an efflux pump expression in biofilms as demonstrated for tobramycin, gentamicin, and ciprofloxacin resistance [14].

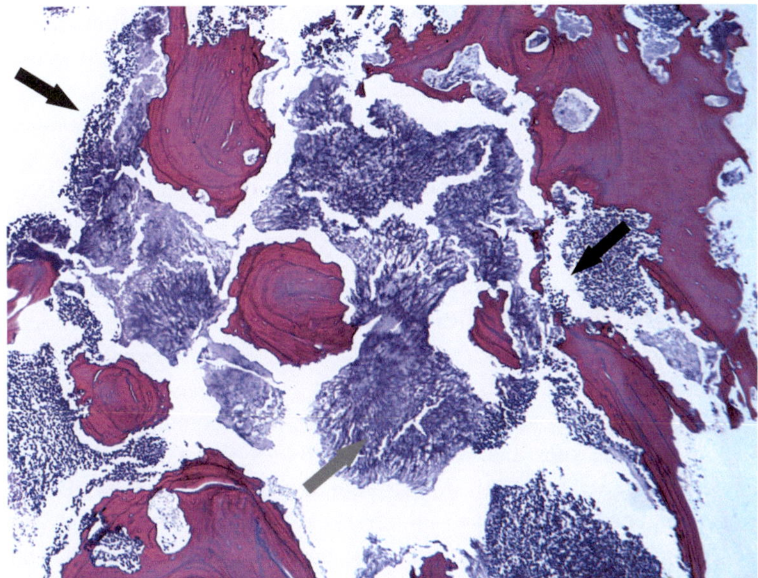

**Fig. 11.1** Histological sample of necrotic bone of an MRONJ patient with intravenous bisphosphonates. Areas with bacteria surrounded by acute inflammatory infiltrate (*black arrows*). In the middle are the typical signs of *Actinomyces* (*gray arrow*) colonies (H&E stain, 100×)

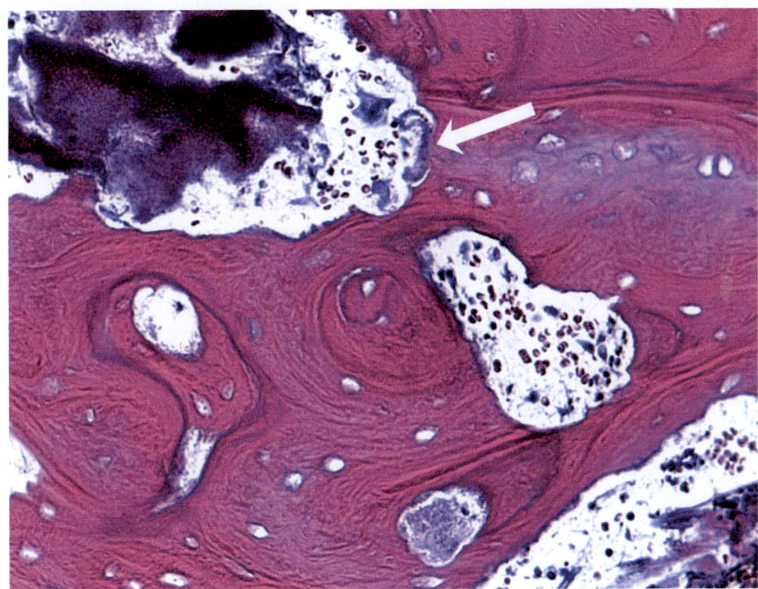

**Fig. 11.2** Histological sample of an MRONJ patient. Close to the bony surface, a biofilm is visible (*arrow*). Necrotic bone visible with empty osteocytic lacunae (H&E stain; 400×)

It has also been reported that bisphosphonates enhance bacterial adhesion to bone hydroxyapatite. Kos et al. demonstrated an increased bacterial adhesion in the presence of pamidronate on hydroxyapatite. They tested *Staphylococcus aureus* and *Pseudomonas aeruginosa* strains. These observations emphasize the infectious aspect of osteonecrosis of the jaw, once again [15]. Ganguli et al. found significantly higher adherence of bacteria on hydroxyapatite-coated ceramic artificial hip joints, if these were coated with pamidronate when compared to clodronate or control [16]. This suggests that bacterial adhesion to bone coated with bisphosphonates may be mediated by proteins termed "microbial surface components" which recognize adhesive matrix molecules. The amino-terminal domain binds by direct electrostatic interactions through a direct surface protein interaction or by providing an amino acid on the surface of the bony hydroxyapatite, which interacts with these molecules and mediates increased bacterial adhesion [17]. In vitro and in vivo experiments showed that a combination of pamidronate and *Fusobacterium nucleatum* caused the death of gingival fibroblasts and the downregulation of growth factors of keratinocytes, responsible for epithelial cell growth and migration [18].

## Regularly Observed Microbiological Findings

Though oral infection is a common finding, the therapist should know the special characteristics of the oral cavity and its local microflora. A distinct number of aerobic and anaerobic species are regularly observed and described. The bacteria identified in the bone specimens comprised Gram-positive and Gram-negative organisms. These also include aerobes, although anaerobes and facultative anaerobes dominate [8]. Anaerobic species are from the *Peptostreptococcus, Prevotella, Fusobacterium, Gemella,* and *Porphyromonas* genera. Aerobic species are *Streptococcus, Staphylococcus,* and *Corynebacterium.* Each of these microorganisms occupies a different microniche, but the prevailing balance is easily disturbed. Especially pathogenic or opportunistic bacteria (*Actinomyces, Prevotella intermedia*), yeasts (*Candida sp. Histoplasma capsulatum*), viruses, and parasites profit from any disturbance of the equilibrium and can then harm the organism [10]. Denaturing gradient gel electrophoresis profile and dice coefficient described 3 predominant genera in MRONJ, namely, *Streptococcus, Eubacterium,* and *Pseudoramibacter* [3].

The biofilms in these patients have a distinct combination of species/phylotypes, segregating a population with compositional changes but maintaining functional similarity of acid production [2]. The development of biofilms on the surface of the exposed bone may account for the poor response to systemic antimicrobial therapy as described above [19]. Bone specimens from MRONJ-affected sites showed large areas of occluded biofilms comprising mainly bacteria, and occasionally yeast, embedded in extracellular polymeric substance. The number of bacteria in these biofilms ranged from 2 to 15 and included species from genera *Fusobacterium, Bacillus, Actinomyces, Staphylococcus, Streptococcus,* and *Selenomonas* and 3 different types of treponemes [8]. The phyla described by Ji et al. found in MRONJ lesions are *Acinetobacter, Bacteroidetes, Chloroflexi, Cyanobacteria, Firmicutes, Fusobacteria, Proteobacteria,* and *Synergistetes* [2]. Badros et al. identified *Prevotella, Porphyromonas, Fusobacterium, Peptostreptococcus, Streptococcus sp.,* and *Eikenella species* [20]. MRONJ site biofilm contained predominantly *Fusobacterium, Actinomyces, Staphylococcus, Streptococcus, Selenomonas, and Treponema species* as reported by Sedghizadeh and coworkers [8]. These different research teams demonstrated similarities but also differences in their findings. Though principally microbial cultures from the areas of infected exposed bone will show normal oral microbes, it must be taken into consideration that in cases with extensive soft-tissue involvement, microbial culture data may facilitate the selection of an appropriate antibiotic [19]. Awareness, however, must be drawn to the length of time the bone was exposed to the oral cavity as nonpermanent bacteria species may infect the bone as the nature of the biofilm is expected to change and adapt within time [8]. Interestingly, some histopathological examinations have even indicated that edentulous jaws contain regions of necrotic bone and microbial biofilm formation even after one year of tooth extraction and mucosal healing resulting eventually in MRONJ formation [21].

Though microbiology findings in MRONJ bone are dependent on the local oral flora, the spectrum may vary considerably. Some authors do not recommend microbial testing in principal, but nevertheless, it is the prerequisite for an adequate antibiotic regime and must be therefore recommended.

## Actinomyces

*Actinomyces* species are frequently observed in MRONJ. *Actinomyces* is regularly observed in histological bone specimens (Fig. 11.1) of

MRONJ patients. In 70 to 100 % of all cases, *Actinomyces* is present [22–24]. In the beginning of the MRONJ discussion, *Actinomyces* was considered to be a particular complication [24] and to be an underestimated agent in the pathogenesis of MRONJ [11].

*Actinomyces* is a non-spore-forming, anaerobic, or microaerophilic bacterial species of the genus *Actinomyces*. *Actinomyces* spp. are Gram-positive, pleomorphic, and commonly delicately filamentous microbes. *Actinomyces* can be commonly found in gingivodental crevices [11, 24] and must be suspected as an opportunistic infection [10, 24, 25]. Mucosal disruption is also the key step in pathogenesis. Histologically *Actinomyces* can form clumps called sulfur granules [11]. Even though *Actinomyces* spp. were frequently found in exposed necrotic bone, however, the development of MRONJ also occurs in its absence [22, 24].

tified consistently included *Candida* spp. [8, 10, 26]. Analysis of oral lesions demonstrated a correlation between higher *Candida* colonization and the severity of the lesion [27].

It must be taken into consideration that most of the addressed bacteria are strictly dependent on the culture-dependent methods used. Though most of the infectious diseases of the oral and maxillofacial regions are caused by polymicrobial infections of anaerobes and all causative bacteria may not be cultivable by the method used, they cannot be excluded or denied. Therefore, critical analysis of the identified bacteria and yeasts must be compared with the clinical success by antibiotic and antiyeast therapy. An antibiotic regime that does not support the microbiology findings could show a good clinical success and vice versa. Therefore, the clinical outcome is the leading sign for the antibiotic regime.

## Candida, Fungal Infection, and Principal Considerations

Infections with *Candida* spp. are also described regularly. Infections with other fungal spores and hyphae have been observed also frequently (Fig. 11.3) [24], but yeasts that have been iden-

## Antibiotic Therapy

Early in 2005, Bamias et al. described that treatment with antibiotics resulted in transient improvement of MRONJ after multiple courses of antibiotics. It is possible to improve the infectious symptoms in the majority of cases with

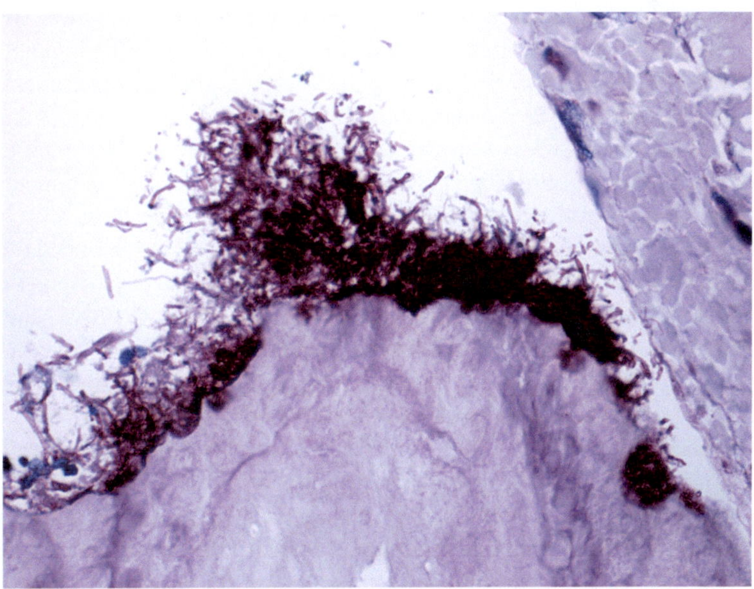

**Fig. 11.3** Fungal spores and hyphae adjacent to the bone (PAS stain, 400×)

antibiotics. It is also evident in most cases that the purulent discharge and pain recurred after discontinuation of the antibiotics [28]. The time till the relapse and worsening of the infectious symptoms may vary.

## Antibiotics Recommended

The "best antibiotic of choice" should be bactericidal, have no side effects, and be economic. The antibiotic should include the resident bacteria but also cope to the considered changed bacteria by the disease and time of exposure.

Recommended antibiotics include penicillin, amoxicillin, metronidazole, quinolones, clindamycin, doxycycline, erythromycin, and ciprofloxacin [2, 4, 6]. The German S3 guideline addresses amoxicillin and clindamycin [25].

Analysis of 391 cases reported in literature demonstrated that most patients were given a combination of antibiotics, either in association or iteratively. Beta-lactam antibiotics were prescribed most frequently. These antibiotics included aminopenicillins (39 %), aminopenicillins with beta-lactamase inhibitor (28 %), methoxyphenyl penicillin (26 %), clindamycin (33 %), metronidazole (13 %), tetracyclines (11 %), and fluoroquinolones (1 %).

The sensitivity of bacteria located in the oral cavity to antimicrobials however is on the decline with a marked trend towards resistance. *Prevotella* and *Porphyromonas* are genera resistant frequently to a higher number of antibiotics and subsequently 80 % sensitive to amoxicillin plus clavulanate, clindamycin, and metronidazole. Oral streptococci and *Eikenella corrodens* have a resistance to special antimicrobial agents, particularly macrolides (35–70 %) and to penicillin and clindamycin (10–15 %). Resistance to metronidazole, macrolides, and first- and second-generation cephalosporins is also described. In contrast, *Eikenella corrodens* is sensitive to amoxicillin [10].

Surgery should always be supported by an antibiotic regime, as recommended by the German S3 guideline [25]. This antibiotic regime is generally advised as prophylactic support in elective surgery (e.g., extraction), surgery of MRONJ, or conservative treatment of MRONJ. The time recommended for therapy noticeably varies in literature.

Eckert and coworkers recommend ampicillin plus clavulanic acid 7 days postoperatively [29], and Bagan et al. advised a minimum of 10 to 30 days [30]. In case of allergies, clindamycin is recommended as an alternative [30]. Penicillin and metronidazole given intermittently or continuously for 1 week intravenously and then orally for the next 3 weeks were also described [31, 32]. Therapy with amoxicillin plus clavulanic acid for 10 days followed by 3 weeks of doxycycline has also been recommended [33]. Stanton et al. prescribed levofloxacin before surgery and in combination with metronidazole for 4–6 weeks postoperatively [34].

Table 11.1 gives an overview of the antibiotics recommended for MRONJ treatment and prophylaxis.

Systemic antibiotic therapy is indicated to treat infection and prevent a more widespread inflammatory condition [19]. A prolonged antibiotic regime before surgery of MRONJ lesions turned out to have a significant influence on the long-term result [6]. Interestingly, only few oncological patients developed serious side effects during long-term antibiotic therapy [6].

An antibiotic therapy alone has only limited abilities to heal MRONJ completely. Studies with limited sample sizes indicated that oral antibiotic therapies have only a low efficiency on bacterial populations associated with MRONJ lesions. No significant differences in bacterial diversity of patients who are taking antibiotics and those who are not have been observed. Species included 69 % Gram-positive and 32 % Gram-negative in the antibiotic group and 75 % Gram-positive and 25 % Gram-negative in non-antibiotic groups. Patients on antibiotics showed a higher count of phylum Firmicutes with the bacterial species *Streptococcus intermedius*, *Lactobacillus gasseri*, *Mogibacterium timidum*, and *Solobacterium moorei*, whereas patients not taking antibiotics had larger populations of *Parvimonas micra* and *Streptococcus anginosus*. These findings suggest marked

**Table 11.1** Systemic antibiotic therapy recommended for MRONJ treatment (for additional information, see text)

| Penicillins (methoxyphenyl penicillin) | Penicillin (benzylpenicillin) |
|---|---|
| Aminopenicillin | Ampicillin/amoxicillin |
| Aminopenicillins with beta-lactam inhibitors | Ampicillin with sulbactam (sultamicillin) |
| | Amoxicillin/ampicillin with clavulanic acid |
| Cephalosporins | Cefazolin |
| | Cefuroxime |
| Carbapenem | Imipenem, meropenem |
| Quinolone (fluoroquinolones) | Ciprofloxacin, levofloxacin, moxifloxacin |
| Aminoglycoside | Gentamicin |
| Tetracycline | Doxycycline |
| Macrolide | Roxithromycin, clarithromycin, azithromycin, erythromycin |
| Lincosamide | Clindamycin |
| Nitroimidazole | Metronidazole |
| Antimycotic (polyene, azole) | Nystatin, miconazole, amphotericin B |

effect on the microbial population but also demonstrated not to be sufficient enough to reduce or even eliminate the infection [2]. These findings explain the poor success rates when only an antimicrobial therapy is used in a conservative treatment of osteonecrosis of the jaw [2, 6]. This contrast may also support the idea of combining antibiotic therapy and surgery in order to improve therapy success rates (see treatment chapter) [6].

Extension of the antibiotic therapy may vary according to the underlying disease of the patient. Patients receiving an immunosuppressive therapy may lack a functional immune response and must be supported with antibiotics in a larger extent and longer period of time than other patients [23, 24]. This may account for a wide variety of antibiotics and time of prescriptions mentioned above. Analyzing reports on comorbidities in MRONJ patients demonstrated a high frequency of immunomodulating therapies: it was found that 55 % of patients received a chemotherapy and 32 % a corticotherapy [22]. Generally, it should be taken into consideration that in all patients with immunosuppressive chemotherapies and MRONJ, an acute leukocyte depression can worsen the stage (infection) of MRONJ. With expected leukocyte deficiencies during chemotherapy, an antibiotic temporary regime is useful to prevent an exacerbation of the infection. In such cases, the use of antimicrobial mouth rinses in or without combination with systemic antibiotic therapy is rec-

ommended to stabilize MRONJ and reduce the clinical symptoms. Less severe MRONJ cases will be able to heal completely [4]. In conclusion, any antibiotic treatment requires an individual sensitivity study (antibiogram typing) to select the most efficient antibiotic regime for each patient.

## Mouth Rinses as Local Therapy

Local therapy turned out to be an important factor as well. This local therapy includes mouth rinses. In consequence, osteonecrotic lesions can be controlled by local antiseptic mouth rinses (chlorhexidine 0.12–0.2 %) and other similar mouth rinses [35, 36]. Chlorhexidine mouth rinses produced better results concerning supra- and subgingival microorganisms compared to other mouth rinses like cetylpyridinium chloride or fluoride in contrast [37].

Other studies observed inhibitory effects of a number of different plant extracts on pathogenic bacteria. These substances included extracts from *Zingiber officinale* (ginger), *Salvia officinalis* (sage), *Chamomilla recutita* (chamomile), *Rosmarinus officinalis* (rosemary), *Syzygium aromaticum* (clove), *Krameria lappacea* (ratanhia), and *Commiphora abyssinica* (myrrh). These extracts proved to be sufficient against *Aggregatibacter actinomycetemcomitans*, *Enterococcus faecalis*, *Porphyromonas gingivalis,* and *Fusobacterium nucleatum* [38]. Especially green tea, *Camellia sinensis,* seems to have special antiseptic, antioxidant, anti-inflammatory properties and support wound healing [36, 39, 40]. The use of plant extracts should not replace antiseptic "traditional medical" mouth rinses. Clinical experience showed that patients gratefully accepted the additional offer of phytotherapeutic mouth rinses.

## Side Effects of Antibiotic Therapies

Long-term antibiotic regimes optimize surgery success rates and are therefore recommended [1, 4]. On the other hand, long-term antibiotic regimes increase the risk of intestinal side effects like colitis or *Clostridium difficile* infections. Attention must be paid to these diarrheic side effects or intestinal problems under antibiotic (long-term) therapies [6].

It must be taken also into consideration that – as Ji et al. mentioned by using a molecular technique – the use of systemic antibiotics failed to restrict the bacterial colonization without effective healing of the MRONJ lesion [2].

### Conclusion

The bone affected by antiresorptive drug-induced osteonecrosis of the jaw shows regularly certain species of microorganisms. Over the time of bone exposure, the microbial profile of the lesions might change. Therefore, microbiological examination and antibiograms are essential to find the appropriate antibiotic therapy. Microbial infections play a crucial role in the etiology of MRONJ and the development of the osteonecrotic lesions, which in turn means that antibiotics remain one of the important pillars of therapy. The antibiotic therapy as a singular therapy is only able to heal osteonecrosis of the jaw in few cases. If no antibiogram is available, the antibiotic regime should cover the oral flora and the regularly observed bacteria of odontogenic infections or the bacteria described above.

## References

1. Egan PJ, Carding SR. Downmodulation of the inflammatory response to bacterial infection by gammadelta T cell cytotoxic for activated macrophages. J Exp Med. 2000;191(12):2145–58.
2. Ji X, Pushalkar S, Li Y, Glickman R, Fleischer K, Sexana D. Antibiotic effects on bacterial profile in osteonecrosis of the jaw. Oral Dis. 2012;18(1):85–95.
3. Wei X, Pushalkar S, Estilo C, Wong C, Farooki A, Fornier M, Bohle G, Huryn J, Li Y, Doty S, Saxena D. Molecular profiling of oral microbiota in jaw bone samples of bisphosphonate related osteonecrosis of the jaw. Oral Dis. 2012;18(6):602–12.
4. Vescovi P, Nammour S. Bisphosphonate-related osteonecrosis of the jaw (BRONJ) therapy. A critical review. Minerva Stomatol. 2010;59(4):181–203; 204–213.
5. Kumar V, Sinha RK. Evolution and etiopathogenesis of bisphosphonates induced osteonecrosis of the jaw. N Am J Med Sci. 2013;5(4):260–5.
6. Hoefert S, Eufinger H. Relevance of a prolonged preoperative antibiotic regime in the treatment of bisphosphonate-related osteonecrosis of the jaw. J Oral Maxillofac Surg. 2011;69(2):362–80.
7. Hoefert S, Wierich W, Eufinger H, Krempien B. BP-associated avascular necrosis (AN) of the jaws: histological findings. Bone. 2006;38(Suppl):76.
8. Sedghizadeh PP, Kumar SK, Gorur A, Schaudinn C, Shuler CF, Costerton JW. Identification of microbial biofilms in osteonecrosis of the jaws secondary to bisphosphonate therapy. J Oral Maxillofac Surg. 2008;66(4):767–75.
9. Ruggiero SL, Didson TB, Assael LA, Landesberg R, Marx RE, Mehrotra B. American Association of Oral and Maxillofacial Surgeons Position Paper on Bisphosphonate-related osteonecrosis of the jaws-2009 update. J Oral Maxillofac Surg. 2009;67 Suppl 1:2–12.
10. Prieto-Prieto J, Calvo A. Microbiological basis of oral infections and sensitivity to antibiotics. Med Oral Patol Oral Cir Bucal. 2004;9(Suppl):11–8.
11. Naik NH, Russo TA. Bisphosphonate-related osteonecrosis of the jaw: the role of actinomyces. Clin Infect Dis. 2009;49(11):1729–32.
12. Thumbigere-Math V, Michalowicz BS, Hodges JS, Tsai ML, Swenson KK, Rockwell L, Gopalakrishnan R. Periodontal disease as a risk factor for bisphosphonate-related osteonecrosis of the jaw. J Periodontol. 2014;85(2):226–33.
13. Tsurushima H, Kokuryo O, Sakaguchi J, Tanaka J, Tominaga K. Bacterial promotion of bisphosphonate-induced osteonecrosis in wistar rats. Int J Oral Maxillofac Surg. 2013;42(11):1481–7.
14. Hall-Stoodely L, Stoodley P. Evolving concepts in biofilm infection. Cell Microbiol. 2009;11(7):1034–43.
15. Kos M, Junka A, Smutnicka D, Bartoszewicz M, Kurzynowski T, Gluza K. Pamidronate enhances bacterial adhesion to bone hydroxyapatite. another puzzle in the pathology of bisphosphonate-related

osteonecrosis of the jaw? J Oral Maxillofac Surg. 2013;71(6):1010–6.

16. Ganguli A, Steward C, Butler L, Philips J, Meikle ST, Lloyd AW, Grant MH. Bacterial adhesion to bisphosphonate coated hydroxyapatite. J Mater Sci Mater Med. 2005;16(4):283–7.

17. Kos M, Luczak K. Bisphosphonates promote jaw osteonecrosis through facilitating bacterial colonisation. Bioscience Hypotheses. 2009;2(9):34–6.

18. Mawardi H, Giro G, Kajiya M, Ohta K, Armazrrooa A, Alshwaimi E, Woo SB, Nishimura I, Kawai T. A role of oral bacteria in bisphosphonate-induced osteonecrosis of the jaw. J Dent Res. 2011;90(11):1339–145.

19. Ruggiero S. An office-based approach to the diagnosis and management of osteonecrosis. Atlas Oral Maxillofac Surg Clin North Am. 2013;21(2):167–73.

20. Badros A, Weikel D, Salama A, Goloubeva O, Schneider A, Rapoport A, Fenton R, Gahres N, Sausville E, Ord R, Meiller T. Osteonecrosis of the jaw in multiple myeloma patients: clinical features and risk factors. J Clin Oncol. 2006;24(6):945–52.

21. Kassolis JD, Scherper M, Jham B, Reynolds MA. Histopathologic findings in bone from edentulous alveolar ridges: a role in osteonecrosis of the jaw? Bone. 2010;47(1):127–30.

22. Filleul O, Crompot E, Saussez S. Bisphosphonate-induced osteonecrosis of the jaw: a review of 2,400 patient cases. J Cancer Res Clin Oncol. 2010;136(8):1117–24.

23. Thumbigere-Math V, Sabino MC, Gopalakrishnan R, Huckabay S, Dudek AZ, Basu S, Hughes PJ, Michalowicz BS, Leach JW, Swenson KK, Swift JQ, Adkinson C, Basi DL. Bisphosphonate-related osteonecrosis of the jaw: clinical features, risk factors, management, and treatment outcome of 26 patients. J Oral Maxillofac Surg. 2009;67(9):1904–13.

24. Hansen T, Kunkel M, Springer E, Walter C, Weber A, Siegel E, Kirkpatrick CJ. Actinomyces of the jaws – histopathological study of 45 patients shows significant involvement in bisphosphonate-associated osteonecrosis and infected osteoradionecrosis. Virchows Arch. 2007;451(6):1009–17.

25. AWMF-Register Nr. 007/091. Bisphosphonat-assoziierte Kiefernekrosen (BP-MRONJ) und andere Medikamenten-assoziierte Kiefernekrosen. 2012. http://www.awmf.org/uploads/tx_szleitlinien/007-0911_S3_Bisphosphonat-assoziierte_Kiefernekrose_2012-04.pdf (Stand 3/2014).

26. Rautemaa R, Ramage G. Oral candidosis-clinical challenge of a biofilm disease. Crit Rev Microbiol. 2011;37(4):328–36.

27. Hebbar PB, Pai A. Mycological and histological associations of Candida in oral mucosal lesions. J Oral Sci. 2013;55(2):157–60.

28. Bamias A, Kastritis E, Bamia C, Moulopoulos LA, Melakopoulos I, Bozas G, Koutsoukou V, Gika D, Anagnostopoulos A, Papadimitriou C, Terpos E, Dimopoulos MA. Osteonecrosis of the jaw in cancer after treatment with bisphosphonates: incidences and risk factors. J Clin Oncol. 2005;23(34):8580–7.

29. Eckert AW, Maurer P, Meyer L. Bisphosphonate-related jaw necrosis – severe complication in maxillofacial surgery. Cancer Treat Rev. 2007;33(1):58–63.

30. Bagan J, Blade J, Cozar JM. Recommendations for the prevention, diagnosis, and treatment of osteonecrosis of the jaws (MRONJ) in cancer patients treated with bisphosphonates. Med Oral Pathol Oral Bucal. 2007;12(4):E336–40.

31. Vescovi P, Merigo E, Meleti M, Menfredi M. Bisphosphonate-associated osteonecrosis (BON) of the jaws: a possible treatment? J Oral Maxillofac Surg. 2006;64(9):1460–2.

32. Alons K, Kuijpers SCC, DeJong E, Van Merkesteyn JPR. Treating low- and medium potency bisphosphonate-related osteonecrosis of the jaw with a protocol for the treatment of chronic suppurative osteomyelitis: a report of 7 cases. Oral Surg Oral Med Oral Pathol Oral Radiol Endod. 2009;107(2):E1–7.

33. Van den Wyngaert T, Claeys T, Huizing MT, Vermorken JB, Fossion E. Initial experience with conservative treatment in cancer patients with osteonecrosis of the jaw (MRONJ) and predictors of outcome. Ann Oncol. 2008;20(2):331–6.

34. Stanton D, Balasanian E. Outcome of surgical management of bisphosphonate-related osteonecrosis of the jaw. J Oral Maxillofac Surg. 2009;67(5):943–50.

35. Yarom N, Yahalom R, Shoshani Y, Hamed W, Regev E, Elad S. Osteonecrosis of the jaw induced by orally administered bisphosphonates: incidence, clinical features, predisposing factors and treatment outcome. Osteoporos Int. 2007;18(10):1363–70.

36. Hoefert S. Prothesendruckstellen als Risiko einer Bisphosphonat-assoziierten Kiefernekrose. ZWR. 2012;121(11):564–71.

37. Kneist S, Gebelein K, Küpper H. Zur antimikrobiellen Wirkung von Mundspüllösungen. ZWR. 2013;122(2):8–15.

38. Staudte H, Sigusch W. Die Wirkung von Pflanzenstoffen auf parodontalpathogene Bakterien. ZWR. 2013;122(2):18–24.

39. Kim HK, Kawazoe T, Han DW, Matsumara K, Suzuki S, Tsutsumi S, Hyon SH. Enhanced wound healing by an epigallocatechin gallate-incorporated collagen sponge in diabetic mice. Wound Repair Regen. 2008;16(5):714–20.

40. Lee JH, Shim JS, Chung MS, Lim ST, Kim KH. In vitro anti-adhesive activity of green tea extract against pathogen adhesion. Phytother Res. 2009;23(12):460–6.

# Histopathology of Medication-Related Osteonecrosis of the Jaw

**12**

Risa Chaisuparat and Bruno C. Jham


**Abstract**

Osteonecrosis of the jaw in the patients receiving bisphosphonate or denosumab treatment is a serious condition. Despite several terminologies have been used for this condition, bisphosphonate-related osteonecrosis of the jaw (BRONJ) and medication-related osteonecrosis of the jaw (MRONJ) are applied throughout this chapter. BRONJ/MRONJ clinically presents as exposed bone of the mandible or the maxilla with further symptoms such as pain, drainage, or swelling. Histopathological confirmation is strongly recommended to prove the clinical diagnosis whenever surgical intervention is performed. This chapter describes the macroscopic and microscopic features of BRONJ/MRONJ and discusses the histopathologic differential diagnosis of this condition.


## Introduction

Bisphosphonate-related osteonecrosis of the jaw (BRONJ) is a complication seen in patients under bisphosphonate treatment for various diseases, such as cancer, bone metastasis, and osteoporosis [1, 2]. The disease was first described and reported in the literature in the early years of the twenty-first century [3–5]. Since then, an increasing number of case reports and reviews of BRONJ have been published. However, clear explanation for pathogenesis of this condition remains unknown. Current theories are discussed in detail in the pathogenesis (see Chap. 13). Clinically, BRONJ is usually characterized by exposed and necrotic bone affecting the alveolar part of the jaws. Patients present with or without pain, local infection, loosening of teeth, and draining fistulas [1]. As already described in the previous chapters, the diagnosis of BRONJ/MRONJ is achieved based on bone exposure in the maxillofacial region in the patients under current or previous treatment with bisphosphonates or denosumab with no history of radiation therapy to the jaws [6].

Microscopic confirmation of BRONJ is not always possible, as a biopsy is sometimes avoided due to the poor healing capacity of those patients. Hence, it has been recommended that a biopsy is performed only when there is


R. Chaisuparat, DDS, PhD
Department of Oral Pathology,
Faculty of Dentistry, Chulalongkorn University,
Bangkok, Thailand
e-mail: risa.c@chula.ac.th

B.C. Jham, DDS, MS, PhD
College of Dental Medicine–Illinois,
Midwestern University, Illinois, USA
e-mail: bjham@midwestern.edu



S. Otto (ed.), *Medication-Related Osteonecrosis of the Jaws: Bisphosphonates, Denosumab, and New Agents*, 131
DOI 10.1007/978-3-662-43733-9_12, © Springer-Verlag Berlin Heidelberg 2015

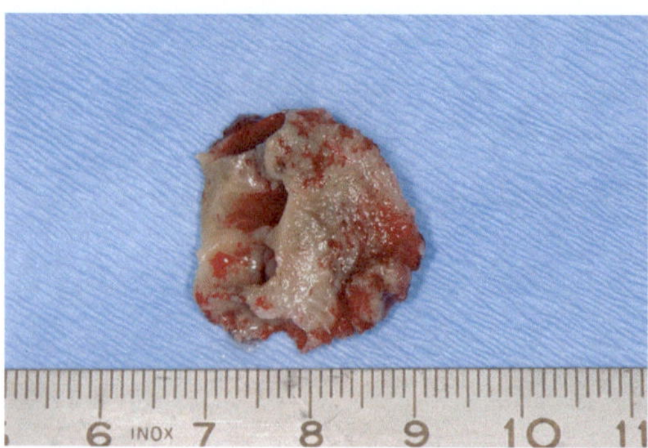

**Fig. 12.1** Specimen from BRONJ patient

high clinical suspicion of cancer metastasis [7]. Nonetheless, surgical removal of the necrotic bone is often required for treating the condition [8]. In these instances, the obtained specimen has to be submitted for microscopic examination to confirm the clinical diagnosis. Therefore, the aim of this chapter is to describe the macroscopic and microscopic features of BRONJ, in addition, discuss the histopathologic differential diagnosis of this condition.

## Macroscopic Features

Received specimens from BRONJ patients can range from multiple bone fragments to a large part of jawbone depending on treatment. The specimens can consist of a mixture of hard tissue and soft tissue. Necrotic bone fragments appear as several small pale whitish gray pieces. Jaw resection specimens are sometimes submitted to biopsy service for analysis [9] (Fig. 12.1).

## Histopathologic Features

Microscopic presentation of BRONJ is characterized by necrotic bony trabeculae demonstrating empty osteocyte lacunae. The necrotic bone is usually surrounded by bacterial colonies and shows irregular peripheral resorption and prominent reversal lines [10] (Fig. 12.2). *Actinomyces* in contact with vital bone has been described as a consistent histologic finding [11–13], and it has been suggested that this microorganism could be responsible for the chronic, nonhealing

inflammatory processes and the purulent discharge seen in BRONJ [11]. Osteoclasts containing numerous intracytoplasmic vacuoles are seen at the periphery and in the intertrabecular spaces of the bony trabeculae. Large and hypernucleated osteoclasts have been reported in patients who received long-term oral bisphosphonate treatment [10]. The empty Howship's lacunae at the periphery of the bone are frequently seen. It has been suggested that this microscopic finding depicts that osteoclasts have undergone apoptosis after interalizing bisphosphonates [14]. The intertrabecular space is infiltrated by inflammatory cells including neutrophils, lymphocytes, and plasma cells [15–17]. Pseudoepitheliomatous hyperplasia of the overlying mucosa has also been observed in BRONJ [11].

Bisphosphonates have been found to inhibit endothelial function in vitro and in vivo and to reduce levels of vascular endothelial growth factor [18, 19]. In spite of these known antiangiogenic effects, data on the histologic changes of the vessels in BRONJ are scarce. In a rat model, a decreased rate of capillary formation could be observed [18]. In humans, obliteration of larger arterial vessels accompanied by an increased cellular proliferation of the intima and media and relative reduction of blood vessels in BRONJ has been reported [11, 20]. Others have found intact vasculature and no significant reduction of the capillaries on histologic examination [11, 21].

Few studies have investigated the histopathologic changes in the uninvolved bone of patients undergoing bisphosphonate therapy. Specimens from areas without bone exposure that are contiguous with areas of ONJ are characterized by hypervascular fibrous tissue and inflammatory infiltrate filling large intertrabecular spaces, an appearance similar to that of chronic osteomyelitis [22]. The newly formed bone present in non-necrotic areas is mostly composed of large masses of bone tissue showing centrifugal deposition and variable degrees of calcification (mature and recent woven bones), devoid of Haversian canals, and surrounded by prominent collagen deposition apparently entering the bone at right angles. Islands of woven bone contained plump osteoblasts, while osteoclastic activity is absent in such areas [23].

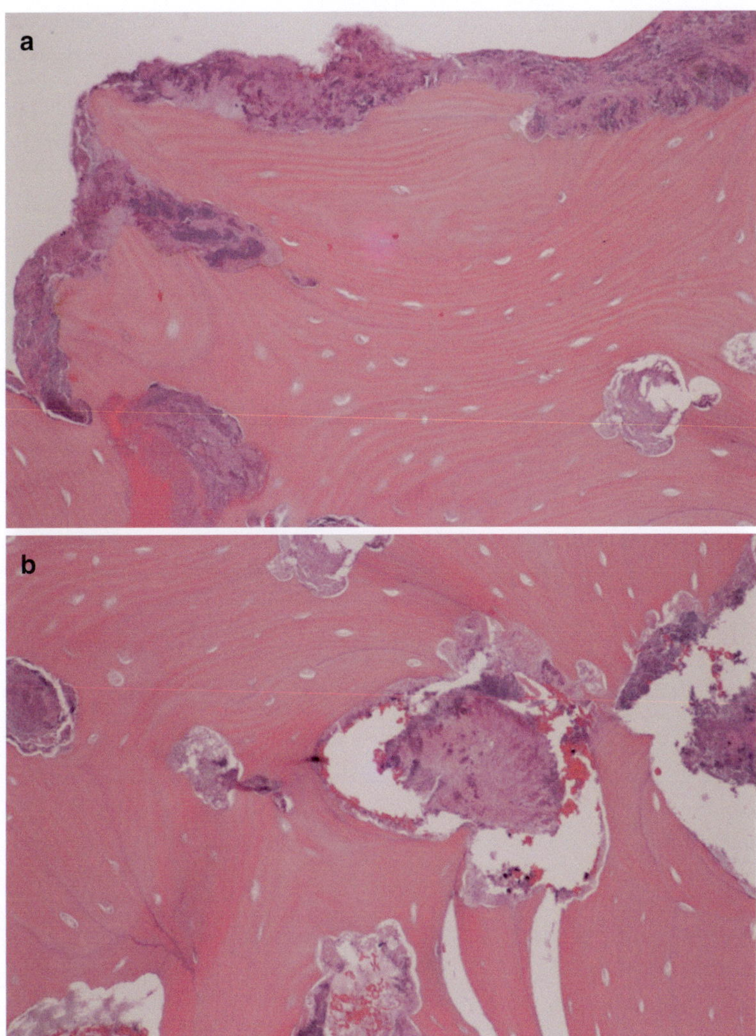

**Fig. 12.2** Bisphosphonate-related osteonecrosis

## Differential Histopathologic Diagnosis

### Osteomyelitis

Osteomyelitis is an inflammatory condition of the bone, which generally begins as an infection of the marrow cavity, rapidly involves the Haversian canals, and eventually extends to the periosteum [9]. Histopathologic features of BRONJ and osteomyelitis may not be distinguishable, with both lesions showing non-vital bone with empty osteocyte lacunae. One difference is that the detachment of osteoclasts from the bone surface is seen in BRONJ, whereas in osteomyelitis, the osteoclasts are attached to the bone [16]. BRONJ cases have been shown to present with a mosaic pattern with a multiple compartment configuration, which is absent in osteomyelitis [24]. Osteomyelitis consistently shows viable inflammatory cells in the marrow spaces (Fig. 12.3). By contrast, BRONJ shows empty marrow spaces devoid of all cellular elements and normal cellular products [14].

### Osteoradionecrosis

Osteoradionecrosis (ORN) is one of the most serious complications in the treatment of head and neck malignancies and is defined as the ischemic necrosis of the irradiated bone, which becomes

**Fig. 12.3** Osteomyelitis

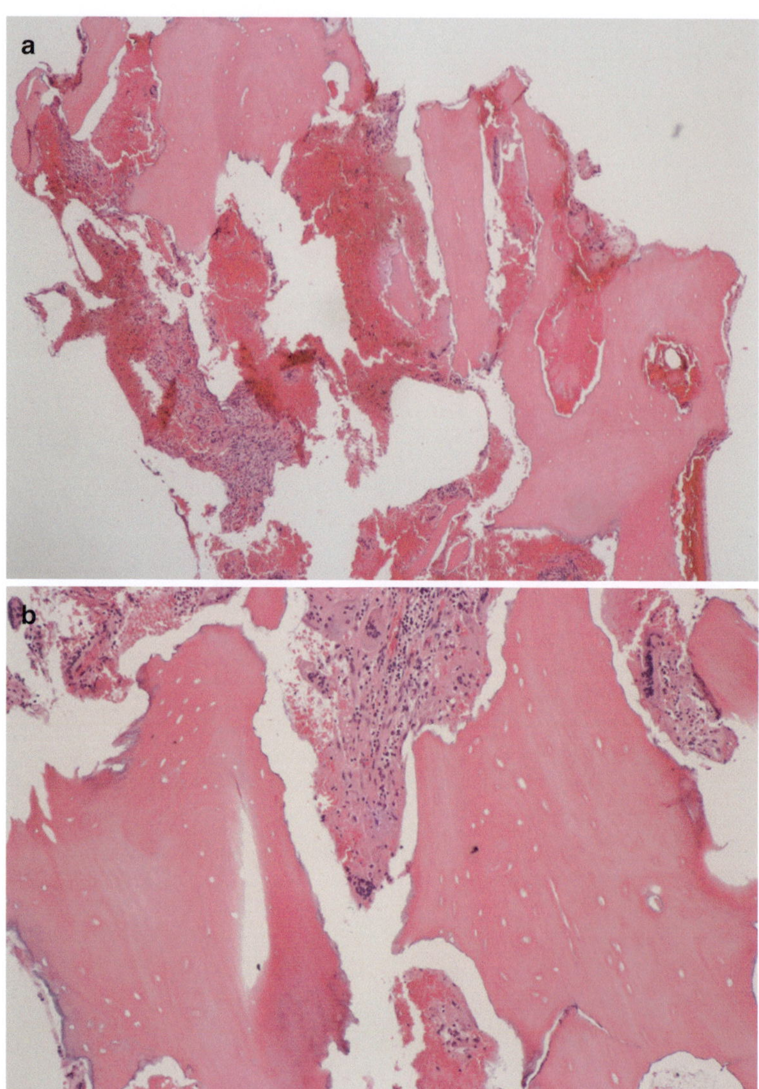

hypovascular, hypocellular, and hypoxic [25, 26]. The histopathologic jaw findings in BRONJ are similar to ORN [4, 5, 27]. Microscopic presentation of ORN shows necrotic bone without osteoblastic and osteoclastic activities (Fig. 12.4). The bone marrow spaces are replaced with fibrosis. Inflammatory cell infiltration is limited [27]. The ghosts of old blood vessels are also seen [14]. The presence of *Actinomyces* has been described in both BRONJ and ORN [11]. It has been described that the areas of osteonecrosis seem to be patchier in tissue specimens of bisphosphonate-treated patients when compared with larger necrotic bone areas in ORN [11]. ORN demonstrates a nonviable periosteum and

no evidence of reactive bone, whereas BRONJ may show viable periosteum and even reactive bone in many cases [14].

## Medication-Related Osteonecrosis of the Jaws

Recently, cases of osteonecrosis of the jaws (ONJ) associated with the use of a non-bisphosphonate antiresorptive agent (denosumab) have been reported [28–30]. Other antiresorptive agents, including cathepsin K inhibitors, also could prove to be associated with ONJ. In fact, it has been recently proposed that

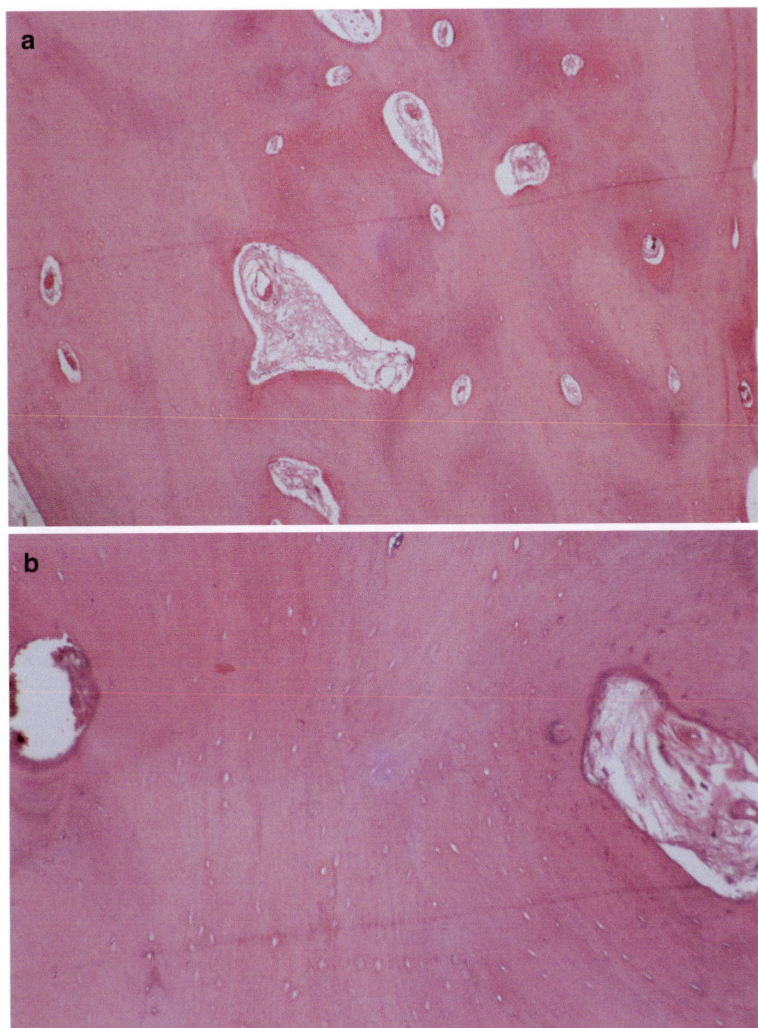

**Fig. 12.4** Osteoradionecrosis

all cases of ONJ related to the administration of antiresorptive therapeutic agents be termed "medication-related ONJ" (MRONJ). This term would encompass cases associated with bisphosphonates, as well as cases associated with the use of other antiresorptive and antiangiogenic agents [31]. Information regarding the histopathological changes in ARONJ is lacking and comes mainly from case reports. Necrotic bone demonstrating a scalloped, "moth-eaten" appearance has been described. Adherent bacteria, including filamentous forms and focal acute inflammation, are also present [29, 32]. Similar to BRONJ, *Actinomyces* has also been found in other MRONJ cases [32, 33]. MRONJ cases due to denosumab intake may not be distinguishable from ONJ due to bisphosphonate intake in terms of histopathology since both conditions are potentially the same entity. Additionally, many cases treated with denosumab have had previous bisphosphonate administrations [34].

## Conclusions

BRONJ/MRONJ has a distinctive histopathology, characterized by nonviable bony trabeculae with irregular border, surrounded by massive bacterial colonies. Even though the diagnosis of BRONJ/MRONJ is mainly based on the patient's history of bisphosphonate or denosumab intake and the clinical presentations, histological confirmation may be required.

# References


1. McLeod NM, Brennan PA, Ruggiero SL. Bisphosphonate osteonecrosis of the jaw: a historical and contemporary review. Surgeon. 2012;10(1):36–42.
2. Murakami H, Takahashi N, Sasaki T, Udagawa N, Tanaka S, Nakamura I, et al. A possible mechanism of the specific action of bisphosphonates on osteoclasts: tiludronate preferentially affects polarized osteoclasts having ruffled borders. Bone. 1995;17(2):137–44.
3. Carter GD, Goss AN. Bisphosphonates and avascular necrosis of the jaws. Aust Dent J. 2003;48(4):268.
4. Marx RE. Pamidronate (Aredia) and zoledronate (Zometa) induced avascular necrosis of the jaws: a growing epidemic. J Oral Maxillofac Surg. 2003;61(9):1115–7.
5. Migliorati CA. Bisphosphonates and oral cavity avascular bone necrosis. J Clin Oncol. 2003;21(22): 4253–4.
6. Ruggiero SL, Dodson TB, Assael LA, Landesberg R, Marx RE, Mehrotra B. American Association of Oral and Maxillofacial Surgeons position paper on bisphosphonate-related osteonecrosis of the jaws–2009 update. J Oral Maxillofac Surg. 2009; 67(5 Suppl):2–12.
7. Phal PM, Myall RW, Assael LA, Weissman JL. Imaging findings of bisphosphonate-associated osteonecrosis of the jaws. AJNR Am J Neuroradiol. 2007;28(6):1139–45.
8. Janovska Z, Mottl R, Slezak R. Experience with the treatment of bisphosphonate-related osteonecrosis of the jaw. Biomed Pap Med Fac Univ Palacky Olomouc Czech Repub. 2013 [Epub ahead of print].
9. Bruder EJ, Jundt G, Eyrich G. Pathology of osteomyelitis. Osteomyelitis of the jaws. Heidelberg: Springer; 2009.
10. Weinstein RS, Roberson PK, Manolagas SC. Giant osteoclast formation and long-term oral bisphosphonate therapy. N Engl J Med. 2009;360(1):53–62.
11. Hansen T, Kunkel M, Weber A, James Kirkpatrick C. Osteonecrosis of the jaws in patients treated with bisphosphonates – histomorphologic analysis in comparison with infected osteoradionecrosis. J Oral Pathol Med. 2006;35(3):155–60.
12. Lugassy G, Shaham R, Nemets A, Ben-Dor D, Nahlieli O. Severe osteomyelitis of the jaw in long-term survivors of multiple myeloma: a new clinical entity. Am J Med. 2004;117(6):440–1.
13. Melo MD, Obeid G. Osteonecrosis of the maxilla in a patient with a history of bisphosphonate therapy. J Can Dent Assoc. 2005;71(2):111–3.
14. Marx RE, Tursun R. Suppurative osteomyelitis, bisphosphonate induced osteonecrosis, osteoradionecrosis: a blinded histopathologic comparison and its implications for the mechanism of each disease. Int J Oral Maxillofac Surg. 2012;41(3):283–9. doi:10.1016/j.ijom.2011.12.016.
15. Ali SM, Esteva FJ, Hortobagyi G, Harvey H, Seaman J, Knight R, et al. Safety and efficacy of bisphosphonates beyond 24 months in cancer patients. J Clin Oncol. 2001;19(14):3434–7.
16. Bagan JV, Murillo J, Jimenez Y, Poveda R, Milian MA, Sanchis JM, et al. Avascular jaw osteonecrosis in association with cancer chemotherapy: series of 10 cases. J Oral Pathol Med. 2005;34(2):120–3.
17. Sutherland KA, Rogers HL, Tosh D, Rogers MJ. RANKL increases the level of Mcl-1 in osteoclasts and reduces bisphosphonate-induced osteoclast apoptosis in vitro. Arthritis Res Ther. 2009;11(2):R58.
18. Fournier P, Boissier S, Filleur S, Guglielmi J, Cabon F, Colombel M, et al. Bisphosphonates inhibit angiogenesis in vitro and testosterone-stimulated vascular regrowth in the ventral prostate in castrated rats. Cancer Res. 2002;62(22):6538–44.
19. Santini D, Vincenzi B, Avvisati G, Dicuonzo G, Battistoni F, Gavasci M, et al. Pamidronate induces modifications of circulating angiogenetic factors in cancer patients. Clin Cancer Res. 2002;8(5):1080–4.
20. Migliorati CA, Schubert MM, Peterson DE, Seneda LM. Bisphosphonate-associated osteonecrosis of mandibular and maxillary bone: an emerging oral complication of supportive cancer therapy. Cancer. 2005;104(1):83–93.
21. Compston J. Pathophysiology of atypical femoral fractures and osteonecrosis of the jaw. Osteoporos Int. 2011;22(12):2951–61.
22. Bedogni A, Blandamura S, Lokmic Z, Palumbo C, Ragazzo M, Ferrari F, et al. Bisphosphonate-associated jawbone osteonecrosis: a correlation between imaging techniques and histopathology. Oral Surg Oral Med Oral Pathol Oral Radiol Endod. 2008;105(3):358–64.
23. Favia G, Pilolli GP, Maiorano E. Histologic and histomorphometric features of bisphosphonate-related osteonecrosis of the jaws: an analysis of 31 cases with confocal laser scanning microscopy. Bone. 2009;45(3):406–13.
24. Paparella ML, Brandizzi D, Santini-Araujo E, Cabrini RL. Histopathological features of osteonecrosis of the jaw associated with bisphosphonates. Histopathology. 2012;60(3):514–6.
25. Sciubba JJ, Goldenberg D. Oral complications of radiotherapy. Lancet Oncol. 2006;7(2):175–83.
26. Teng MS, Futran ND. Osteoradionecrosis of the mandible. Curr Opin Otolaryngol Head Neck Surg. 2005;13(4):217–21.
27. Reuther T, Schuster T, Mende U, Kubler A. Osteoradionecrosis of the jaws as a side effect of radiotherapy of head and neck tumour patients–a report of a thirty year retrospective review. Int J Oral Maxillofac Surg. 2003;32(3):289–95.
28. Aghaloo TL, Felsenfeld AL, Tetradis S. Osteonecrosis of the jaw in a patient on Denosumab. J Oral Maxillofac Surg. 2010;68(5):959–63.

29. Malan J, Ettinger K, Naumann E, Beirne OR. The relationship of denosumab pharmacology and osteonecrosis of the jaws. Oral Surg Oral Med Oral Pathol Oral Radiol. 2012;114(6):671–6.
30. Rachner TD, Platzbecker U, Felsenberg D, Hofbauer LC. Osteonecrosis of the jaw after osteoporosis therapy with denosumab following long-term bisphosphonate therapy. Mayo Clin Proc. 2013;88(4):418–9.
31. Hellstein JW, Adler RA, Edwards B, Jacobsen PL, Kalmar JR, Koka S, et al. Managing the care of patients receiving antiresorptive therapy for prevention and treatment of osteoporosis: executive summary of recommendations from the American Dental Association Council on Scientific Affairs. J Am Dent Assoc. 2011;142(11):1243–51.
32. Estilo CL, Fornier M, Farooki A, Carlson D, Bohle 3rd G, Huryn JM. Osteonecrosis of the jaw related to bevacizumab. J Clin Oncol. 2008;26(24):4037–8.
33. Koch FP, Walter C, Hansen T, Jager E, Wagner W. Osteonecrosis of the jaw related to sunitinib. Oral Maxillofac Surg. 2011;15(1):63–6.
34. Otto S, Baumann S, Ehrenfeld M, Pautke C. Successful surgical management of osteonecrosis of the jaw due to RANK-ligand inhibitor treatment using fluorescence guided bone resection. J Craniomaxillofac Surg. 2013;41(7):694–8.

# Pathogenesis of Medication-Related Osteonecrosis of the Jaw

**13**

Sven Otto, Jose Ignacio Aguirre, Ezher Dayisoylu, and Thomas Ziebart


**Abstract**

Since the first descriptions of bisphosphonate-related osteonecrosis (BRONJ) of the jaw, numerous studies and research articles have focused on the pathophysiology of the disease which has currently been renamed to medication-related osteonecrosis of the jaw (MRONJ). Several possible pathomechanisms including over-suppression of jawbone turnover, specific pathogens, antiangiogenic effects, and soft tissue toxicity have been proposed to be the main drivers of the disease. More recently, theories dealing with the role of local inflammations and consecutive pH changes have been introduced. While the precise aetiology is still under current investigation, it is now widely accepted that medication-related osteonecrosis of the jaw has a multifactorial aetiology. Besides, there is more and more evidence that local inflammations and dento-alveolar infections play a key role in the pathogenesis of the disease. Recently, osteonecrotic lesions in the jaw have been described under the treatment with denosumab as well, an antibody against RANK ligand. A better understanding of this entity and the involvement of the RANK-RANKL-OPG system might offer new insights towards a comprehensive understanding of medication-related osteonecrosis of the jaw (MRONJ).



S. Otto, MD, DMD, FEBOMFS (✉)
Department of Oral and Maxillofacial Surgery,
Ludwig-Maximilians-University of Munich,
Munich, Germany
e-mail: otto_sven@web.de

J.I. Aguirre
Department of Physiological Sciences,
University of Florida, Gainesville, Florida, USA
e-mail: aguirrej@ufl.edu

E. Dayisoylu, DDS, PhD
Department of Oral and Maxillofacial Surgery,
Konya Research Hospital, Baskent University,
Konya 42100, Turkey
e-mail: edayisoylu@gmail.com

T. Ziebart, MD, DDS, PhD
Department of Maxillofacial Surgery,
University Medical Center Mainz,
Augustusplatz 2, Mainz 55131, Germany
e-mail: ziebart@mkg.klinik.uni-mainz.de



S. Otto (ed.), *Medication-Related Osteonecrosis of the Jaws: Bisphosphonates, Denosumab, and New Agents*,
DOI 10.1007/978-3-662-43733-9_13, © Springer-Verlag Berlin Heidelberg 2015

## Theories Regarding the Pathogenesis of BRONJ/MRONJ

Over the past decade research into the pathogenesis of medication-related osteonecrosis of the jaw (MRONJ) has mainly focussed on bisphosphonate-related osteonecrosis of the jaw (BRONJ). The precise pathogenesis of BRONJ/MRONJ is under current investigation. However, some main theories speculating about the pathogenesis of this disease prevail. A potential main driver is over-suppression of jawbone turnover which should occur after a special accumulation of bisphosphonates in the jawbone [1–3]. Bisphosphonates accumulate in the bone and inhibit bone resorption by inducing apoptosis of osteoclasts. Therefore, bone remodelling is suppressed [4]. It is speculated that over-suppression of bone turnover after a special accumulation of bisphosphonates in the jawbone might induce necrosis [1, 2, 5]. Indeed, jawbone turnover is known to be higher when compared with other bones [2, 6, 7]. Besides the inhibitory effect of osteoclasts, bisphosphonates interact also with other cell systems of the hard and soft tissues: Especially nitrogen-containing bisphosphonates can reduce the biological activity and viability of osteoblasts, keratinocytes and fibroblasts [8, 9]. However, till now, no scientific evidence for an over-accumulation of bisphosphonates in the jawbone or that remodelling of the jaw is affected to a higher degree when compared to other bone sites is available. An animal study could confirm that there was no special accumulation of bisphosphonates in the jaw compared to other bones [1, 2, 10].

Based on the regular presence of Actinomyces species in the histopathological and microbiological specimen of affected jawbone areas, there were also speculations that BRONJ/MRONJ might be due to a specific infection [2, 11, 12]. Actinomyces species are also regularly present in cases of osteoradionecrosis so that a crucial pathogenetical role seems to be unlikely. However, as bisphosphonates are known to modulate the activity of different cell types involved in the immune response [2, 13, 14], this might also alleviate the response towards biofilms and pathogens such as Actinomyces species in particular [1, 2, 11, 12].

It is also assumed that the anti-angiogenetic properties of bisphosphonates after accumulation might play an important part in the pathogenesis of ONJ. With regard to the fact that BRONJ was first described as avascular necrosis and that bisphosphonates could prove anti-angiogenetic effects in tumour tissue vascularity might play an important role [2, 11, 15, 16]. Bisphosphonates interact on different levels of the angiogenesis. In vitro and in vivo data showed that bisphosphonates reduce cell number, migration capacity and colony-forming rate of endothelial progenitor cell (EPC), which play a key role for neovascularisation and therefore for adult endothelial stem cell mobilisation [9, 17–19]. Additionally the mature cell-based angiogenesis is impaired by bisphosphonates (Fig. 13.1). Cytoskeletal disorder and dysfunction as well as disturbed gene expression are reported after incubation with nitrogen-containing bisphosphonates [20].

On the other hand, angiogenesis during bone formation was not significantly altered by bisphosphonates [2, 21, 22]. However, vascularity might well play a role in the pathogenesis of the disease and especially with regard to the frequency of occurrence in the mandible and the maxilla [23], but it is not likely to be the key factor in the pathogenesis because it cannot be explained why only the jawbones are affected – especially when having in mind that maxilla and mandible have a completely different pattern of vascularity – while there are only few cases reported in other bones of the human body [2, 24–26].

Furthermore, it has been discussed that after local accumulation of bisphosphonates and combined with other cancer medications, bisphosphonates might exert direct soft tissue toxicity towards the oral mucosa. This could lead to mucosal injury and jawbone exposure as seen in MRONJ [2, 27–29]. Also soft tissue toxicity might play a role in the pathogenesis of MRONJ, and mucosal healing is delayed after dento-alveolar surgeries in patients receiving bisphosphonates, but jawbone exposure is not constantly present in all cases of BRONJ/MRONJ proven by histology especially not in early stages (stage 0 according to

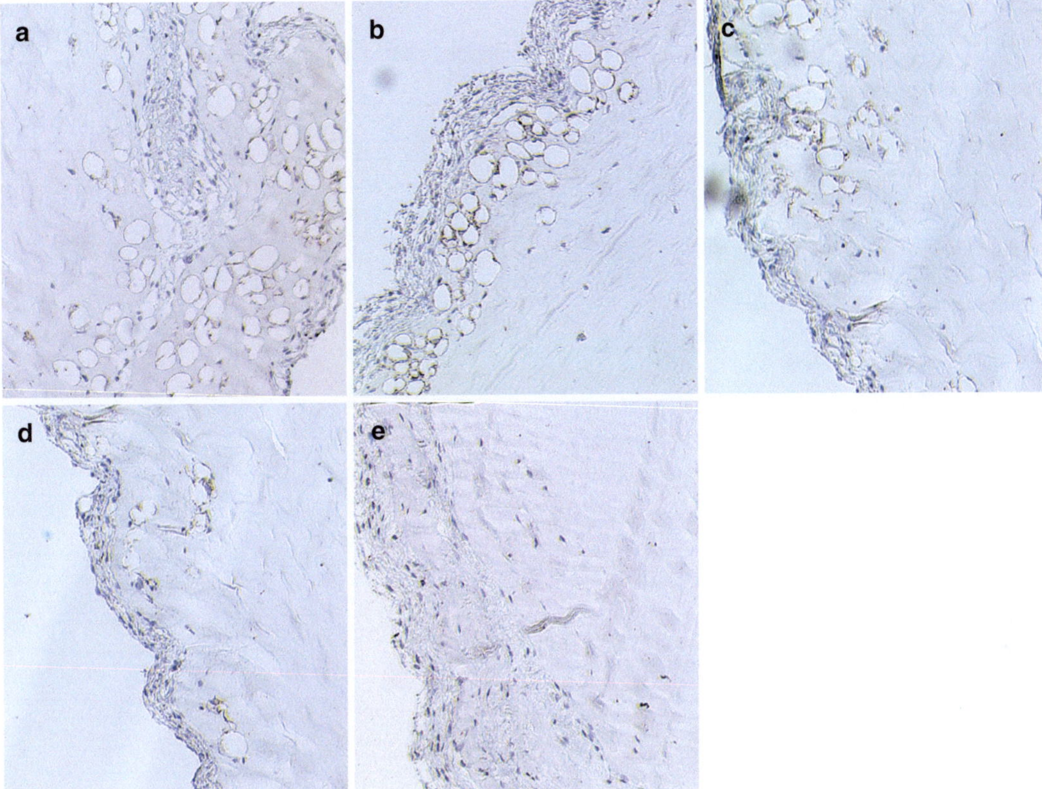

**Fig. 13.1** Influence of different bisphosphonates on angiogenesis in a murine Matrigel angiogenesis model: (**a**) control group, (**b**) treatment with clodronate, (**c**) ibandronate, (**d**) pamidronate, and (**e**) zoledronate. Especially nitrogen-containing bisphosphonates reduce angiogenesis

AAOMS 2009 and 2014), and some radiological and clinical symptoms like pain and impairment of the inferior alveolar nerve function can occur when mucosal integrity is still intact [1, 2, 30, 31].

While all of these theories might play a role in the pathogenesis of BRONJ/MRONJ, none of them neither in isolation nor in combination are able to provide satisfactory answers for questions of paramount importance:

Why is the jawbone almost exclusively the target for BRONJ/MRONJ?

Why are nitrogen-containing bisphosphonates associated with a much higher risk for the development of BRONJ/MRONJ when compared to non-nitrogen-containing bisphosphonates?

What is the role of the proposed risk factors and the so-called "trigger events" in the development of BRONJ/MRONJ? [1, 2, 23].

## Effects of Local Inflammations and pH on BRONJ/MRONJ Pathogenesis

In order to be able to answer the above-mentioned questions, one has to deal with the special features of bisphosphonates on the one hand and of the jawbone on the other hand. Bisphosphonates have the special property of selective uptake by their target organ, namely, the bone. While bisphosphonates bind to the hydroxyapatite at neutral pH values, they are released and activated in acidic milieus [2]. This well-known mechanism takes place physiologically in Howship's lacunae when the bone is resorbed by osteoclasts when the dissociation between the bone (hydroxyapatite) and bisphosphonates is increased in acidic pH values [1, 2, 23, 32]. Up

**Fig. 13.2** Schematic diagram of the potential pathogenesis of bisphosphonate-related osteonecrosis of jaw (BRONJ) with the pH-value reduction as a crucial activator. The minus signs symbolise inhibition of the following processes or tissues; the question marks identify the cursorily investigated pathogenesis theories. The *asterisks* depict the points where risk factors (smoking, diabetes, steroids, chemotherapy, poor oral hygiene, co-morbidity) might aggravate the BRONJ pathogenesis [2] (Reprinted from Otto et al. [2] with kind permission of Elsevier)

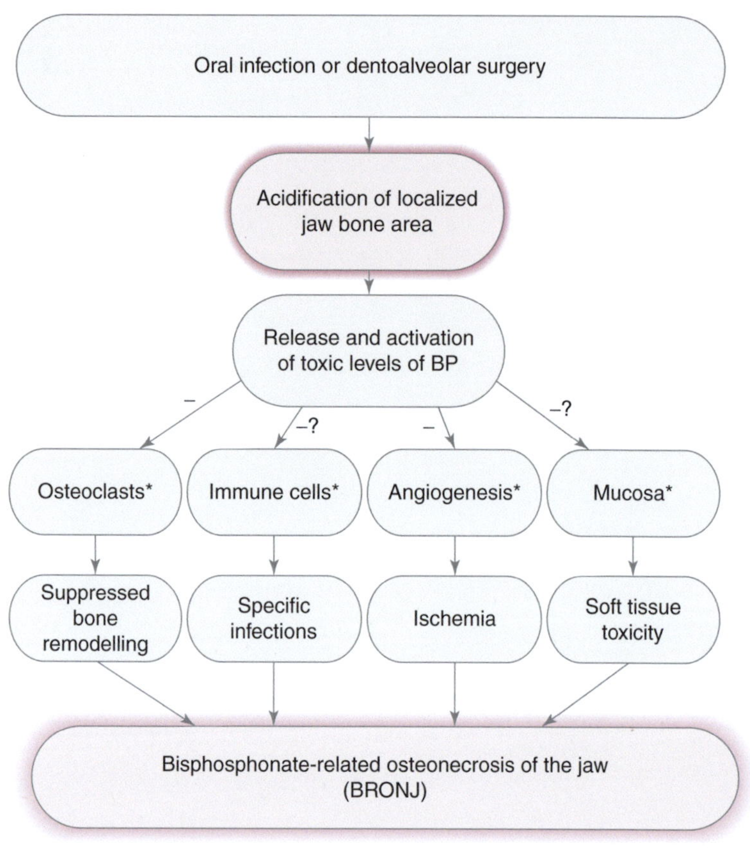


until now, this known mechanism has not been brought into connection with the pathophysiology of bisphosphonate-related osteonecrosis of the jaws although it might play a substantial role in the multi-factorial aetiology of BRONJ/MRONJ. Supporting this, it was already shown in 1991 by Sato and colleagues that alendronate is released in acidic milieus in a rat model [2, 33]. Clinically, acidic milieus commonly occur in the course of infections and during wound healing after surgical procedures [34, 35]. Such conditions occur more often in the jawbones due to the frequency of marginal and apical infections and dento-alveolar surgeries, especially tooth extractions. Thus, these infections can lead to the acidification of localised jawbone areas, resulting in the release and activation especially of nitrogen-containing bisphosphonates into potentially toxic levels which can finally lead to BRONJ/MRONJ (see Fig. 13.2) [1, 2, 32, 36]. This cascade of processes might as well occur

after pressure sores and micro-traumata or even "spontaneously" depending on the duration of intake and route of administration (cumulative dose present in the bone) combined with other potential risk factors such as co-morbidities and co-medications. Non-nitrogen-containing bisphosphonates (e.g. clodronate and etidronate) having lower antiresorptive potencies in general are not activated by these processes. This is in line with the fact that despite decades of clinical use, there are only few reported cases of BRONJ due to the intake of non-nitrogen-containing bisphosphonates [1, 2, 37].

Once a critical concentration of bisphosphonates in solution is reached, there is not only an inhibitory effect on the target cells of bisphosphonate treatment, namely, osteoclasts, but there is an inhibitory and potentially even toxic effect on a number of other cell types including mesenchymal stem cells, osteoblasts and osteocytes as well as endothelial cells, mucosal

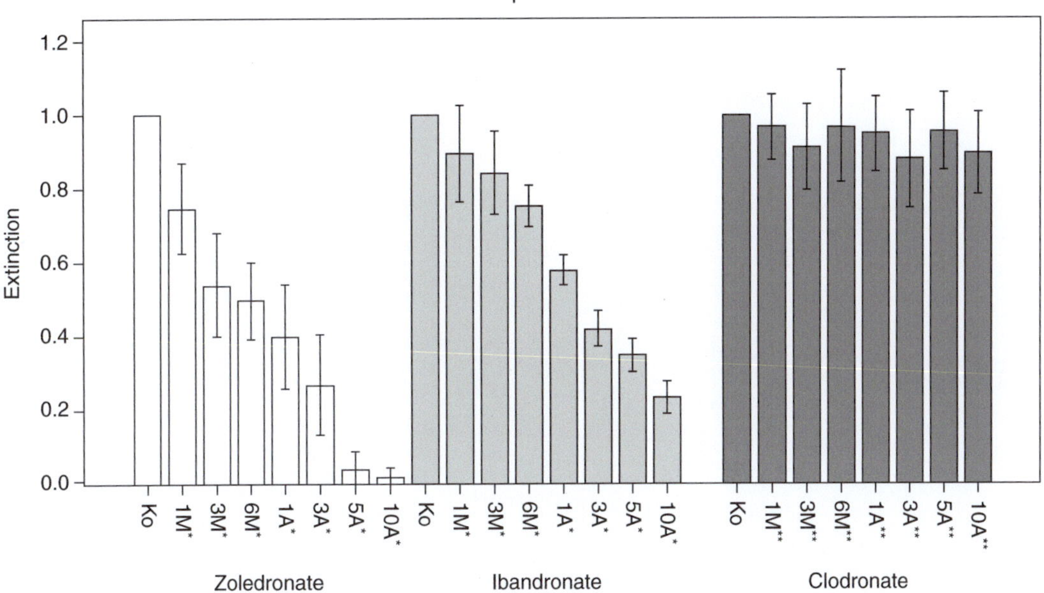



**Fig. 13.3** Quantitative analysis of cell viability and cell activity using WST assay at pH 7.4 for the two N-BPs, zoledronate and ibandronate, and the non-N-BP, clodronate. Zoledronate: control vs. 6-month exposure equivalent $p<0.01$, control vs. 3-year exposure equivalent $p<0.01$ and 6 month- vs. 3-year exposure equivalent $p<0.01$. Ibandronate: control vs. 6-month exposure equivalent $p<0.01$, control vs. 3-year exposure equivalent $p<0.01$ and 6-month vs. 3-year exposure equivalent $p<0.01$. Clodronate: control vs. 6-month exposure equivalent $p=0.214$, control vs. 3-year exposure equivalent $p=0.05$ and 6-month vs. 3-year exposure equivalent $p=0.038$. *Dose-adjusted concentrations equivalent to a treatment in standard oncology dose. **Equimolar concentrations of clodronate as calculated for dose-adjusted concentrations of zoledronate [1] (Reprinted from Otto et al. [1] with kind permission of Elsevier)

cells and immuno-competent cells including macrophages and T-lymphocytes [38, 39]. At this point, all the above-mentioned theories regarding BRONJ/MRONJ development come into play (Fig. 13.2). So, in fact, other existing theories can be linked with this theory [1, 2].

Not only does the above-described theory explain why the jawbone is an almost exclusive target of BRONJ/MRONJ and why apical and marginal infections as well as dento-alveolar surgeries and especially nitrogen-containing bisphosphonates can trigger the occurrence of BRONJ/MRONJ. But it also offers a thorough rationalisation of why chemotherapy, immuno-suppression and systemic disorders such as diabetes can increase the risk for BRONJ/MRONJ. The reason is that these circumstances are associated with a higher risk of wound healing disturbances and local infections [2, 40–42].

## Experimental Data Supporting the Role of Local Inflammations and pH Changes in the Pathogenesis of BRONJ

Indeed, cell cultural data could prove that increasing doses of nitrogen-containing bisphosphonates in solution lead to severe reduction in cell survival and activity of human mesenchymal stem cells while equimolar concentrations of the non-nitrogen-containing bisphosphonate clodronate did not show significant inhibitory effects (see Fig. 13.3) [1]. This is in line with the clinical finding that the majority of BRONJ/MRONJ cases occurred after long-term intravenous treatment with zoledronic acid while there are hardly any cases of ONJ under treatment with non-nitrogen-containing bisphosphonates even though they have been in clinical use for decades [23, 37].

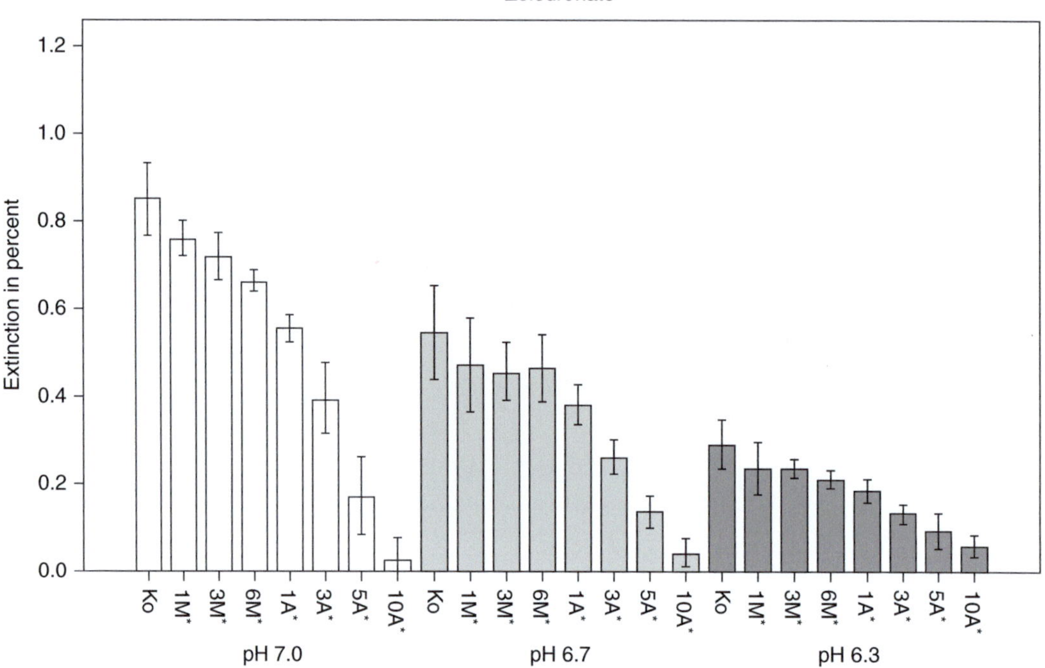


**Fig. 13.4** Quantitative analysis of cell viability and activity using WST assay at pH 7.0, 6.7 and 6.3 for zoledronate. Values are expressed as percentage of activity at pH 7.4, which was set to 1.0 in all cases. *Dose-adjusted concentrations equivalent to a treatment in standard oncology dose. **Equimolar concentrations of clodronate as calculated for dose-adjusted concentrations of zoledronate [1] (Reprinted from Otto et al. [1] with kind permission of Elsevier)

Moreover, these inhibitory effects on cell survival, activity and motility were more pronounced for nitrogen-containing bisphosphonates when pH decreased to 6.2 – comparable to local inflammations in the human body (see Fig. 13.4) [1]. This is in line with the clinical finding that the majority of BRONJ/MRONJ cases are preceded by inflammatory conditions [43].

Furthermore, the group of Agis could prove that once bisphosphonates are bound to the hydroxyapatite, they are completely inert while the same concentration of nitrogen-containing bisphosphonates in solution showed toxic effects towards fibroblasts [44]. The physiological mechanism which brings bisphosphonates which are normally bound to the hydroxyapatite of the bone in solution is local acidification which occurs during inflammatory processes. This condition has a crucial role for the vitality of the jawbone. In addition to inflammatory odontogenic infections, the oral microenvironment becomes acidic with very frequent intake of various foods and drinks [45]. The buffering and washing capacity of saliva plays an important role in the maintenance of the pH level of the oral flora. Although the oral cavity has a naturally low alkaline pH level, it is often influenced by decreases in pH levels in other parts of the body. The buffering capacity of saliva might be insufficient to protect the oral flora-bone-soft tissue junction microenvironment in cases of excessive decreases at pH level which leads to BP release from the bone and probable infection with necrosis in related structures that could explain why BRONJ/MRONJ affects mainly the jawbones [46].

In fact, a recent animal study performed on rats could prove that an alkaline environment achieved using local applications of sodium bicarbonate has a preventive effect with regard to the development of BRONJ/MRONJ after tooth extractions. The authors concluded as well that local inflammations might play a key role for the pathogenesis of BRONJ [46]. Furthermore, Aguirre and co-workers could prove that ONJ like lesions developed in areas with pre-existing periodontitis after the administration of onco-logical doses of zoledronic acid in rats without tooth extractions or other surgical interventions [47]. Recently, a large animal model for BRONJ in mini pigs has been developed, and studies regarding the effect of local infections in large animal models are on the way [48]. Considering the results obtained from these studies, the presence of a damaged gap (either traumatically or periodontally) between the bone and oral flora which causes infection may found to be inductive for the onset of the disease.

## Clinical Data Supporting the Role of Local Inflammations and pH Changes in the Pathogenesis of BRONJ

Besides that there are numerous clinical proofs that local infections play a crucial role for the pathogenesis of medication-related osteonecrosis of the jaws, Dimopoulos et al. showed that implementation of preventive measures prior to the start of bisphosphonate treatment in multiple myeloma patients could significantly reduce the risk of BRONJ [49]. Riplamonti and colleagues could confirm this significant decrease of BRONJ/MRONJ occurrence if preventive measures aiming in avoidance of local infections were implemented prior to the start of bisphosphonate treatment in patients with solid tumours. Even if prophylactic measurements were implemented after the start of bisphosphonate treatment, the risk for BRONJ was lower and lesions could be detected earlier [50].

Besides that, all expert panels and studies recommend to perform dento-alveolar surgeries in patients receiving bisphosphonates in a way that avoids local wound infections in order to prevent the occurrence of BRONJ/MRONJ. If dento-alveolar surgeries in bisphosphonate patients are performed under antibiotic prophylaxis and using local mucosal or mucoperiosteal flaps, the occurrence of BRONJ/MRONJ is significantly reduced.

Furthermore, the progression of the disease can be stopped or at least reduced in the majority of cases simply by local (mouth rinse) and systemic (antibiotics) disinfective measurements, and the treatment of MRONJ cases is basically aimed at the removal of necrotic and infected bone parts accompanied by local mucoperiosteal or flap closure and antibiotic treatment. All of these clinical data give a strong hint for the role of inflammation and infection in the occurrence and progression of the disease.

Besides, there some general considerations that seem to prove the role of pH value with regard to the effects as well as the side effects of bisphosphonates. When taken orally, the main side effect occurs in the gastro-intestinal tract because bisphosphonates are in solution in the strong acidic milieu of the stomach due to gastric acid. When given intravenously, the main side effect occurs in the kidney where once again bisphosphonates are in solution and where there is an acidic milieu of the primary urine close to the tubulus cells.

The increasing numbers of recent publications dealing with the occurrence of osteonecrotic lesions of the external ear channel, a location which is also prone to infections, and the report of occurrence in bone transplants in the jawbone area [51] are more arguments for the crucial role of the local milieu and infections for the development of MRONJ rather than the jawbone or jawbone turnover alone.

## Osteonecrosis Due To RANKL-Inhibitor and VEGF-Inhibitor Treatment

In the last years, new anti-resorptive substances for patients with bone metastases and osteoporotic patients have been used clinically. One class is RANK-ligand inhibitors, namely, denosumab. In normal condition, osteoblasts can activate osteoclast differentiation and clonal expansion via the secretion of RANK ligand. This balance can be disturbed in pathophysiological conditions. Tumour cells can activate osteoblasts via cytokine secretion, increasing

RANK-ligand production. This results in an increased bone resorption by osteoclasts, which plays a key role in the development of bone metastasis. RANK-ligand inhibitors disable this pathophysiologic mechanism. Some anti-angiogenic drugs were also used in cancer patients, alone or in combination with bisphosphonates, and are under the cloud to trigger osteonecrosis of the jaw. The real incidence of medication-related osteonecrosis of the jaw besides bisphosphonate-related osteonecrosis of the jaw is still unknown. Several case series of osteonecrosis of the jaw in patients with cancer who underwent denosumab therapy have been reported in the recent literature, and seemingly, the overall incidence of denosumab-related osteonecrosis of the jaw is similar to that for nitrogen-containing bisphosphonates in this population [52]. The vascular endothelial growth factor (VEGF) receptor plays a major role in neovascularisation, which is a keystone for cancer progression and can be targeted by drugs inhibiting the tyrosine kinase activator or other second messengers. Most neovascularisation inhibitors, such as monoclonal antibody bevacizumab and the kinase inhibitor sunitinib, target the biochemical VEGF signalling pathway and decrease the angiogenic capacity. Unfortunately, cases of bevacizumab-related avascular osteonecrosis of the jaw have been reported in patients in combination therapy with bevacizumab and nitrogen-containing bisphosphonates. There are also few studies reporting sunitinib-related osteonecrosis of the jaw [53, 54]. Therefore, different international guidelines recommend that patients undergoing bisphosphonate treatment, denosumab or bevacizumab therapy, require current dental health and dental examination in frequent intervals [55]. Good oral hygiene status and stopping nicotine abuse should be suggested for all patients requiring such treatments. Given the fact that the processes of infection defense and wound healing in bone are in strong need for remodelling and angiogenesis in the respective bone it is not surprising that the uncoupling of these processes can lead to medication-related osteonecrosis of the jaw.

# References


1. Otto S, Pautke C, Opelz C, Westphal I, Drosse I, Schwager J, Bauss F, Ehrenfeld M, Schieker M. Osteonecrosis of the jaw: effect of bisphosphonate type, local concentration, and acidic milieu on the pathomechanism. J Oral Maxillofac Surg. 2010;68:2837–45.
2. Otto S, Hafner S, Mast G, Tischer T, Volkmer E, Schieker M, Sturzenbaum SR, von Tresckow E, Kolk A, Ehrenfeld M, Pautke C. Bisphosphonate-related osteonecrosis of the jaw: is pH the missing part in the pathogenesis puzzle? J Oral Maxillofac Surg. 2010;68:1158–61.
3. Allen MR. The effects of bisphosphonates on jaw bone remodeling, tissue properties, and extraction healing. Odontology. 2011;99:8–17.
4. McDonald MM, Dulai S, Godfrey C, Amanat N, Sztynda T, Little DG. Bolus or weekly zoledronic acid administration does not delay endochondral fracture repair but weekly dosing enhances delays in hard callus remodeling. Bone. 2008;43:653–62.
5. Reid IR. Osteonecrosis of the jaw: who gets it, and why? Bone. 2009;44:4–10.
6. Vignery A, Baron R. Dynamic histomorphometry of alveolar bone remodeling in the adult rat. Anat Rec. 1980;196:191–200.
7. Huja SS, Fernandez SA, Hill KJ, Li Y. Remodeling dynamics in the alveolar process in skeletally mature dogs. Anat Rec A Discov Mol Cell Evol Biol. 2006;288:1243–9.
8. Walter C, Klein MO, Pabst A, Al-Nawas B, Duschner H, Ziebart T. Influence of bisphosphonates on endothelial cells, fibroblasts, and osteogenic cells. Clin Oral Investig. 2010;14:35–41.
9. Walter C, Pabst A, Ziebart T, Klein M, Al-Nawas B. Bisphosphonates affect migration ability and cell viability of HUVEC, fibroblasts and osteoblasts in vitro. Oral Dis. 2011;17:194–9.
10. Bauss F, Pfister T, Papapoulos S. Ibandronate uptake in the jaw is similar to long bones and vertebrae in the rat. J Bone Miner Metab. 2008;26:406–8.
11. Hansen T, Kunkel M, Weber A, James Kirkpatrick C. Osteonecrosis of the jaws in patients treated with bisphosphonates – histomorphologic analysis in comparison with infected osteoradionecrosis. J Oral Pathol Med. 2006;35:155–60.
12. Sedghizadeh PP, Kumar SK, Gorur A, Schaudinn C, Shuler CF, Costerton JW. Identification of microbial biofilms in osteonecrosis of the jaws secondary to bisphosphonate therapy. J Oral Maxillofac Surg. 2008;66:767–75.
13. Wolf AM, Rumpold H, Tilg H, Gastl G, Gunsilius E, Wolf D. The effect of zoledronic acid on the function and differentiation of myeloid cells. Haematologica. 2006;91:1165–71.
14. Roelofs AJ, Jauhiainen M, Monkkonen H, Rogers MJ, Monkkonen J, Thompson K. Peripheral blood

monocytes are responsible for gammadelta T cell activation induced by zoledronic acid through accumulation of IPP/DMAPP. Br J Haematol. 2009;144:245–50.

15. Scavelli C, Di Pietro G, Cirulli T, Coluccia M, Boccarelli A, Giannini T, Mangialardi G, Bertieri R, Coluccia AM, Ribatti D, Dammacco F, Vacca A. Zoledronic acid affects over-angiogenic phenotype of endothelial cells in patients with multiple myeloma. Mol Cancer Ther. 2007;6:3256–62.

16. Fournier P, Boissier S, Filleur S, Guglielmi J, Cabon F, Colombel M, Clezardin P. Bisphosphonates inhibit angiogenesis in vitro and testosterone-stimulated vascular regrowth in the ventral prostate in castrated rats. Cancer Res. 2002;62:6538–44.

17. Ziebart T, Pabst A, Klein MO, Kammerer P, Gauss L, Brullmann D, Al-Nawas B, Walter C. Bisphosphonates: restrictions for vasculogenesis and angiogenesis: inhibition of cell function of endothelial progenitor cells and mature endothelial cells in vitro. Clin Oral Investig. 2011;15:105–11.

18. Tsai SH, Huang PH, Chang WC, Tsai HY, Lin CP, Leu HB, Wu TC, Chen JW, Lin SJ. Zoledronate inhibits ischemia-induced neovascularization by impairing the mobilization and function of endothelial progenitor cells. PLoS One. 2012;7:e41065.

19. Ziebart T, Ziebart J, Gauss L, Pabst A, Ackermann M, Smeets R, Konerding MA, Walter C. Investigation of inhibitory effects on EPC-mediated neovascularization by different bisphosphonates for cancer therapy. Biomed Rep. 2013;1:719–22.

20. Pabst AM, Ziebart T, Ackermann M, Konerding MA, Walter C. Bisphosphonates' antiangiogenic potency in the development of bisphosphonate-associated osteonecrosis of the jaws: influence on microvessel sprouting in an in vivo 3D Matrigel assay. Clin Oral Investig. 2014;18(3):1015–22.

21. Cetinkaya BO, Keles GC, Ayas B, Gurgor P. Effects of risedronate on alveolar bone loss and angiogenesis: a stereologic study in rats. J Periodontol. 2008;79:1950–61.

22. Deckers MM, Van Beek ER, Van Der Pluijm G, Wetterwald A, Van Der Wee-Pals L, Cecchini MG, Papapoulos SE, Lowik CW. Dissociation of angiogenesis and osteoclastogenesis during endochondral bone formation in neonatal mice. J Bone Miner Res. 2002;17:998–1007.

23. Otto S, Schreyer C, Hafner S, Mast G, Ehrenfeld M, Sturzenbaum S, Pautke C. Bisphosphonate-related osteonecrosis of the jaws – characteristics, risk factors, clinical features, localization and impact on oncological treatment. J Craniomaxillofac Surg. 2012;40:303–9.

24. Kharazmi M, Hallberg P, Warfvinge G. Bisphosphonate-associated osteonecrosis of the external auditory canal. J Craniofac Surg. 2013;24:2218–20.

25. Polizzotto MN, Cousins V, Schwarer AP. Bisphosphonate-associated osteonecrosis of the auditory canal. Br J Haematol. 2006;132:114.

26. Longo R, Castellana MA, Gasparini G. Bisphosphonate-related osteonecrosis of the jaw and left thumb. J Clin Oncol. 2009;27:e242–3.

27. Reid IR, Bolland MJ, Grey AB. Is bisphosphonate-associated osteonecrosis of the jaw caused by soft tissue toxicity? Bone. 2007;41:318–20.

28. Sonis ST, Elting LS, Keefe D, Peterson DE, Schubert M, Hauer-Jensen M, Bekele BN, Raber-Durlacher J, Donnelly JP, Rubenstein EB. Perspectives on cancer therapy-induced mucosal injury: pathogenesis, measurement, epidemiology, and consequences for patients. Cancer. 2004;100:1995–2025.

29. Landesberg R, Cozin M, Cremers S, Woo V, Kousteni S, Sinha S, Garrett-Sinha L, Raghavan S. Inhibition of oral mucosal cell wound healing by bisphosphonates. J Oral Maxillofac Surg. 2008;66:839–47.

30. Otto S, Hafner S, Grotz KA. The role of inferior alveolar nerve involvement in bisphosphonate-related osteonecrosis of the jaw. J Oral Maxillofac Surg. 2009;67:589–92.

31. Ruggiero SL, Mehrotra B, Rosenberg TJ, Engroff SL. Osteonecrosis of the jaws associated with the use of bisphosphonates: a review of 63 cases. J Oral Maxillofac Surg. 2004;62:527–34.

32. Russell RG, Watts NB, Ebetino FH, Rogers MJ. Mechanisms of action of bisphosphonates: similarities and differences and their potential influence on clinical efficacy. Osteoporos Int. 2008;19:733–59.

33. Sato M, Grasser W, Endo N, Akins R, Simmons H, Thompson DD, Golub E, Rodan GA. Bisphosphonate action. Alendronate localization in rat bone and effects on osteoclast ultrastructure. J Clin Invest. 1991;88:2095–105.

34. Hays RC, Mandell GL. PO2, pH, and redox potential of experimental abscesses. Proc Soc Exp Biol Med. 1974;147:29–30.

35. Bertram P, Treutner KH, Klosterhalfen B, Arlt G, Anurov M, Polivoda M, Ottinger A, Schumpelick V [Artificial pressure increase in subcutaneous abscess with evidence of general systemic reaction]. Langenbecks Arch Chir. 1997;382:291–4.

36. Nancollas GH, Tang R, Phipps RJ, Henneman Z, Gulde S, Wu W, Mangood A, Russell RG, Ebetino FH. Novel insights into actions of bisphosphonates on bone: differences in interactions with hydroxyapatite. Bone. 2006;38:617–27.

37. Abu-Id MH, Warnke PH, Gottschalk J, Springer I, Wiltfang J, Acil Y, Russo PA, Kreusch T. "Bis-phossy jaws" – high and low risk factors for bisphosphonate-induced osteonecrosis of the jaw. J Craniomaxillofac Surg. 2008;36:95–103.

38. Kimachi K, Kajiya H, Nakayama S, Ikebe T, Okabe K. Zoledronic acid inhibits RANK expression and migration of osteoclast precursors during osteoclastogenesis. Naunyn Schmiedebergs Arch Pharmacol. 2011;383:297–308.

39. Pazianas M. Osteonecrosis of the jaw and the role of macrophages. J Natl Cancer Inst. 2011;103:232–40.

40. Hess LM, Jeter JM, Benham-Hutchins M, Alberts DS. Factors associated with osteonecrosis of the jaw among bisphosphonate users. Am J Med. 2008;121: 475–483.e3.

41. Bamias A, Kastritis E, Bamia C, Moulopoulos LA, Melakopoulos I, Bozas G, Koutsoukou V, Gika D, Anagnostopoulos A, Papadimitriou C, Terpos E, Dimopoulos MA. Osteonecrosis of the jaw in cancer after treatment with bisphosphonates: incidence and risk factors. J Clin Oncol. 2005;23:8580–7.

42. Hoff AO, Toth BB, Altundag K, Johnson MM, Warneke CL, Hu M, Nooka A, Sayegh G, Guarneri V, Desrouleaux K, Cui J, Adamus A, Gagel RF, Hortobagyi GN. Frequency and risk factors associated with osteonecrosis of the jaw in cancer patients treated with intravenous bisphosphonates. J Bone Miner Res. 2008;23:826–36.

43. Lesclous P, Abi Najm S, Carrel JP, Baroukh B, Lombardi T, Willi JP, Rizzoli R, Saffar JL, Samson J. Bisphosphonate-associated osteonecrosis of the jaw: a key role of inflammation? Bone. 2009;45:843–52.

44. Agis H, Blei J, Watzek G, Gruber R. Is zoledronate toxic to human periodontal fibroblasts? J Dent Res. 2010;89:40–5.

45. Osterberg T, Landahl S, Hedegard B. Salivary flow, saliva, pH and buffering capacity in 70-year-old men and women. Correlation to dental health, dryness in the mouth, disease and drug treatment. J Oral Rehabil. 1984;11:157–70.

46. Dayisoylu EH, Ungor C, Tosun E, Ersoz S, Duman MK, Taskesen F, Senel FC. Does an alkaline environment prevent the development of bisphosphonate-related osteonecrosis of the jaw? An experimental study in rats. Oral Surg Oral Med Oral Pathol Oral Radiol. 2014;117(3):329–34.

47. Aguirre JI, Akhter MP, Kimmel DB, Pingel JE, Williams A, Jorgensen M, Kesavalu L, Wronski TJ. Oncologic doses of zoledronic acid induce osteonecrosis of the jaw-like lesions in rice rats (Oryzomys palustris) with periodontitis. J Bone Miner Res. 2012; 27:2130–43.

48. Pautke C, Kreutzer K, Weitz J, Knodler M, Munzel D, Wexel G, Otto S, Hapfelmeier A, Sturzenbaum S, Tischer T. Bisphosphonate related osteonecrosis of the jaw: a minipig large animal model. Bone. 2012; 51:592–9.

49. Dimopoulos MA, Kastritis E, Bamia C, Melakopoulos I, Gika D, Roussou M, Migkou M, Eleftherakis-Papaiakovou E, Christoulas D, Terpos E, Bamias A. Reduction of osteonecrosis of the jaw (ONJ) after implementation of preventive measures in patients with multiple myeloma treated with zoledronic acid. Ann Oncol. 2009;20:117–20.

50. Ripamonti CI, Maniezzo M, Campa T, Fagnoni E, Brunelli C, Saibene G, Bareggi C, Ascani L, Cislaghi E. Decreased occurrence of osteonecrosis of the jaw after implementation of dental preventive measures in solid tumour patients with bone metastases treated with bisphosphonates. The experience of the National Cancer Institute of Milan. Ann Oncol. 2009;20:137–45.

51. Pautke C, Otto S, Reu S, Kolk A, Ehrenfeld M, Sturzenbaum S, Wolff KD. Bisphosphonate related osteonecrosis of the jaw–manifestation in a microvascular iliac bone flap. Oral Oncol. 2011;47:425–9.

52. Sivolella S, Lumachi F, Stellini E, Favero L. Denosumab and anti-angiogenetic drug-related osteonecrosis of the jaw: an uncommon but potentially severe disease. Anticancer Res. 2013;33:1793–7.

53. Koch FP, Walter C, Hansen T, Jager E, Wagner W. Osteonecrosis of the jaw related to sunitinib. Oral Maxillofac Surg. 2011;15:63–6.

54. Ayllon J, Launay-Vacher V, Medioni J, Cros C, Spano JP, Oudard S. Osteonecrosis of the jaw under bisphosphonate and antiangiogenic therapies: cumulative toxicity profile? Ann Oncol. 2009;20:600–1.

55. Hellstein JW, Adler RA, Edwards B, Jacobsen PL, Kalmar JR, Koka S, Migliorati CA, Ristic H. Managing the care of patients receiving antiresorptive therapy for prevention and treatment of osteoporosis: executive summary of recommendations from the American Dental Association Council on Scientific Affairs. J Am Dent Assoc. 2011;142:1243–51.

Noam Yarom and Stefano Fedele

**Abstract**

Management of Medication-Related Osteonecrosis of the Jaw is challenging and outcomes of treatment are unpredictable. There is wide consensus that risk of ONJ can be, at least in part, reduced through control of a number of factors associated with increased likelihood of ONJ development. Robust evidence however remains limited. The aim of this chapter is to provide a comprehensive summary of available evidence upon risk-reduction measures for patients at risk of ONJ.

## Introduction

Medication-Related Osteonecrosis of the Jaw (ONJ) is a potentially severe adverse side effect associated with the use of several medications, most notably bisphosphonates and denosumab [1]. Treatment of ONJ remains challenging and there remains no definitive curative with the possible exception of surgical resection in selected cases. Considering that the vast majority of patients are also affected by metastatic incurable cancer, therapy of ONJ is often aimed at controlling painful symptoms and infection [2].

Several studies have reported a number of risk factors that increase the likelihood of patients to develop ONJ (see chapter 3, page 27); accordingly, it has been suggested that control of these factors could translate into a reduced risk of ONJ. During the last decade, a number of risk-reduction strategies have been suggested and introduced [3–5]. However, relevant recommendations have been mostly based on expert opinion with little, if any, solid supporting clinical evidence. There remains virtually no well-designed randomised controlled trial and very few small prospective observational studies that have investigated the efficacy of risk-reduction strategies in individuals exposed to anti-resorptive agents. The aim of this chapter is to provide a

N. Yarom, DMD (✉) • S. Fedele, DDS, PhD
Oral Medicine Unit, UCL Eastman Dental Institute,
256 Gray's Inn Road, University College London,
London WC1X 8LD, UK
e-mail: noamyar@post.tau.ac.il

S. Otto (ed.), *Medication-Related Osteonecrosis of the Jaws: Bisphosphonates, Denosumab, and New Agents*,
DOI 10.1007/978-3-662-43733-9_14, © Springer-Verlag Berlin Heidelberg 2015

comprehensive summary of available evidence regarding risk-reduction measures for patients at risk of ONJ. The relevance of genetics and bone turnover markers for the prediction of ONJ will be discussed as well. Considering the different risk profiles of cancer patients with respect to individuals with osteoporosis [6], risk-reduction strategies will be discussed separately for these two populations.

## Risk-Reduction Strategies in Patients with Cancer

### Before Commencement of Anti-resorptive Therapy

There is robust evidence that a significant number of ONJ cases in cancer patients are associated with a history of surgical procedures to the jaw bones (e.g. dental extraction and placement of osteointegrated implants) [7]. Although the exact portion of ONJ cases associated with surgical procedures vs those who develop ONJ "spontaneously" remains unclear, recent studies suggest that at least 50–60 % of all ONJ cases can present jawbone surgery as likely trigger [7]. As consequence, avoidance of surgical procedures during and after anti-resorptive therapy has been suggested to represent a potentially effective risk-reduction strategy. Most recommendations suggest that cancer patients who are due to start anti-resorptive therapy should be examined by an oral health practitioner with the aim of restoring diseased dentition and removing non-restorable teeth before treatment initiation. The ultimate goal is to prevent the clinical scenario where patients may require surgical intervention to manage dental infection during or after anti-resorptive therapy.

It is also important to highlight that available literature has suggested an association between ONJ development and active dental infection. Therefore, resolution of dental infection via restorative therapy is also believed to represent a risk-reduction strategy to be performed before commencement of anti-resorptive therapy, where possible.

It is suggested that oncologists refer patients to oral health practitioner as early as possible in order to allow mucosal and possibly bone healing (about 3–6 weeks) in individuals who receive extraction of non-restorable teeth before initiation of anti-resorptive therapy. It is also important that patients are instructed regarding regular oral hygiene procedures, as well as receive meticulous professional dental plaque and calculus removal 2–4 times per year and have caries and periodontal disease treated as soon as they are diagnosed. This is believed to increase the chances of preventing acute dental infection and the need of surgical extraction during anti-resorptive therapy.

Unfortunately, the real efficacy of the above risk-reduction strategies was only evaluated in a few observational uncontrolled studies. A reduction in the occurrence of ONJ among solid cancer patients was observed after the implementation of a prophylactic dental programme compared with historical controls [3, 4]. Similar findings were found among multiple myeloma patients treated with zoledronic acid [5]. In conclusion, although the above measures are routinely applied in many centres worldwide, robust scientific evidence is lacking as relevant studies are burdened by a number of significant limitations.

### After Commencement of Anti-resorptive Therapy

Risk-reduction strategies in individuals who have commenced anti-resorptive therapy are aimed at avoiding acute dental infection and surgery to the jawbones [2, 8]. This includes elective surgical procedures, such as placement of osteointegrated implants, which should not be performed in these patients.

There is general agreement that individuals who are using anti-resorptive agents should be instructed to keep meticulous oral hygiene habits and receive regular professional dental plaque and calculus removal [2, 8]. Dental caries and periodontal infections that develop during anti-resorptive therapy should be promptly managed with restorative and nonsurgical procedures as soon as the medical status of the patient allows.

Most recommendations suggest that nonrestorable or fractured teeth should not be extracted [8]. Root canal treatment should be the treatment of choice for all infected teeth, including those that are non-restorable whose roots can be left in situ. Similarly, periodontally diseased teeth should be managed conservatively with regular scaling and root planning so as to minimise the risk of acute infection.

Management of existing dental implants should follow similar recommendations, as it has been documented that ONJ may develop around dental implants [9].

Notwithstanding the recommendation that surgical procedures should be avoided, there are instances where dental extraction represents the only reliable treatment. Examples include severe periodontitis causing tooth mobility, root fractures, as well as recurrent infections not responding to conservative procedures. In these cases conventional dental extractions would significantly increase the likelihood of ONJ development. A number of potential strategies have been suggested to minimise the risk of ONJ in these individuals, including antibiotic cover [10], "atraumatic extraction" [11], primary closure of surgical site [12], orthodontic extrusion [13], use of plasma rich in growth factors (PRGF) [14], Nd:YAG low-level laser [15], etc. Unfortunately, there remains very little evidence to support any of these strategies due to the lack of well-designed case-control randomised clinical trials.

Patients' prognosis should be taken into account while planning dental treatment. Patients with grave prognosis should be approached differently from patients with life expectancy of a few years.

Dentists should always keep in mind that those patients are usually on ongoing anti-neoplastic treatment such as chemotherapy and radiotherapy. Therefore, a thorough medical status update should be performed before each dental treatment session.

## Patients with Previous History of Exposure to Anti-resorptive Therapy

Bisphosphonates have high bonding affinity for bone tissue and are released very slowly over time and excreted in urine. The terminal half-life of bisphosphonates is similar to that of bone mineral, approximately 10.5 years, and therefore some of their skeletal effects may last for years after treatment stops [16]. Therefore, it is generally recommended that dento-alveolar surgery in cancer patients who had been exposed to IV BPs should be avoided for many years beyond drug cessation. There is no solid evidence regarding the washout period of BPs from the jaws. Moreover, it is not clear how long it would take for the bony tissues to restore their normal remodelling properties after total or partial clearance of BPs.

## Other Risk-Reduction Strategies

Available preliminary genetics studies report that certain genetic variants may be associated with increased risk of ONJ, therefore suggesting that some individuals may have a genetic predisposition to the toxic effects of anti-resorptive agents. Studies using dedicated gene approach as well as genome-wide association studies (GWAs) have identified a number of potentially associated gene variants that need further validation and replication [17–19]. It is expected that robust identification of an associated predisposing gene variant would lead to personalised strategies and patient stratification so as to reduce the risk of ONJ development after exposure to anti-resorptive medications.

Serum cross-linked C-telopeptide of type I collagen (CTX) is a marker of bone turnover and has been suggested as potential predictor of the risk of ONJ in individuals who have been exposed to anti-resorptive agents [20]. There remains however significant controversy regarding the validity of this marker in estimating the risk of ONJ [21].

## Risk-Reduction Strategies in Patients with Osteoporosis

Similarly to ONJ development in cancer patients, there is robust evidence that a significant number of ONJ cases in osteoporosis patients are associated with a history of surgical procedures to the jaw bones (e.g. dental extraction and placement of osteointegrated implants) [6]. Similarly, available literature has suggested an association between ONJ development and active dental infection.

However, the risk of ONJ development in this population is significantly lower than that observed in the cancer setting [2], and therefore most recommendations suggest that risk-reduction strategies are not as crucial [2]. The rationale is that ONJ development in osteoporosis patients exposed to anti-resorptive therapy is so uncommon (approximately 0.1 %) that no particular effort is required in attempting to minimise the two most important risk factors, namely, surgical procedures and acute dental infection. Most authors agree that these individuals do not need urgent referral before commencing anti-resorptive therapy in order to receive surgical therapy and start conservative dental treatment of diseased dentition. Provision of routine dental check-ups and dental treatment should be recommended, albeit with no significant differences with respect to individuals who are not on anti-resorptive medications. Similarly, surgical procedures, including elective surgery (e.g. implant placement), are not contraindicated in individuals with osteoporosis who are using anti-resorptive medications. Nevertheless, prior to any surgical procedure, the patient should be informed regarding the low risk for ONJ. The healing process should be monitored and early intervention is recommended for any signs and symptoms associate with ONJ.

Indeed the same dental recommendations that are targeted at healthy individuals with respect to oral hygiene procedures, regular dental check-ups, and professional plaque and calculus removal can also apply to the population of individuals with osteoporosis who are due to start or are using anti-resorptive therapy.

Attempts to stratify this population into risk categories (e.g. using a cut-off of 3 years of anti-resorptive therapy or serum CTX values) have never been validated and represent expert opinion rather than robust evidence.

### Conclusions

Management of Medication-Related Osteonecrosis of the Jaw is challenging and outcomes of treatment are unpredictable. There is wide consensus that risk of ONJ can be, at least in part, reduced through control of a number of factors associated with increased likelihood of ONJ development. There is some weak and limited evidence that prevention of dental infection and avoidance of dento-alveolar surgery can reduce the risk of ONJ development in cancer patients using intravenous bisphosphonates. Therefore, potentially effective risk-reduction measures in the cancer setting would include provision of prophylactic dentistry before the start of bisphosphonate therapy, including restorative dental treatment and extraction of non-restorable dentition. Provision of regular dental reviews and restorative dental treatment is also recommended during anti-resorptive therapy so as to avoid dento-alveolar infections and need for surgical intervention. In those instances where dental extractions cannot be avoided, there are no clear indications of effective risk-reduction measures.

Because the risk of ONJ in osteoporosis patients taking oral BP is very low, there is a general consensus that no particular risk-reduction measure is warranted beyond regular dental check-ups and routine dental treatment before and during anti-resorptive therapy.

Genetic and serum biomarkers predictive of the risk of developing ONJ are being investigated.

## References


1. Yarom N, Elad S, Madrid C, Migliorati CA. Osteonecrosis of the jaws induced by drugs other than bisphosphonates – a call to update terminology in light of new data. Oral Oncol. 2010;46:e1.
2. Ruggiero SL, Dodson TB, Assael LA, Landesberg R, Marx RE, Mehrotra B. Task Force on Bisphosphonate-Related Osteonecrosis of the Jaws, American Association of Oral and Maxillofacial Surgeons. American Association of Oral and Maxillofacial Surgeons position paper on bisphosphonate-related osteonecrosis of the jaw – 2009 update. J Oral Maxillofac Surg. 2009; 67:2–12.
3. Ripamonti CI, Maniezzo M, Campa T, Fagnoni E, Brunelli C, Saibene G, Bareggi C, Ascani L, Cislaghi E. Decreased occurrence of osteonecrosis of the jaw after

implementation of dental preventive measures in solid tumour patients with bone metastases treated with bisphosphonates. The experience of the National Cancer Institute of Milan. Ann Oncol. 2009;20:137–45.

4. Vandone AM, Donadio M, Mozzati M, Ardine M, Polimeni MA, Beatrice S, Ciuffreda L, Scoletta M. Impact of dental care in the prevention of bisphosphonate-associated osteonecrosis of the jaw: a single-center clinical experience. Ann Oncol. 2012;23:193–200.

5. Dimopoulos MA, Kastritis E, Bamia C, Melakopoulos I, Gika D, Roussou M, Migkou M, Eleftherakis-Papaiakovou E, Christoulas D, Terpos E, Bamias A. Reduction of osteonecrosis of the jaw (ONJ) after implementation of preventive measures in patients with multiple myeloma treated with zoledronic acid. Ann Oncol. 2009;20:117–20.

6. Yarom N, Yahalom R, Shoshani Y, Hamed W, Regev E, Elad S. Osteonecrosis of the jaw induced by orally administered bisphosphonates: incidence, clinical features, predisposing factors and treatment outcome. Osteoporos Int. 2007;18:1363–70.

7. Lazarovici TS, Yahalom R, Taicher S, Elad S, Hardan I, Yarom N. Bisphosphonate-related osteonecrosis of the jaws: a single-center study of 101 patients. J Oral Maxillofac Surg. 2009;67:850–5.

8. Khosla S, Burr D, Cauley J, Dempster DW, Ebeling PR, Felsenberg D, Gagel RF, Gilsanz V, Guise T, Koka S, McCauley LK, McGowan J, McKee MD, Mohla S, Pendrys DG, Raisz LG, Ruggiero SL, Shafer DM, Shum L, Silverman SL, Van Poznak CH, Watts N, Woo SB, Shane E, American Society for Bone and Mineral Research. Bisphosphonate-associated osteonecrosis of the jaw: report of a task force of the American Society for Bone and Mineral Research. J Bone Miner Res. 2007;22:1479–91.

9. Lazarovici TS, Yahalom R, Taicher S, Schwartz-Arad D, Peleg O, Yarom N. Bisphosphonate-related osteonecrosis of the jaw associated with dental implants. J Oral Maxillofac Surg. 2010;68:790–6.

10. Ferlito S, Puzzo S, Liardo C. Preventive protocol for tooth extractions in patients treated with zoledronate: a case series. J Oral Maxillofac Surg. 2011;69:e1–4.

11. Regev E, Lustmann J, Nashef R. Atraumatic teeth extraction in bisphosphonate-treated patients. J Oral Maxillofac Surg. 2008;66:1157–61.

12. Heufelder MJ, Hendricks J, Remmerbach T, Frerich B, Hemprich A, Wilde F. Principles of oral surgery for prevention of bisphosphonate-related osteonecrosis of the jaw. Oral Surg Oral Med Oral Pathol Oral Radiol. 2014;117(6):e429–35.

13. Smidt A, Lipovetsky-Adler M, Sharon E. Forced eruption as an alternative to tooth extraction in long-term use of oral bisphosphonates: review, risks and technique. J Am Dent Assoc. 2012;143:1303–12.

14. Scoletta M, Arduino PG, Pol R, Arata V, Silvestri S, Chiecchio A, Mozzati M. Initial experience on the outcome of teeth extractions in intravenous bisphosphonate-treated patients: a cautionary report. J Oral Maxillofac Surg. 2011;69:456–62.

15. Vescovi P, Meleti M, Merigo E, Manfredi M, Fornaini C, Guidotti R, Nammour S. Case series of 589 tooth extractions in patients under bisphosphonates therapy. Proposal of a clinical protocol supported by Nd:YAG low-level laser therapy. Med Oral Patol Oral Cir Bucal. 2013;18:e680–5.

16. Black DM, Schwartz AV, Ensrud KE, Cauley JA, Levis S, Quandt SA, Satterfield S, Wallace RB, Bauer DC, Palermo L, Wehren LE, Lombardi A, Santora AC, Cummings SR, FLEX Research Group. Effects of continuing or stopping alendronate after 5 years of treatment: the Fracture Intervention Trial Long-term Extension (FLEX): a randomized trial. JAMA. 2006;296:2927–38.

17. Sarasquete ME, García-Sanz R, Marín L, Alcoceba M, Chillón MC, Balanzategui A, Santamaria C, Rosiñol L, de la Rubia J, Hernandez MT, Garcia-Navarro I, Lahuerta JJ, González M, San Miguel JF. Bisphosphonate-related osteonecrosis of the jaw is associated with polymorphisms of the cytochrome P450 CYP2C8 in multiple myeloma: a genome-wide single nucleotide polymorphism analysis. Blood. 2008;112:2709–12.

18. Nicoletti P, Cartsos VM, Palaska PK, Shen Y, Floratos A, Zavras AI. Genomewide pharmacogenetics of bisphosphonate-induced osteonecrosis of the jaw: the role of RBMS3. Oncologist. 2012;17:279–87.

19. Katz J, Gong Y, Salmasinia D, Hou W, Burkley B, Ferreira P, Casanova O, Langaee TY, Moreb JS. Genetic polymorphisms and other risk factors associated with bisphosphonate induced osteonecrosis of the jaw. Int J Oral Maxillofac Surg. 2011;40:605–11.

20. Lazarovici TS, Mesilaty-Gross S, Vered I, Pariente C, Kanety H, Givol N, Yahalom R, Taicher S, Yarom N. Serologic bone markers for predicting development of osteonecrosis of the jaw in patients receiving bisphosphonates. J Oral Maxillofac Surg. 2010;68:2241–7.

21. Kim JW, Kong KA, Kim SJ, Choi SK, Cha IH, Kim MR. Prospective biomarker evaluation in patients with osteonecrosis of the jaw who received bisphosphonates. Bone. 2013;57:201–5.

# Animal Models of Medication-Related Osteonecrosis of the Jaw

**15**

Matthew R. Allen


**Abstract**

Bisphosphonates have been extensively studied with hundreds of studies describing how they affect various skeletal parameters using animal models. Despite this extensive body of literature, when the clinical description of osteonecrosis of the jaw emerged in 2003/2004, the relative paucity of data describing how bisphosphonates affect the maxillofacial skeletal became clear. Over the past 10 years, there have been several dozen publications showing various aspects of ONJ in mice, rats, dogs, and swine treated with bisphosphonates. Recent work has extended these findings to treatment with RANK-L inhibitors. The establishment of these models will be essential in propelling the field forward to understand the underlying pathophysiology of ONJ and ultimately finding a way to prevent or cure this debilitating condition.


Bisphosphonates, a class of anti-osteoporotic agents that work by reducing osteoclast activity, have been extensively studied in the preclinical bone literature [1]. Since the initial description by Schenk and colleagues of etidronate-induced increased metaphyseal bone volume in the growing rats [2], hundreds of studies have been published describing how bisphosphonates affect various skeletal parameters using animal models. Despite this extensive body of literature, when the clinical description of osteonecrosis of the jaw (ONJ) emerged in 2003/2004 [3, 4], the relative paucity of data describing how bisphosphonates affect the maxillofacial skeletal became clear. Questions regarding the pathophysiology of ONJ were centered on basic questions that in most cases could only be answered using animal models. Were bisphosphonates having a unique effect on the oral cavity compared to the axial/appendicular skeleton; was dose/duration of bisphosphonate influencing the manifestation of exposed bone; what role was altered vasculature/microbial environment playing in the disease manifestation; and could ONJ be treated or prevented [5]? It was clear that an animal model of ONJ would be essential for answering these questions [6].


M.R. Allen
Department of Anatomy and Cell Biology,
Indiana University School of Medicine,
635 Barnhill Drive MS 5035, Indianapolis,
IN 46202, USA
e-mail: matallen@iupui.edu



S. Otto (ed.), *Medication-Related Osteonecrosis of the Jaws: Bisphosphonates, Denosumab, and New Agents*,
DOI 10.1007/978-3-662-43733-9_15, © Springer-Verlag Berlin Heidelberg 2015

**Table 15.1** Common animal models in skeletal research

| Species | Advantages | Limitations |
| --- | --- | --- |
| Mice | Ease of genetic manipulation | Lack of intracortical remodeling<br>Small size for surgical manipulation |
| Rats | Most widely used model of OVX-induced bone loss | Lack of intracortical remodeling |
| Large animals (dogs, pigs, sheep) | Intracortical remodeling<br>Large size<br>Biopsies possible | Expensive<br>Limited/variable response to OVX |
| Nonhuman primates | Intracortical remodeling<br>OVX-induced bone loss<br>Large size<br>Biopsies possible | Expensive<br>Limited access for many labs |

Perhaps not surprisingly, progress toward an animal model of ONJ was slow. Evidence of necrotic bone in dogs treated for 3 years with bisphosphonates was published in 2008 [7], yet the absence of exposed bone (the key clinical criteria of ONJ) called into question how applicable these findings were to the clinical condition. One year later, a highly influential paper was published showing exposed bone in rats resulting from the combination of dental surgery, bisphosphonates, and dexamethasone [8]. In the 4 years to follow, there have been several dozen publications showing various aspects of ONJ in mice, rats, dogs, and swine. Some of these reports focus on basic aspects of "model development," others aim to answer questions regarding the pathophysiology of ONJ, and still others focus on basic effects of bisphosphonates on the oral cavity without trying to produce an animal model.

This chapter reviews the current state of ONJ animal models. Because of fundamental differences in the physiology of the cortical bone, large animal models are discussed separate from rodent models. If you are short on time, the take-home message is simple – there are numerous models, each with strength and weaknesses and each which probably provides unique insight into the pathophysiology of the disease.

## Animal Models in Skeletal Biology

Several different animals are commonly used in preclinical skeletal research (Table 15.1). Rodents are by far the most popular. They have numerous advantages as a research model including having well-characterized responses to estrogen withdrawal (and thus a model of postmenopausal osteoporosis) and well-established methods for genetic manipulation. One significant limitation of the rodent from a skeletal physiology standpoint is the lack of remodeling within the cortical bone (called intracortical remodeling) [9]. Intracortical remodeling, a prominent physiological process in humans to renew cortical bone tissue, does not occur in rats/mice under normal conditions although it can be stimulated by various interventions (estrogen withdrawal, calcium restriction, induction of microdamage) [10, 11]. Thus, when a research question is aimed at understanding cortical bone dynamics, the use of rodents has limitations. Larger animals, such as rabbits, sheep, dogs, and pigs, undergo intracortical remodeling and thus have cortical bone physiology more similar to humans [12]. These positives are offset to some degree by both social views and economical limitation of using these models.

## Large Animal Models of Osteonecrosis of the Jaw

The first reports of oral bone necrosis associated with bisphosphonate treatment came from an experiment in our laboratory that was focused on investigating how bisphosphonates affect bone mechanical properties [13, 14]. The design of these experiments was such that skeletally mature female beagle dogs were treated with daily oral

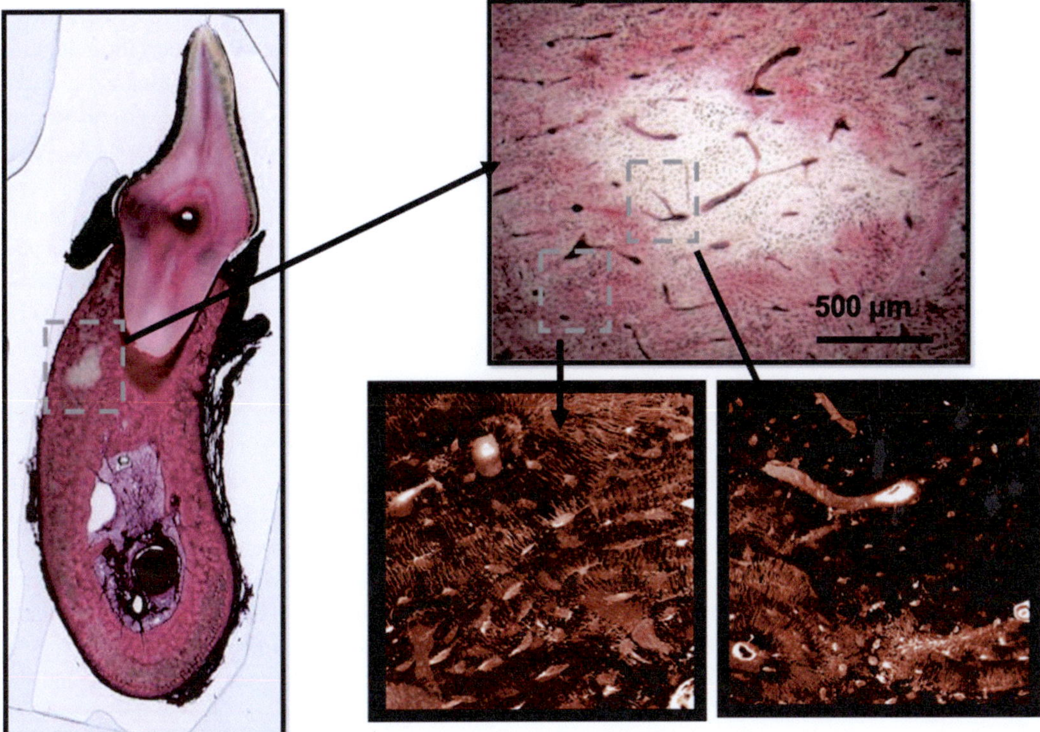

**Fig. 15.1** Bone matrix necrosis associated with bisphosphonate treatment in beagle dogs. Following 1 or 3 years of treatment, basic fuchsin staining of samples revealed regions of nonviable bone that were notably absent in control animals. Regions of nonviable bone appear white in fuchsin-stained bone due to the absence of penetration of the stain into regions that lack patent canaliculi. These can be observed using either bright-field or confocal microscopy (Adapted from Allen and Burr [7])

alendronate at a dose consistent with that used for treatment of postmenopausal osteoporosis (on a mg/kg basis) or a dose 5× higher (approximating the dose used in Paget's disease). An age-matched control treated with oral saline was also part of the experiment. Groups of dogs were treated for 1, 2, or 3 years in duration. Although the effects of alendronate on the oral skeleton were not part of original analysis plan, the mandibles were saved "just in case" at the recommendation of a collaborator.

Following several years of clinical ONJ reports, we began to investigate the utility of our stored tissue to understand ONJ. Historical precedence existed for studying bone necrosis histologically. Using basic fuchsin staining, which our lab was quite familiar with based on our interest in microdamage, regions of necrotic bone could be histologically identified by an absence of stain penetration [15]. Using this method, we showed that animals treated with oral alendronate for three years had a significantly higher incidence of matrix necrosis within the mandible compared to vehicle-treated controls [7]. Our sampling method, which examined four different regions of bone throughout the mandible, revealed no regions of nonviable matrix in vehicle animals while 30 % of alendronate-treated animals had at least one necrotic region. Necrotic regions, which represented areas lacking viable lacuna-canalicular networks (Fig. 15.1), were fundamentally different from what was being seen clinically with ONJ – exposed bone in the oral cavity. Follow-up analyses of animals that had been treated for 1 year with these same doses of oral alendronate showed a similar pattern of matrix necrosis with alendronate-treated animals, but not vehicle controls, having regions of nonviable bone in the mandible matrix [16]. While the matrix necrosis did not match the clinical manifestation of ONJ, it was hypothesized that these necrotic regions could be the early stages of bone death that would eventually manifest into exposed bone if combined with other factors. These studies also documented, for the first time, that daily oral alendronate at clinically meaningful doses significantly suppressed intracortical remodeling within the mandible cortex. This was important as suppression of remodeling within the oral cortical bone, which normally occurs at a high rate, was hypothesized to be a key factor in the etiology of ONJ but had not been previously shown to occur in a model with intracortical remodeling.

Subsequent to these experiments, our group designed a series of studies to further investigate the utility of the beagle dog as a model for ONJ. As the majority of the emerging ONJ reports were in patients treated with bisphosphonate doses consistent with those in cancer patients (intravenous zoledronic acid), we asked the question of whether there was a difference in matrix necrosis between IV zoledronic acid and oral alendronate. In short-term experiments (3 and 6 months), we showed that while IV zoledronic acid produced a more rapid and profound suppression of remodeling in the mandible compared to oral alendronate, neither agent produced regions of bone matrix necrosis (assessed using basic fuchsin staining) [17]. The working hypothesis that emerged from this study was that the matrix necrosis necessitated longer than 6 months to manifest even in the face of potent remodeling suppression such as occurs with intravenous dosing regimens for cancer treatment.

Two additional experiments aimed at understanding the interaction between bisphosphonates and dental extraction. Early clinical reports suggested (and subsequent reports have strongly confirmed) that dental intervention precipitated exposed bone in patients at a significantly higher rate than occurred spontaneously. In an acute experiment (3 months in duration), we observed one case of exposed bone in animals treated with IV zoledronic acid and then subjected to dental extraction [18]. This exposed bone matched several of the clinical criteria for ONJ including the production of a sequestrum (Fig. 15.2).

Our follow-up experiment, where animals were treated for 7 months with IV zoledronic acid prior to dental extraction (9 months' total experimental duration), failed to produce exposed bone in any animal, even in those animals in which zoledronic acid was combined with dexamethasone (a common cofactor in clinical ONJ) [19]. Despite the lack of exposed bone, high-resolution CT revealed two animals with high-dose zoledronic acid had significantly compromised extraction socket healing. Furthermore, the majority of animals treated with bisphosphonates, but not those treated with vehicle, had periosteal reaction (new bone formation on the periosteal surface) associated with the extraction site. Similar to our earlier studies, these extraction studies revealed that IV zoledronic acid potently suppressed (and in some cases completely abolished) cortical bone remodeling in the mandible.

A handful of other experiments have investigated the interaction between bisphosphonates and the oral skeleton in dogs, although not always focused on producing ONJ. A small-scale experiment was conducted to look at extraction healing in the presence of zoledronic acid with or without bone morphogenic protein treatment [20]. These results showed significant bisphosphonate effects on remodeling and healing but made no measures of necrotic bone. In a similar way, studies examining extraction and/or implant healing in animals treated with zoledronic acid failed to produced exposed bone, although remodeling suppression and matrix necrosis (assessed using lactate dehydrogenase histochemistry) were both noted in treated animals [21, 22]. Collectively, these studies in a dog model produce a consistent picture of potent suppression of intracortical remodeling and negatively affect osseous healing. However, the model does not produce a robust manifestation of exposed bone.

The other large animal species investigated as a model of ONJ is the swine with two reports showing manifestation of exposed bone. Skeletally mature male Gottingen mini pigs were treated with either weekly zoledronic acid or vehicle for 16 weeks with multiple dental extractions (6 in total) at week 6 [23]. All bisphosphonate-treated animals developed exposed bone at three or more of the extraction sockets, while the vehicle

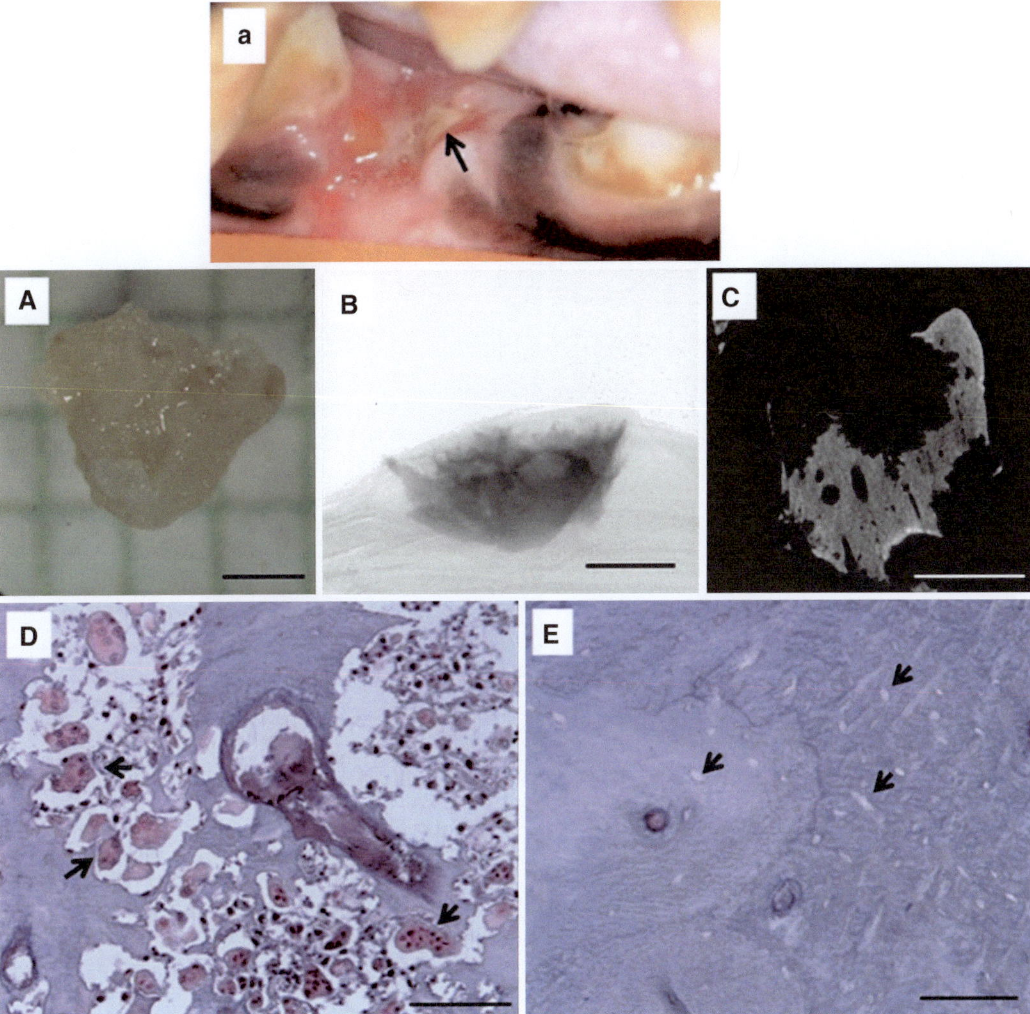

**Fig. 15.2** Exposed bone in a zoledronate-treated beagle dog following dental extraction (**a**). The exposed bone eventually formed a sequestrum. (**A**) Photograph; (**B**) two-dimensional micro-CT image through the center of the sequestrum showing highly scalloped surfaces; (**C**) two-dimensional micro-CT projection image of the entire specimen; (**D**) photomicrograph of histological section through the sequestrum stained with tartrate-resistant acid phosphatase (TRAP) to visualize osteoclasts (select, but not all, osteoclasts identified with *black arrowheads*); (**E**) photomicrograph of histological section through the sequestrum stained with TRAP showing empty osteocyte lacunae (select, but not all, empty osteocyte lacunae identified with *black arrowheads*). Scale bars = 1 mm for (**A–C**) and 100 μm for (**D, E**) (Reproduced with permission from Allen et al. [18])

animals all had epithelial coverage within 2 weeks (Fig. 15.3). This study conducted a robust analysis of several factors related to necrosis – effectively showing visual, histological, and CT-based evidence of ONJ. This represents the most thoroughly documented evidence of clinically consistent ONJ in a large animal model. A second study, using a different strain of swine (Wuzhishan mini pigs), also documented the development of exposed bone when zoledronic acid treatment was superimposed with extraction [24]. Again, control animals showed complete healing at the time point assessed. Neither of these studies measured intracortical bone turnover rates nor commented on the amount of osteonal bone within the mandible tissue of mini pigs.

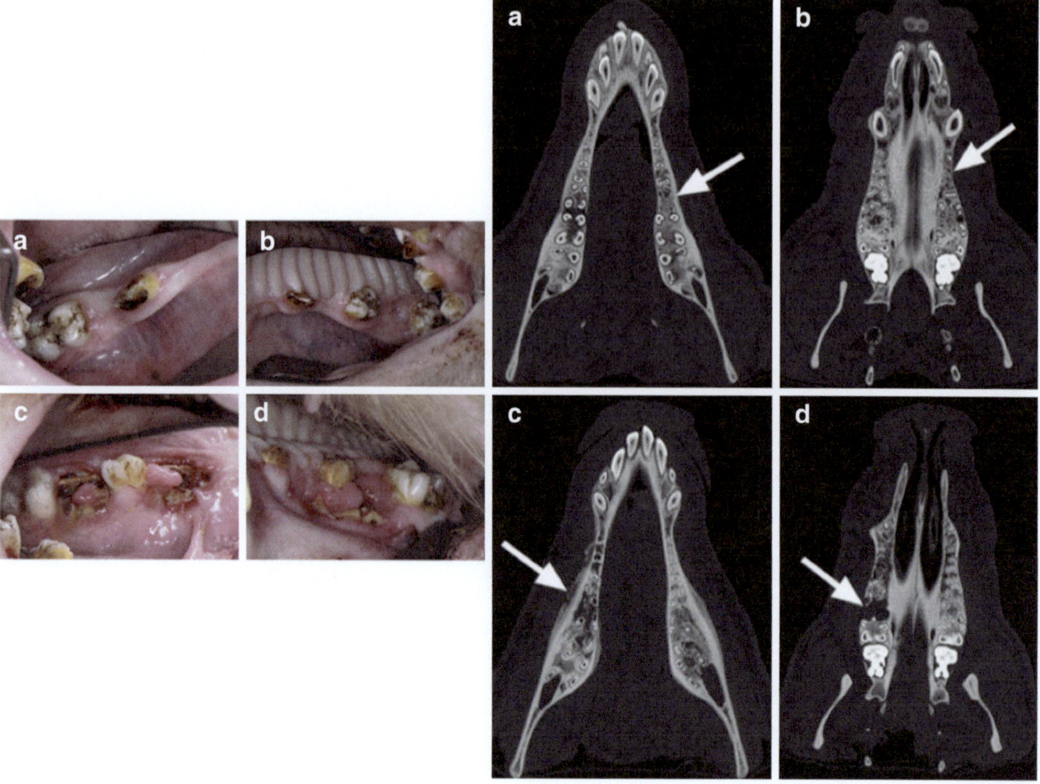

**Fig. 15.3** Exposed bone and disrupted healing post-extraction in a mini pig model. Intraoral views of the animals 10 weeks after tooth extractions with uneventful wound healing in the control group (**a**: mandible; **b**: maxilla). In contrast, all animals in the bisphosphonate group showed impaired healing and exposed bone (**c**: mandible; **d**: maxilla). Computed tomography images (*axial views*) of the lower and upper jaw of animals in the control group (**a, b**) as well as of the bisphosphonate group (**c, d**). The extraction sites are indicated by *white arrows*. Bony healing and no periosteal reaction were observed in the control animals (**a, b**). In contrast, the bisphosphonate group exhibited no bone remodeling of extraction sockets, and typical radiological hallmarks of a bisphosphonate-related osteonecrosis were observed (cortical erosion, periosteal calcification, hypo- and hyperdensities) (**c, d**) (Reproduced with permission from Pautke et al. [23])

Although rabbits are not necessarily a "large animal," they are often grouped in this category for skeletal research because like other larger animals (and different from rodents), they undergo intracortical remodeling. There are no published reports focused on ONJ in rabbits, although the rabbit is a common model for studying dental perturbations such as distraction osteogenesis. A potentially interesting aspect of rabbits is that although they do undergo intracortical remodeling, qualitative analysis revealed it was not common in the mandible [16].

The underlying mechanism driving the disconnect between the two large animal models, canine and swine, with respect to producing exposed bone following bisphosphonate/dental extraction is not clear. Doses of bisphosphonates were roughly comparable between the studies in these two models, as was the time post-extraction that the animals were assessed. Yet, out of confusion arises opportunity. The disparate results in these two large animal models set the stage for potentially useful comparative studies, examining either bone/mucosal-specific factors or bacterial profiles in the oral cavity that differ between mini pigs and dogs. Such factors that exist in swine but not dogs may provide insight into key factors involved in the manifestation of exposed bone in the setting of bisphosphonates.

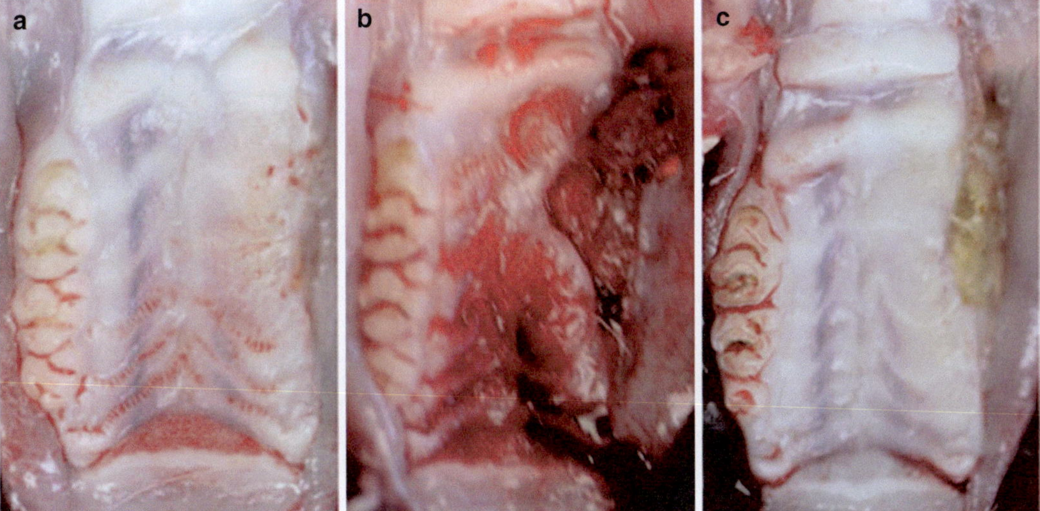


**Fig. 15.4** Exposed bone following dental extraction in the first rat model of ONJ. Representative photographs of gross clinical appearance of maxillary ridges in animals with intact epithelium (**a**, day 28 following extraction) or ulcerated mucosa overlying necrotic bone at days 14 (**b**) and 28 (**c**) following extraction. Ulcerative areas were characterized by rolled mucosa, lack of drainage, and, by day 28 post-extraction, central areas of *yellow/gray* necrosis (Reproduced with permission from Sonis et al. [8])

## Rodent Models of Osteonecrosis of the Jaw

In 1981, Gotcher and Jee produced, in retrospect, the first animal model of ONJ [25]. They treated young, rapidly growing rats with high doses of clodronate for up to 18 weeks and observed bone protruding into the oral cavity that upon histological analysis was found to be void of viable cells and considered devitalized. These studies utilized the rice rat, a model known for developing periodontal disease. Interestingly, the exposed bone occurred in the absence of any dental intervention. Because the animals were young and received high doses of drug, the results were, at the time, considered to have limited clinical relevance.

Nearly three decades later, the first animal model to emerge following the clinical description of ONJ was published. Sonis and colleagues designed their study specifically to try and produce changes in the oral cavity consistent with the clinical and radiographic criteria of ONJ [8]. Three-month-old rats were treated with a combination of zoledronic acid and dexamethasone and then subjected to extraction of three molars in the mandible or maxilla. The results were striking (Fig. 15.4), with many treated animals developing mucosal ulceration at the extraction sites, and those treated with both drugs had persistent ulcerations even 28 days postsurgery. Despite the oral examination showing clear lack of healing in treated animals, most of the other analyses (radiographic, histological) were qualitative. Yet this study is considered one of the most of important preclinical contributions to the field of ONJ as it provided a foundation for future work in animals.

Since the work of Sonis and colleagues, over three dozen publications have described how bisphosphonates, with or without dental perturbation or coadministration of other drugs, lead to the manifestation (or lack) of ONJ in rodents (Table 15.2). The majority of these have utilized the rat as a model although both rats and mice have been shown to develop exposed bone and related oral manifestations. The remainder of this section will highlight some generalizations and key rodent papers, rather than detailing specific strengths/weaknesses about each study. Those

**Table 15.2** ONJ studies in rodents

| First author (year) | Species | Bisphosphonate | Dental insult | Exposed bone |
|---|---|---|---|---|
| Sonis (2009)[A] | Rat | Zoledronate (SC) | All molars from one maxilla | Yes |
| Hikita (2009)[B] | Rat | Alendronate injections in oral cavity | Second molar from one maxilla | No |
| Biasotto (2010)[C] | Rat | Zoledronate (IV) | One upper molar plus an additional 4 mm defect | Yes |
| Hokugo (2010)[D] | Rat | Zoledronate (IV) | All molars from one maxilla | Yes |
| Lopez-Jornet (2010)[E] | Rat | Pamidronate (IP) | All molars from one maxilla | Yes |
| Maahs (2010)[F] | Rat | Alendronate (oral) or zoledronate (IP) | All molars from one maxilla | Yes |
| Senel (2010)[G] | Rat | Zoledronate (IP) or pamidronate (IP) | None | Yes |
| Aguirre (2010)[H] | Rat | Alendronate (SC) | Mandibular first molar | No |
| Xiong (2010)[I] | Rat | Alendronate (SC) | Periapical lesion at the mandibular first molar | No |
| Jee (2010)[J] | Rat | Alendronate (SC) | First molar from one maxilla | No |
| Kobayashi (2010)[K] | Mouse | Zoledronate (SC) | First molar from one maxilla | No |
| Yamashita (2010)[L] | Rat | Zoledronate (SC) | Denuded palatal mucosa between the first molar and great palatine canal | No |
| Kikuiri (2010)[M] | Mouse | Zoledronate (IV) | First molar from one maxilla | Yes |
| Bi (2010)[N] | Mouse | Zoledronate (IP) | First molar from one maxilla | No |
| Aghaloo (2011)[O] | Rat | Zoledronate (IP) | Ligature-induced periodontal disease | Yes |
| Lopez-Jornet (2011)[P] | Rat | Pamidronate (IP) | All molars from one maxilla or mandible | Yes |
| Marino (2012)[Q] | Rat | Zoledronate (IV) | Mandibular first molar | Yes |
| Aguirre (2012)[R] | Rat | Alendronate (SC) or zoledronate (IV) | Diet-induced periodontitis | Yes |
| Abtahi (2012)[S] | Rat | Alendroante | First molar from one maxilla | Yes |
| Said (2012)[T] | Rat | Etidroante (SC) | None | No |
| Zhao (2012)[U] | Mouse | Zoledronate (IV) | First molar from one maxilla | Yes |
| Conte Neto (2013)[V] | Rat | Alendronate (SC) | Mandibular first molar | Yes |
| Abtahi (2013)[W] | Rat | Alendronate (SC) | First molar from one maxilla | Yes |
| Hokugo (2013)[X] | Rat | Zoledronate (IV) | First molar from one maxilla | No |
| Bonnet (2013)[Y] | Mouse | Zoledronate (SC) | Diet-induced periodontitis | No |
| Abtahi (2013)[Z] | Rat | Alendronate (SC) | First molar from one maxilla | Yes |
| Berti-Couto (2013)[AA] | Rat | Alendronate (SC) | All molars from one maxilla | Yes |
| Kuroshima (2013)[BB] | Rat | Zoledronate (SC) | Left and right maxillary second molars | No |
| Zhang (2013)[CC] | Mouse | Zoledronate (IV) | Maxillary first molar | Yes |
| Kang (2013)[DD] | Mouse | Zoledronate (IP) | Pulpal exposure | Yes |
| Tsurushima (2013)[EE] | Rat | Zoledronate (SC) | Drill hole | No |
| Dayisoylu (2013)[FF] | Rat | Zoledronate (IP) | Mandibular first molar | Yes |
| Kuroshima (2013)[GG] | Mouse | Zoledronate (SC) | Left and right maxillary first molars | Yes |
| Aghaloo (2014)[HH] | Mouse | RANK-Fc or OPG-Fc (IP) | Pulpal exposure | Yes |

References: A [8], B [26], C [27], D [28], E [29], F [30], G [31], H [32], I [33], J [34], K [35], L [36], M [37], N [38], O [39], P [40], Q [41], R [42], S [43], T [44], U [45], V [46], W [47], X [48], Y [49], Z [50], AA [51], BB [52], CC [53], DD [54], EE [55], FF [56], GG [57], HH [58]

interested in specifics are encouraged to use Table 15.2 as a guide to work through the relevant literature.

The original model published by Gotcher and Jee utilized a special strain of rat (the marsh rice rat) [25] that was susceptible to periodontitis when fed soft food. Aguirre et al. revisited the model using modernized analysis techniques and modifications to several aspects of the study design including the use of nitrogen-containing bisphosphonates (as opposed to etidronate) [42]. These studies showed prominent periodontal lesions in both treated and control animals after 12, 18, or 24 weeks of treatment, but only zoledronate-treated animals had exposed bone. Similar results have been shown in Sprague-Dawley rats that were induced to have periodontitis using a ligature model [39]. Specifically, treatment of animals having periodontal disease with zoledronate resulted in the development of exposed bone, sequestrum formation, and histological necrosis. These studies have important implications, as the general view in the field is that dental surgery is key in the pathophysiology of ONJ. These controlled preclinical studies show that periodontal disease and the local changes associated with this disease (such as inflammation) are sufficient when combined with potent bisphosphonates (intravenous zoledronate) to manifest ONJ lesions.

A handful of other papers have similarly shown that dental extraction is not necessary to produce ONJ lesions. Some of these are difficult to interpret because nothing was done to the animal besides dosing with bisphosphonate – yet exposed bone was noted [31]. This is not consistent with the majority of studies, nor the clinical epidemiology. Others have simply done various insults to the oral cavity, but not extracted teeth. Localized bacterial injections [55], induction of periapical lesions [33, 54], and denuting the palatal bone gingiva [36] have all been shown to produce various degrees of bone necrosis ranging from matrix necrosis to exposed bone. These effects were all more prominent in bisphosphonate-treated rats/mice compared to vehicle-treated controls.

The far more common approach investigators have taken to study ONJ is to extract teeth in bisphosphonate-treated animals. Dozens of studies have utilized this approach, in both rats and mice, with variable outcomes (Table 15.2). The reason for conflicting results, with some studies showing exposed bone while others do not, is unclear. The easiest outcome to compare across studies is exposed bone based on visual examination (Fig. 15.5). Other outcomes, such as histological necrosis, are more vague and could depend on how the authors define such necrosis (size, criteria for number of nonviable osteocytes, etc.). Another challenge for the interpretation of all these animal studies is the use of different bisphosphonates (alendronate, zoledronate, pamidronate), administered through different routes (IP, SC, IV) at different doses (or dosing schedules). Any or all of these could affect the results, and unfortunately, the most basic experiments, comparing different drugs/routes/doses, have not been undertaken in a systematic way. This has hindered the field by leading to extreme heterogeneity among studies and, from a translational point of view, has not informed clinicians on the most important aspects of dosing to reduce the risk of ONJ.

Recently, an animal model of ONJ was produced using analogs for denosumab, the only other antiremodeling agent that has shown clinical manifestation of ONJ [59]. Treatment of mice with either RANK-Fc or OPG-Fc (binding domains of RANK and OPG are bound to the fusion compound (Fc) of IgG) produced bone exposure following pulpal exposure in 20–30 % of treated animals [58]. All treated animals displayed histological osteonecrosis and periosteal bone formation. This paper represents a significant advancement to the field as, similar to the work of Sonis and colleagues, it provides a starting point of a model for how manipulation of the RANK/RANK-L/OPG system can lead to ONJ. Future work in the field will now be able to, at least in mice, compare and contrast bisphosphonates and RANK-L inhibition as it relates to the pathophysiology of ONJ.

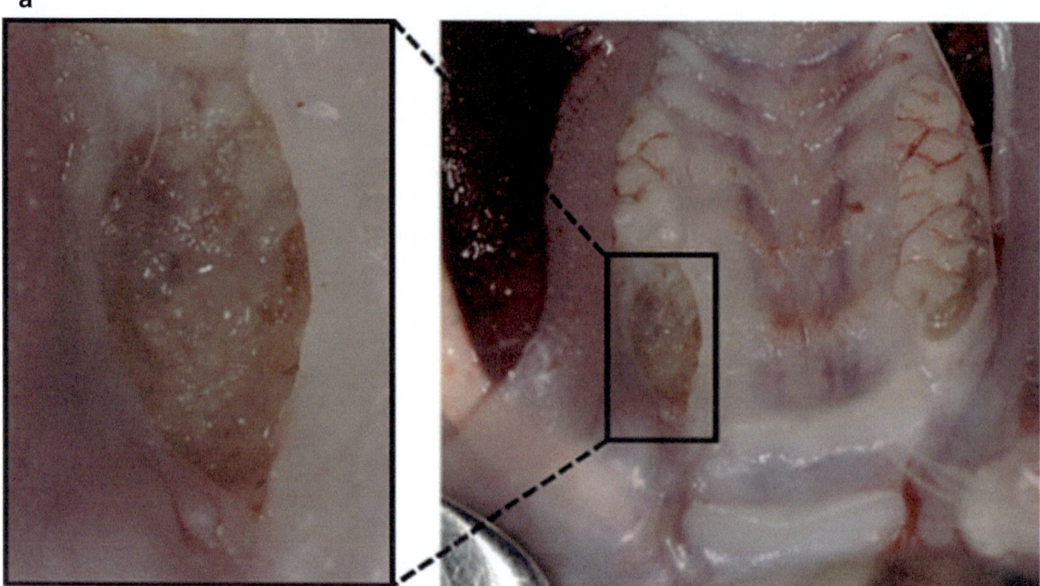

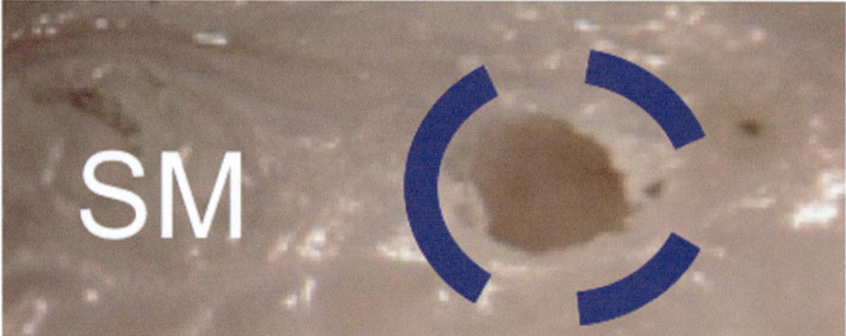


**Fig. 15.5** Typical bone exposure in rat (**a**) and mouse (**b**) following dental extraction (Reproduced with permission from Abtahi et al. [50] and Kikuiri et al. [37])

## Future Directions

The field has made great strides in developing animal models of ONJ. Not only have models been developed, but they have begun being used to examine potential ways to reduce the risk or treat ONJ. One challenge moving forward is determining, for an individual study, what animal model to use. The rodent models appear most robust and, given the ease of access for most investigators, likely represent the initial model of choice. Yet because of fundamental differences in remodeling of the cortical bone between rodents and larger species and the exciting emergence of the swine model (and to a lesser degree dog), those findings that appear most promising from rodents should be confirmed in a larger animal model. Finally, several papers from across all animal models (mice, rats, dogs, swine) have documented new periosteal bone formation that is most prominent in animals treated with antiresorptive agents (both bisphosphonates and RANK inhibitors) (Fig. 15.6). This has also been documented in several clinical ONJ papers. The reason for this new bone formation is not clear, but it is an area that is ripe for exploration as a

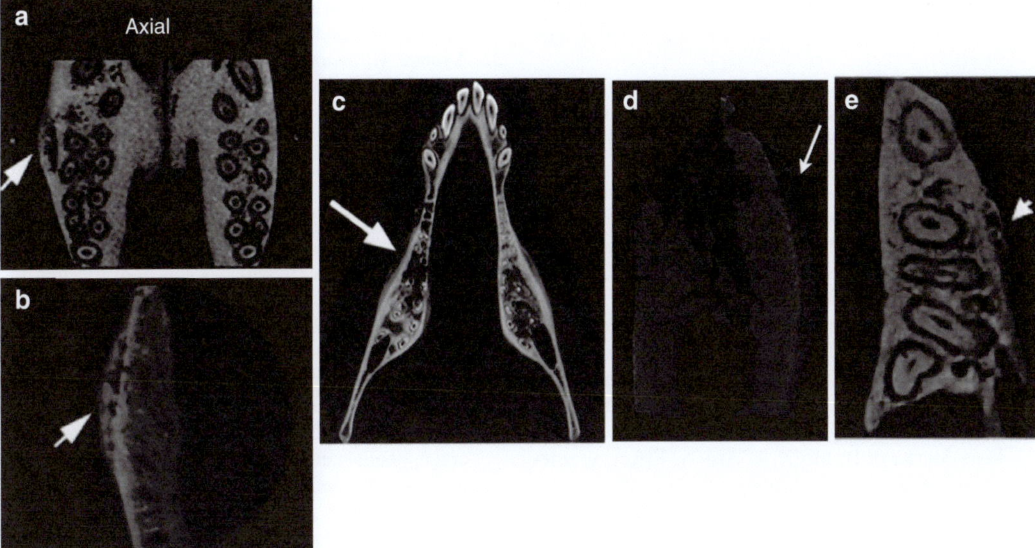



**Fig. 15.6** Several studies have documented new bone formation on the periosteal surface. This has been shown in rats (**a**), humans (**b**), mini pigs (**c**), dogs (**d**), and mice (**e**) (Reproduced with permission from (**a, b**; Aghaloo et al. [39]), (**c**; Pautke et al. [23]), (**d**; Allen et al. [19]))

potential marker of ONJ. The ability for in vivo imaging of animals, and animal models in general, is the perfect setting for such exploration.

# References


1. Russell RGG. Bisphosphonates: the first 40 years. Bone. 2011;49(1):2–19.
2. Schenk R, Merz W, Mühlbauer R, Russell RGG, Fleisch H. Effect of ethane-1-hydroxy-1, 1-diphosphonate (EHDP) and dichloromethylene diphosphonate (Cl 2 MDP) on the calcification and resorption of cartilage and bone in the tibial epiphysis and metaphysis of rats. Calcif Tissue Int. 1973;11(3):196–214.
3. Ruggiero S, Mehrotra B, Rosenberg T. Osteonecrosis of the jaws associated with the use of bisphosphonates: a review of 63 cases. J Oral Maxillofac Surg. 2004; 62(5):527–34.
4. Marx R. Pamidronate (Aredia) and zoledronate (Zometa) induced avascular necrosis of the jaws: a growing epidemic. J Oral Maxillofac Surg. 2003;61(9):1115.
5. Allen MR, Burr DB. The pathogenesis of bisphosphonate-related osteonecrosis of the jaw: so many hypotheses, so few data. J Oral Maxillofac Surg. 2009;67(5):61–70.
6. Allen M. Animal models of osteonecrosis of the jaw. J Musculoskelet Neuronal Interact. 2007;7(4):358.
7. Allen MR, Burr DB. Mandible matrix necrosis in beagle dogs after 3 years of daily oral bisphosphonate treatment. J Oral Maxillofac Surg. 2008;66(5):987–94.
8. Sonis ST, Watkins BA, Lyng GD, Lerman MA. Bony changes in the jaws of rats treated with zoledronic acid and dexamethasone before dental extractions mimic bisphosphonate-related osteonecrosis in cancer patients. Oral Oncol. 2009;45(2):164–72.
9. Jowsey J. Studies of Haversian systems in man and some animals. J Anat. 1966;100(Pt 4):857–64.
10. Kubek D, Burr D, Allen M. Ovariectomy stimulates and bisphosphonates inhibit intracortical remodeling in the mouse mandible. Orthod Craniofac Res. 2010; 13(4):214–22.
11. Bentolila V, Boyce T, Fyhrie D, Drumb R, Skerry T, Schaffler MB. Intracortical remodeling in adult rat long bones after fatigue loading. Bone. 1998;23(3):275–81.
12. Reinwald S, Burr D. Review of nonprimate, large animal models for osteoporosis research. J Bone Miner Res. 2008;23(9):1353–68.
13. Allen M, Iwata K, Phipps R, Burr D. Alterations in canine vertebral bone turnover, microdamage accumulation, and biomechanical properties following 1-year treatment with clinical treatment doses of risedronate or alendronate. Bone. 2006;39(4):872–9.
14. Allen M, Burr D. Three years of alendronate treatment results in similar levels of vertebral microdamage as after one year of treatment. J Bone Miner Res. 2007;22(11):1759–65.
15. Frost H. Micropetrosis. J Bone Joint Surg Am. 1960; 42(1):144.
16. Burr DB, Allen MR. Mandibular necrosis in beagle dogs treated with bisphosphonates. Orthod Craniofac Res. 2009;12(3):221–8.
17. Allen M, Kubek D, Burr D. Cancer treatment dosing regimens of zoledronic acid result in near-complete

suppression of mandible intracortical bone remodeling in beagle dogs. J Bone Miner Res. 2010;25(1): 98–105.

18. Allen MR, Kubek DJ, Burr DB, Ruggiero SL. Compromised osseous healing of dental extraction sites in zoledronic acid-treated dogs. Osteoporos Int. 2011;22(2):693–702.

19. Allen MR, Chu T-MG, Ruggiero SL. Absence of exposed bone following dental extraction in beagle dogs treated with 9 months of high-dose zoledronic acid combined with dexamethasone. J Oral Maxillofac Surg. 2013;71(6):1017–26. Elsevier.

20. Gerard DA, Carlson ER, Gotcher JE, Pickett DO. Early inhibitory effects of zoledronic acid in tooth extraction sockets in dogs are negated by recombinant human bone morphogenetic protein. J Oral Maxillofac Surg. 2013;72(1):61–6.

21. Huja SS, Kaya B, Mo X, D'Atri A. Effect of zoledronic acid on bone healing subsequent to mini-implant insertion. Angle Orthod. 2011;81(3):363–9.

22. Huja SS, Mason A, Fenell C, Mo X, Hueni S, D'Atri A, et al. Effects of short-term zoledronic acid treatment on bone remodeling and healing at surgical sites in the maxilla and mandible of aged dogs. J Oral Maxillofac Surg. 2010;69(2):418–27.

23. Pautke C, Kreutzer K, Weitz J, Knödler M, Münzel D, Wexel G, et al. Bisphosphonate related osteonecrosis of the jaw: a minipig large animal model. Bone. 2012;51(3):592–9 (Elsevier B.V.).

24. Li Y, Xu J, Mao L, Liu Y, Gao R, Zheng Z, et al. Allogeneic mesenchymal stem cell therapy for bisphosphonate-related jaw osteonecrosis in swine. Stem Cells Dev. 2013;22(14):2047–56.

25. Gotcher J, Jee W. The progress of the periodontal syndrome in the rice rat. J Periodontal Res. 1981; 16(3):275–91.

26. Hikita H, Miyazawa K, Tabuchi M, Kimura M. Bisphosphonate administration prior to tooth extraction delays initial healing of the extraction socket in rats. J Bone Miner Metab. 2009;27(6):663–72.

27. Biasotto M, Chiandussi S, Zacchigna S, Moimas S, Dore F, Pozzato G, et al. A novel animal model to study non-spontaneous bisphosphonates osteonecrosis of jaw. J Oral Pathol Med. 2010;39(5):390–6.

28. Hokugo A, Christensen R, Chung E, Sung E, Felsenfeld A, Sayre J, et al. Increased prevalence of bisphosphonate-related osteonecrosis of the jaw with vitamin D deficiency in rats. J Bone Miner Res. 2010;25(6):1337–49.

29. López-Jornet P, Camacho-Alonso F, Molina-Miñano F, Gómez-García F, Vicente-Ortega V. An experimental study of bisphosphonate-induced jaws osteonecrosis in Sprague–Dawley rats. J Oral Pathol Med. 2010; 39(9):697–702. Blackwell Publishing Ltd.

30. Maahs MP, Azambuja AA, Campos MM, Salum FG, Cherubini K. Association between bisphosphonates and jaw osteonecrosis: a study in Wistar rats. Head Neck. 2011;33(2):199–207. Wiley Subscription Services, Inc., A Wiley Company.

31. Senel F, Duman M, Muci E, Cankaya M, Pampu A, Ersoz S, et al. Jaw bone changes in rats after treatment with zoledronate and pamidronate. Oral Surg Oral Med Oral Pathol Oral Radiol Endod. 2010;109(3):385–91.

32. Aguirre JI, Altman MK, Vanegas SM, Franz SE. Effects of alendronate on bone healing after tooth extraction in rats. Oral Dis. 2010;16(7):674–85.

33. Xiong H, Wei L, Hu Y, Zhang C, Peng B. Effect of alendronate on alveolar bone resorption and angiogenesis in rats with experimental periapical lesions. Int Endod J. 2010;43(6):485–91.

34. Jee J-H, Lee W, Lee BD. The influence of alendronate on the healing of extraction sockets of ovariectomized rats assessed by in vivo micro-computed tomography. Oral Surg Oral Med Oral Pathol Oral Radiol Endod. 2010;110(2):e47–53.

35. Kobayashi Y, Hiraga T, Ueda A, Wang L, Matsumoto-Nakano M, Hata K, et al. Zoledronic acid delays wound healing of the tooth extraction socket, inhibits oral epithelial cell migration, and promotes proliferation and adhesion to hydroxyapatite of oral bacteria, without causing osteonecrosis of the jaw, in mice. J Bone Miner Metab. 2010;28(2):165–75.

36. Yamashita J, Koi K, Yang DY, McCauley LK. Effect of zoledronate on oral wound healing in rats. Clin Cancer Res. 2011;17(6):1405–14.

37. Kikuiri T, Kim I, Yamaza T, Akiyama K, Zhang Q, Li Y, et al. Cell-based immunotherapy with mesenchymal stem cells cures bisphosphonate-related osteonecrosis of the jaw–like disease in mice. J Bone Miner Res. 2010;25(7):1668–79.

38. Bi Y, Gao Y, Ehirchiou D, Cao C, Kikuiri T, Le A, et al. Bisphosphonates cause osteonecrosis of the jaw-like disease in mice. Am J Pathol. 2010;177(1): 280–90.

39. Aghaloo TL, Kang B, Sung EC, Shoff M, Ronconi M, Gotcher JE, et al. Periodontal disease and bisphosphonates induce osteonecrosis of the jaws in the rat. J Bone Miner Res. 2011;26(8):1871–82.

40. López-Jornet P, Camacho-Alonso F, Martínez-Canovas A, Molina-Miñano F, Gómez-García F, Vicente-Ortega V. Perioperative antibiotic regimen in rats treated with pamidronate plus dexamethasone and subjected to dental extraction: a study of the changes in the jaws. J Oral Maxillofac Surg. 2011;69(10): 2488–93.

41. Marino KL, Zakhary I, Abdelsayed RA, Carter JA, O'Neill JC, Khashaba RM, et al. Development of a rat model of bisphosphonate-related osteonecrosis of the jaw (BRONJ). J Oral Implantol. 2012;38 Spec No:511–8.

42. Aguirre JI, Akhter MP, Kimmel DB, Pingel JE, Williams A, Jorgensen M, et al. Oncologic doses of zoledronic acid induce osteonecrosis of the jaw-like lesions in rice rats (Oryzomys palustris) with periodontitis. J Bone Miner Res. 2012;27(10): 2130–43.

43. Abtahi J, Agholme F, Sandberg O, Aspenberg P. Bisphosphonate-induced osteonecrosis of the jaw in a rat model arises first after the bone has become exposed. No primary necrosis in unexposed bone. J Oral Pathol Med. 2012;41(6):494–9.

44. Said F, Ghoul-Mazgar S, Khemiss F, El Ayeb H, Saidane D, Berdal A, et al. The effect of etidronate on

the periodontium of ovariectomized rats. J Periodontol. 2012;83(8):1063–8.

45. Zhao Y, Wang L, Liu Y, Akiyama K, Chen C, Atsuta I, et al. Technetium-99 conjugated with methylene diphosphonate ameliorates ovariectomy-induced osteoporotic phenotype without causing osteonecrosis in the jaw. Calcif Tissue Int. 2012;91(6):400–8.

46. Conte Neto N, Spolidorio LC, Andrade CR, S Bastos A, Guimarães M, Marcantonio Jr E. Experimental development of bisphosphonate-related osteonecrosis of the jaws in rodents. Int J Exp Pathol. 2013;94(1):65–73.

47. Abtahi J, Agholme F, Sandberg O, Aspenberg P. Effect of local vs. systemic bisphosphonate delivery on dental implant fixation in a model of osteonecrosis of the jaw. J Dent Res. 2013;92(3):279–83.

48. Hokugo A, Sun S, Park S, Mckenna CE, Nishimura I. Equilibrium-dependent bisphosphonate interaction with crystalline bone mineral explains anti-resorptive pharmacokinetics and prevalence of osteonecrosis of the jaw in rats. Bone. 2013;53(1):59–68. Elsevier Inc.

49. Bonnet N, Lesclous P, Saffar JL, Ferrari S. Zoledronate effects on systemic and jaw osteopenias in ovariectomized periostin-deficient mice. PLoS One. 2013;8(3): e58726. Isales CM, editor.

50. Abtahi J, Agholme F, Aspenberg P. Prevention of osteonecrosis of the jaw by mucoperiosteal coverage in a rat model. Int J Oral Maxillofac Surg. 2013;42(5):632–6.

51. Berti-Couto SA, Vasconcelos ACU, Iglesias JE, Figueiredo MAZ, Salum FG, Cherubini K. Diabetes mellitus and corticotherapy as risk factors for alendronate-related osteonecrosis of the jaws: a study in Wistar rats. Head Neck. 2013;36(1):84–93.

52. Kuroshima S, Yamashita J. Chemotherapeutic and antiresorptive combination therapy suppressed lymphangiogenesis and induced osteonecrosis of the jaw-like lesions in mice. Bone. 2013;56(1):101–9.

53. Zhang Q, Atsuta I, Liu S, Chen C, Shi S, Shi S, et al. IL-17-mediated M1/M2 macrophage alteration contributes to pathogenesis of bisphosphonate-related osteonecrosis of the jaws. Clin Cancer Res. 2013;19(12):3176–88.

54. Kang B, Cheong S, Chaichanasakul T, Bezouglaia O, Atti E, Dry SM, et al. Periapical disease and bisphosphonates induce osteonecrosis of the jaws in mice. J Bone Miner Res. 2013;28(7):1631–40.

55. Tsurushima H, Kokuryo S, Sakaguchi O, Tanaka J, Tominaga K. Bacterial promotion of bisphosphonate-induced osteonecrosis in Wistar rats. Int J Oral Maxillofac Surg. 2013;42(11):1481–7.

56. Dayisoylu EH, Şenel FÇ, Üngör C, Tosun E, Cankaya M, Ersoz S, et al. The effects of adjunctive parathyroid hormone injection on bisphosphonate-related osteonecrosis of the jaws: an animal study. Int J Oral Maxillofac Surg. 2013;42(11):1475–80.

57. Kuroshima S, Mecano RB, Tanoue R, Koi K, Yamashita J. Distinctive Tooth Extraction Socket Healing: Bisphosphonate vs. Parathyroid Hormone Therapy. J Periodontol. 2014;85:24–33.

58. Aghaloo TL, Cheong S, Bezouglaia O, Kostenuik P, Atti E, Dry SM, et al. RANK-L inhibitors induce osteonecrosis of the jaw in mice with periapical disease. J Bone Miner Res. 2014;29(4):843–54.

59. Aghaloo T, Felsenfeld A, Tetradis S. Osteonecrosis of the Jaw in a Patient on Denosumab. J Oral Maxillofac Surg. 2010;68(5):959–63.

# Dental Rehabilitation in Patients Receiving Antiresorptive Drugs

# 16


Sebastian Hoefert, Feraydoon Sharghi, and Eva Engel



**Abstract**

Oral rehabilitation is a major issue in patients with severe oncological diseases or osteoporosis in order to ensure a better quality of life. Whenever possible, oral rehabilitation should be considered. However, new prostheses and sore spots are often underestimated in regard to their risk of triggering medication-related osteonecrosis of the jaw (MRONJ) lesions. Dental care with monitoring oral hygiene and preserving teeth is essential in MRONJ prophylaxis. Prosthetic treatment should avoid the need of invasive dentoalveolar procedures during antiresorptive therapy if possible because these situations are associated with a risk to trigger MRONJ onset. Clinicians and patients should be aware of these risks. Planning of prostheses and continuous recalls adapted to the individual risk of MRONJ will reduce the patients' risk considerably. The chapter describes the planning of prosthetic oral rehabilitation of patients receiving oral and intravenous bisphosphonate administrations as well as rehabilitation of patients with a history of MRONJ.


## How Does Oral Rehabilitation Affects Oral Health-Related Quality of Life?

Patients under bisphosphonate or denosumab medication are frequently affected by an immense loss of their overall quality of life due to the underlying oncological disease [1] or by a severe osteoporosis [2]. Oncological patients suffer in general from distress, pain, fatigue, anxiety, depression, and practical and psychosocial problems. Cross-sectional studies have documented that approximately 35–45 % of cancer patients of North America experience significant levels


S. Hoefert, DMD, MD (✉)
Department of Oral and Maxillofacial Surgery,
University Hospital Tuebingen,
Osianderstrasse 2-8, Tuebingen, BW, Germany
e-mail: sebastian.hoefert@med.uni-tuebingen.de

F. Sharghi, DMD • E. Engel, DMD
Department of Prosthodontics and Section
"Medical Materials and Technology",
University Hospital Tuebingen,
Osianderstrasse 2-8, Tuebingen,
BW 72076, Germany
e-mail: feraydoon.sharghi@med.uni-tuebingen.de;
eva-maria.engel@med.uni-tuebingen.de



S. Otto (ed.), *Medication-Related Osteonecrosis of the Jaws: Bisphosphonates, Denosumab, and New Agents*,
DOI 10.1007/978-3-662-43733-9_16, © Springer-Verlag Berlin Heidelberg 2015

of distress, and in advanced cancer population, the prevalence of distress may even be as high as 60 % (distress: a multifactorial unpleasant emotional experience of psychological, social, and/or spiritual nature that may interfere with the ability to cope effectively with cancer, its physical symptoms, and its treatment) [1]. Intraoral rehabilitation improves and maintains oral health-related quality of life. Therefore, oral rehabilitation is one of the primary treatment targets of dentists. Additionally, impaired chewing ability, which is also perceived as serious oral health impairment, is related to many other oral health problems especially in those patient groups [3].

In cross-sectional studies of a general population, it was shown that wearing conventional complete dentures improves patients' satisfaction and quality of life [3–5]. Garret et al. reported that even 55 % of patients with poorly fitting dentures are moderately to completely satisfied with their treatment [6]. The patient-reported effects of treatments with fixed or removable partial or complete dentures were associated with reduction of problems which were most frequently complained before insertion of the new prosthesis [7] especially by improving the psychosocial well-being of the rehabilitated patients.

The overall satisfaction with implant-supported dentures is generally higher compared to conventional complete dentures. Interestingly, some authors found no differences in quality of life and satisfaction when conventional maxillary complete dentures were compared with maxillary implant-supported dentures. In contrast, lower complete dentures reach inferior oral health-related quality-of-life functional outcomes compared to even simple implant-supported overdentures [5]. Better results can be obtained by implant-supported fixed partial dentures or long-bar, respectively, telescopic removable partial dentures. According to guidelines for medication-related osteonecrosis, implants are not recommended for patients with regular intravenous bisphosphonate medication [8]. A detailed implant discussion can be found in the chapter Dental implants in the Context of Antiresorptive Drugs and Medication-Related Osteonecrosis of the Jaw (see Chap. 17).

> Oral rehabilitation with fixed or removable prosthesis helps emotionally patients with severe diseases with antiresorptive medication. Oral rehabilitation supports quality of life and may reduce distress.

## How Does Oral Rehabilitation Affect MRONJ?

Patients treated with antiresorptives like bisphosphonates or denosumab who undergo dentoalveolar treatments have a risk for MRONJ. This risk is 5–21-fold enhanced when patients receive intravenous compared to orally administered bisphosphonates [9]. Therefore, it has been postulated that therapeutical interventions which involve direct osseous injury should be avoided as far as possible. Prophylaxis with antibiotics and/or disinfectant agents seems to be essential.

Preventive care consists of caries control and conservative periodontal and restorative as well as appropriate endodontic treatment. Even non-restorable teeth are recommended to be treated by removal of the crown or restoration, doing root canal treatment of the residual root with an adhesive closure of the access hole, and leaving the root in place similar to a sleeping implant [8–10].

Root canal treatment is principally connected with a risk of MRONJ. But overall incidence and therefore the risk is estimated to be low [11, 12]. In patients with high risk for MRONJ, an antibiotic prophylaxis may be considered.

As described in previous chapters, extractions of teeth are the most frequent trigger events for MRONJ [13, 14]. Interestingly, sore spots of dentures bases have been found to be in 10–18 % the cause of MRONJ [13–15]. Highest rates with up to 30 % of incidence and prevalence were reported by Fehm and Vahtsevanos et al. [6, 13, 16]. Analyzing 195 patients with MRONJ demonstrated in 55 % tooth extractions and in 22 % sore spots of the denture base to cause MRONJ [17]. Hasegawa et al. found in patients wearing dentures a shorter duration until onset of MRONJ. The incidence of the area of MRONJ

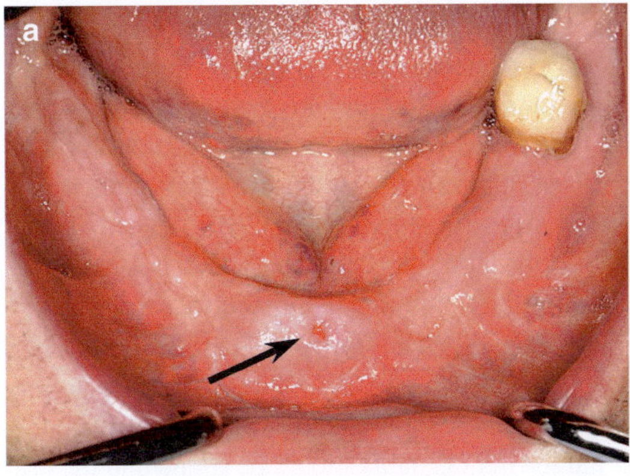

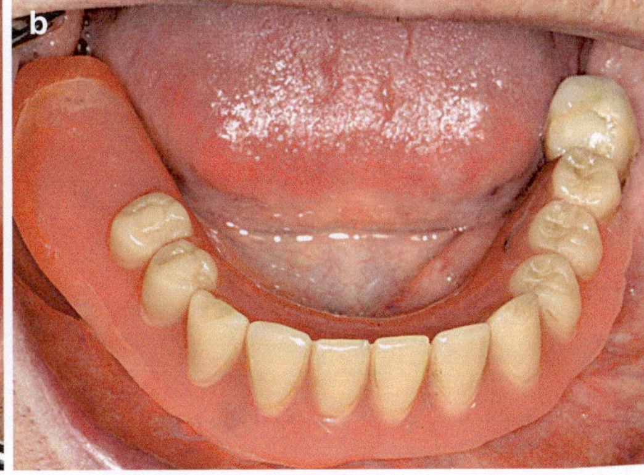

**Fig. 16.1** (**a**) A female patient with intravenous bisphosphonate (zoledronate) with minimum area of exposed bone (*arrow*) after sore spots of her denture (**b**). She complained about sore spots 2 months ago. The blood spot was provoked by probing with a blunt probe

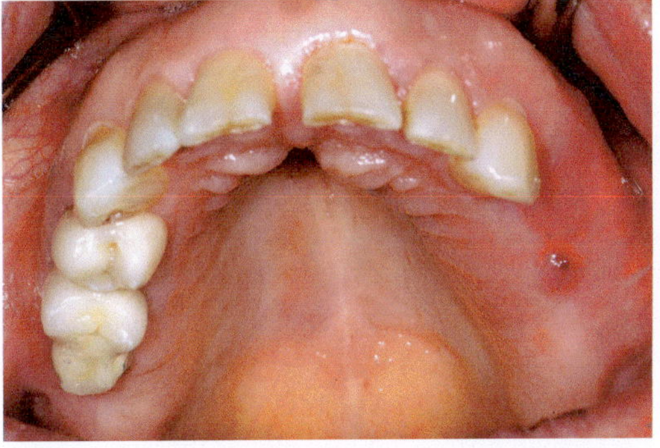

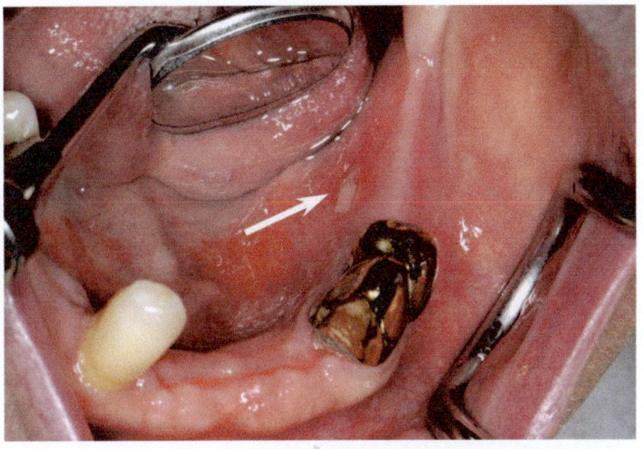

**Fig. 16.2** Purulent fistula of the left upper jaw of a patient with breast cancer and denosumab therapy. Non restorable teeth were extracted before denosumab therapy. The patient complained about a non-fitting prosthesis. The patient was free of complaints and the fistula was discovered at a recall appointment

**Fig. 16.3** Small ONJ lesion caused by a pressure sore (*arrow*) at typical site in the lower jaw. This patient with metastatic prostate cancer received zoledronate intravenously. The exposed bone is located at the lingual boarder of the removable prosthesis

increased from the anterior (Fig. 16.1a, b) to the premolar and the molar region. The upper jaw (Fig. 16.2) was more affected than the lower jaw (Fig. 16.3) [18]. These pressure-related ulcers can also occur at the hard palate [16]. Other studies confirmed a statistically significant increased frequency of MRONJ in cancer patients with intravenous bisphosphonates, if they were wearing removable dentures [11, 12, 18].

Generally spoken, ill-fitting dentures and sore spots are the second most mentioned reasons for MRONJ by opening a pathway for the oral flora to the bone [11] because of the injury of the oral mucosa [12]. Additionally, they contribute to MRONJ through the observed inhibitory or toxic effects on keratinocytes that impair the habitual mucous repair mechanisms and later lead to MRONJ [19, 20]. After this tissue breakdown, the damaged mucosa and the underlying bone are in danger to be infected by the local oral flora [21]. MRONJ could manifest thereafter.

The typical location of the mucosal lesions is similar to sore spots caused by any denture base in any patient. Therefore, it is found either underneath the denture base in the nonmobile oral mucosa or at the base margin where the mucosa is mobile during functional movement of the oral muscles [22]. A decubital lesion in BP patients is usually round or oval with a diameter of 1–8 mm. A deep red color typifies a moderate case, whereas a grayish or white lesion surrounded by a reddish inflammation is characteristic of more serious cases. Persistent lesions which led to the exposed bone can be very pale without any reddish inflammation around and not easy to spot (Fig. 16.1a). A blunt probe is therefore a useful instrument.

Even simple measurements like forced probing of the periodontal ligament are reported to have a certain risk of MRONJ. Gallego et al. described an MRONJ caused by a rubber dam clasp [10].

> Surgical extraction of teeth is regarded to be the most frequent trigger event for MRONJ.
>
> Sore spots of denture bases are important prosthodontic risk factors for MRONJ.
>
> Every injury or damage to the soft tissues (mucosa) close to bone could cause MRONJ.

## Prosthetic Techniques and Recommendations

Guidelines for bisphosphonate-related osteonecrosis (BRONJ) define three levels of risk [8]. In this classification, considerations regarding denosumab were added in brackets:

*Low risk*: Oral bisphosphonate medication or intravenous bisphosphonate once a year (or subcutaneous denosumab) for primary osteoporosis

*Medium risk*: Intravenous bisphosphonate (or subcutaneous denosumab) medication twice a year for secondary osteoporosis (therapy-induced osteoporosis)

*High risk*: Intravenous bisphosphonate (or subcutaneous denosumab) medications monthly for oncological reasons

It should be stated that orally administered antiresorptive medication for more than 3–4 years, as well as concomitant chronic long-term steroid therapy or immunosuppressives like methotrexate may rise the risk [23] to a higher (risk) group. For those patients receiving once-a-year intravenous dose of zoledronate, the risk of necrosis could be higher after 3 years of treatment. In assessing these patients, it is important that oral bisphosphonates before intravenous BP or denosumab therapy should be taken into account estimating the risk [23].

Metastatic cancer patients and patients with multiple myeloma usually receive antiresorptive medications for a long time. These patients could be staged as "high-risk" patients at the beginning of their antiresorptives therapy. This implements that the dental status should be sound and the oral health is in good condition. If decayed teeth have to be removed, generally spoken, if these patients have the need of dentoalveolar surgery, these surgeries should be performed before antiresorptive treatment starts. The start of the antiresorptive therapy should be delayed, if possible, until the dental health is optimized, especially, nonrestorable teeth and those with poor prognosis are extracted. Antiresorptive therapy can be started after a stable wound situation is reached. In general, a 10–14-day delay after surgery should be considered as adequate for wound healing [23]. However, every therapy not compromising the gingiva close to the bone can be performed during antiresorptives therapy.

So far, only a few references in literature with a low impact of evidence are available regarding evidence-based treatment guidelines/recommendations for bisphosphonate or denosumab patients.

The following guidelines are suggested by the available literature and the personal experience of the authors (including personal communications) and therefore must be critically reviewed. Principally, these guidelines are referred to patients with a high MRONJ risk:

- *"Long-term successfully worn" dentures with no history of sore spots should not be changed, if possible.*

  Although relining or renewal of existing dentures are thought to improve occlusion, stability, retention, and facial support [24, 25], replacement should be evaluated critically especially when dealing with elderly patients who have worn their removable dentures successfully over a long time. Normally with new dentures, patients perceive an enhanced oral health-related quality of life [25], *but* new dentures

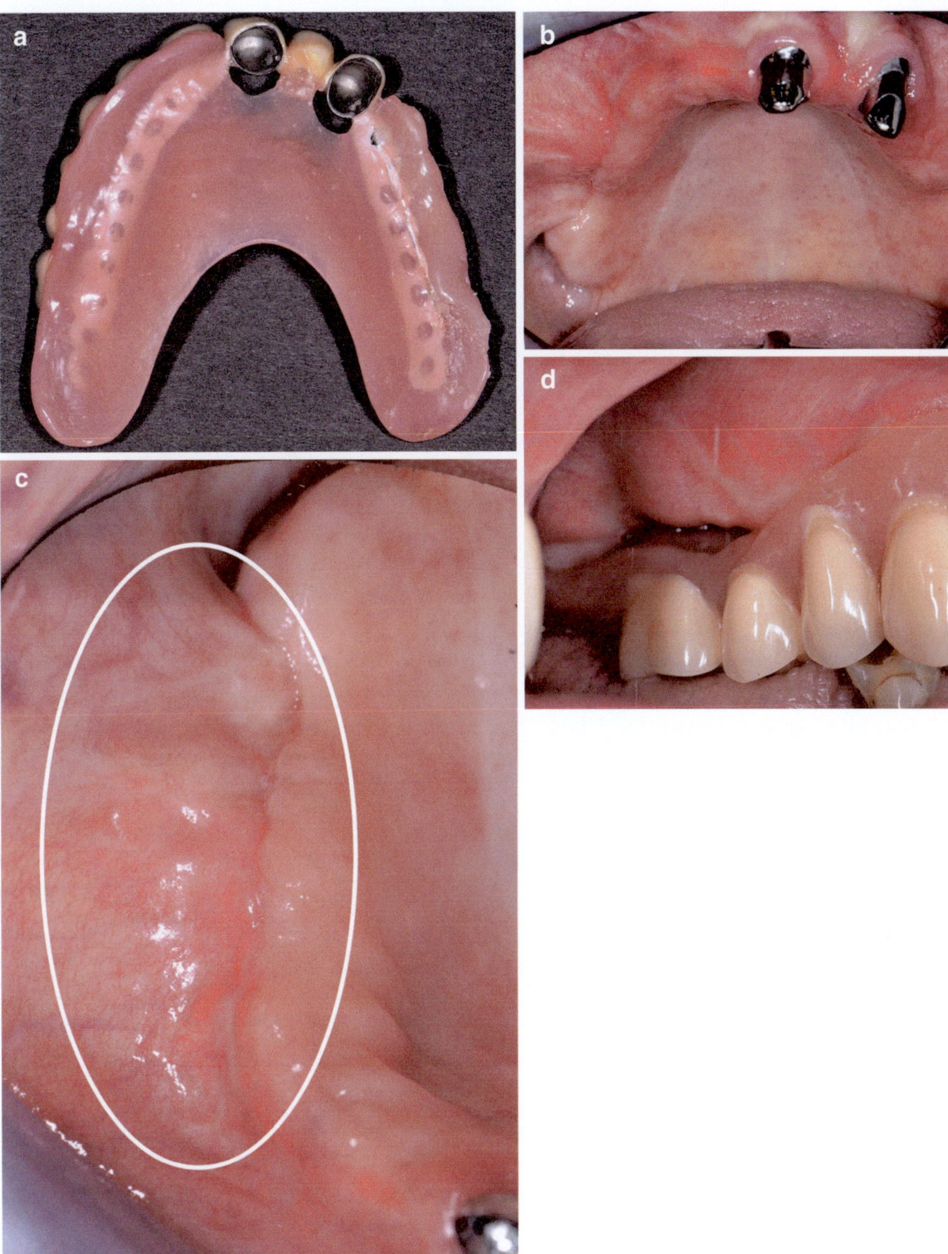

**Fig. 16.4** (**a**) New overdenture of a female patient with multiple myeloma and successful MRONJ treatment (surgical resection). Shortly after therapy, zoledronate was restarted combined with lenalidomide (chemotherapy). The intra-oral situation (**b**) shows a prominent buccal flap covering the defect at the right alveolar jaw. No sign of fistula or exposed bone. Detail (**c**) of this region (photo taken with mirror). The area (**c**) with vulnerable, thin, and non-fixed gingival is marked. This area is very sensitive to sore spots and therefore at risk for a relapse of MRONJ. Special attention was drawn to this area with the prostheses (**d**). A soft lining material covers the vulnerable area. The gap is resulting from retraction of the buccal tissue flap. To reduce the pressure forces, only the first molar was lined up

require that patients adapt to its new function and they are also known to have problems with sore spots after prosthesis delivery: Kivovics et al. observed denture-induced mucosal injuries in 87 % in the first, 50 % in the second, and 7 % in the third week after placement of complete dentures [22]. Therefore, there might be an elevated risk for MRONJ development.

- *If new dentures or prosthesis with gingival support have to be inserted, a soft lining could be considered.*
  Most authors recommend a soft lining technique to reduce sore spots (Fig. 16.4a, d). They also line the surface of dentures to dissipate and distribute forces by their cushioning effect [24, 26]. Soft lining materials are principally applied temporarily to the underling denture base to distribute the pressure uniformly on the supporting tissues under the denture. The viscoelastic properties of these materials are important for their cushioning effect, which allows a more homogeny pressure distribution, and maintaining the shape of the materials [27–29].

  Soft lining materials are very sensitive to contamination with candida or other microorganisms. Soft linings should be controlled regularly and renewed if contamination with candida or other microorganism is obvious [26, 30, 31]. Soft liners should remain for 3 years maximum but usually have to be exchanged earlier [30]. A minimum thickness of 1.5–2 mm is necessary to distribute the pressure to the supporting tissues underneath the denture base [28]; some authors even claim 3 mm [27, 29].

  On the other hand, some authors observed additional irritations of the mucosa with soft liners leading to ulcers [32].
- Regardless of any prosthodontic therapy or treatment concept, *maintenance of dentures, dental prophylaxis, caries control, and conservative restorative dentistry have to be performed continuously* [8, 9, 11, 33].
- *For less stress transference to the bone and reduction of undesirable horizontal forces, acrylic cuspless/monoplane teeth were recommended in dentures* [24].
- *Preprosthetic surgery should be performed, if possible, before any antiresorptive treatment, in order to remove any bony spikes and spicules, which act as foci of stress concentration during denture function* [24].
- *If extraction of fractured teeth is very risky, endodontic treatment, coronectomy, and a lock is possible* [33]. These remnant roots can be covered (without contact) with bridges or denture bases [33].

- *Endodontic treatment is not connected with a high risk for* MRONJ. If a diversion of bacteria over the apices into the bone is expected, an antibiotic prophylaxis can be considered [9–11, 32, 33].
- *In contrast to the general recommendation to wear the new prosthesis 24 h* [33], *breaks of 12 h – normally during night time – are considered to reduce the risk of (minimum to severe) sore spots* [24]. High polished denture bases in the lower jaw are also recommended.
- *If crowns (regardless whether they support fixed or removable partial dentures) are insufficient,* rescue *fillings should be considered,* if the prostheses are functional.
- *Fixed partial dentures seem to be associated with a lower MRONJ risk when compared to removable partial ones with mucosal support.*
- *Mucosal support should be avoided in critical areas of vulnerable tissues or areas of healed MRONJ or lately extraction sites* (Fig. 16.4c).
- *High water design of bridge pontics enables the possibility to control the mucosa underneath,* especially if a tooth was extracted under BP medication in this area previously. The bridge could also be inserted temporarily to control this area before using a permanent luting agent. An esthetic loss should be considered.
- *Supra- and para-marginal preparation for crowns minimize the possibility of severe gingival tissue damage.* In a critical situation, antibiotics and moderate local mouth rinses (chlorhexidine) could be considered [26]. This critical situation (estimated personal risk) could additionally be considered during preparation and impression taking. Retraction fiber could also harm the marginal gingiva and the underlying bone.
- *The patient must be informed about the risk of MRONJ in general and the risk especially associated with extensive prosthodontic rehabilitation* [9, 24, 34].
  A recall program should be adapted to the individual patient's risk. The patient should be recalled at intervals of 2–3 months to monitor health of the denture-bearing tissue, clinically (and radiographically) [24, 34]. This is in contrast to the general guidelines for care and maintenance of dentures on an annual basis [33].

- *Some authors mention that oral hygiene is an important factor contributing to the remission of MRONJ in denture-wearing patients* [18].
- *The follow-up care of fixed and removable partial or complete prosthesis has to be established as a continuous care.* Patients have to be instructed regarding the maintenance needed considering their possibilities in handling, seeing, and understanding. Assistance should be given according to their special needs. Removable prostheses need more maintenance than fixed ones [34].
- *It should be taken into consideration that the maintenance can be interrupted by pain, oncological setbacks, and the accompanying distress and intensified therapies.*

Any dental treatment that affects the gum has a risk to harm tissues and can cause MRONJ.

Patients should be aware of the risk of MRONJ by sore spots.

Prosthodontic rehabilitation concepts should be adapted to:

- The disease
- The possibilities of the patient to handle the dental prosthesis
- The possibility to detect sore spots
- The capability for recall visits
- The risk to develop MRONJ

## How to Handle Sore Spots

As described before, sore spots are one of the major risk factors for MRONJ. Therefore, every sore spot presenting them with and without beginning tissue injury must be considered as a serious event and treated immediately. The following procedures turned out to be useful:

- The patients must be informed about the potential risk of MRONJ and sore spots.
- In case of sore spots, the patient has to consult the dentist immediately in order to remove the causes of the sore spots.
- If this is not possible in due time, the dentures should not be worn anymore, even if those areas cannot be identified later.
- Patients with high anti-pain medications must be aware that they probably will not feel sore spots adequately.

- Sore spots can be controlled by dental care of the prosthesis and moderate local antiseptic mouth rinses (chlorhexidine 0.1–0.2 %) and mouth rinses with tee. Lower concentrations with 0.1 % turned out to be more accepted. Especially green tea is thought to have special antiseptic qualities [15, 17]. In serious cases, an antibiotic therapy should be considered [17].

## MRONJ Caused by Sore Spots

MRONJ lesions caused by sore spots (Figs. 16.1, 16.2, and 16.3) can be kept under control by the daily use of local mouth rinses. Areas of exposed and necrotic bone may remain asymptomatic for a long time. The lesions are most frequently symptomatic when surrounding tissues become inflamed or clinical signs of infection are visible [23]. This can be observed under chemotherapy causing a decrease in leukocyte count. For this reason, special awareness must be drawn to the immune function. Depressed leukocytes or immunosuppressive situations can worsen the affected area in a short time. An antibiotic prophylaxis, especially in immunosuppressive (expected) conditions, turned out to be effective to prevent progression. Continuous antibiotic medication can be administered during expected leukocyte depressions.

## Oral Rehabilitation After MRONJ Treatment

After a successful treatment of MRONJ, the dentist and sometimes the patient are afraid of a relapse caused by a new prosthesis. Some clinicians recommend not to touch an MRONJ-affected area with any prosthesis regardless whether it was treated successfully or still has exposed necrotic bone (personal communications). But, because oral rehabilitation supports the quality of life especially under general health concerns, the decision making in favor or against an oral rehabilitation should be considered carefully. Individual conditions of every single patient should be taken into account on an individual basis.

Oral rehabilitation needs a good expertise and experience of the clinician, because sometimes,

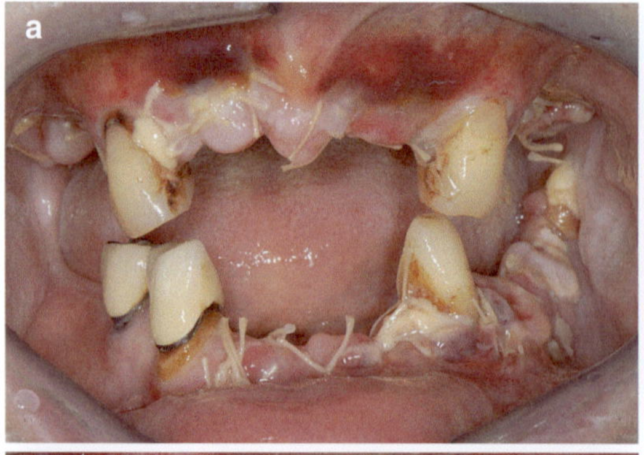
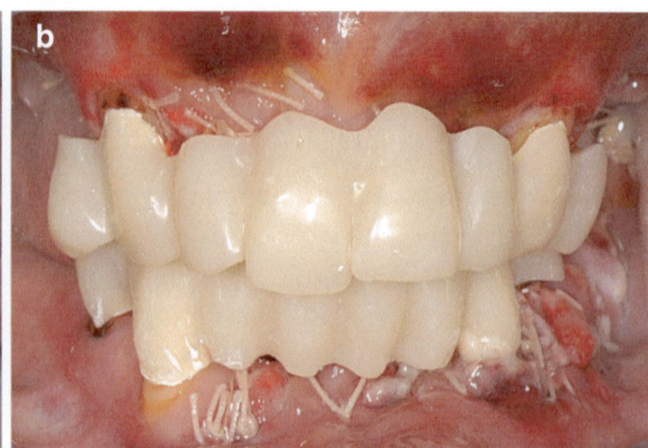
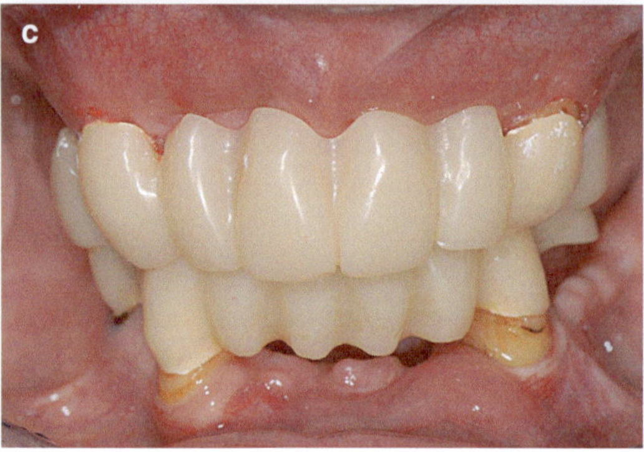

**Fig. 16.5** (**a**) Situation shortly after extraction of teeth under bisphosphonate medication and anticoagulation. The patient wanted an interim prosthesis. The situation (**b**) of the interim prosthesis showing a distance to the wound (high water design). The prosthesis provided acceptable esthetic results and allows the wound to heal undisturbed and uncompromised below the prosthesis (**c**)

these patients end up with enormous bony defects of the jaw or even open maxillary sinuses. Special attention must be drawn to the sensitive and vulnerable regions after (surgical) treatment of these patients (Fig. 16.4a–d). If the patient is able to cope with regular recalls, proper daily cleaning, and handling the prosthesis, has the ability to detect sore spots, and his or her general health condition is good enough to endure the sometimes even for healthy patients exhausting prosthodontic treatment procedure, the oral rehabilitation should be considered.

Göllner et al. reported a noninvasive prosthetic therapy with telescopic overdentures and heat-polymerized resilient liner [26] and observed no complications in a 2-year follow-up.

Patients with maxillofacial defects after MRONJ stage III therapy or sequestrectomy can benefit from obturator prosthesis. Even though an obturator prosthesis has a risk for new MRONJ lesion, it can provide the patient a good function and quality of life. Obturator prosthesis should be considered and discussed with the individual situation of each patient. Depprich et al. demonstrated a good global quality of life after prosthodontic therapy with obturator prosthesis of 65 % on average regarding non-MRONJ patients [35].

## Temporary Prosthesis

Provisional removable prosthesis are more likely to cause sore spots and consecutively MRONJ lesions when compared to permanent dentures, because they are normally not very stable and less supported by the remaining teeth or the gums after extractions. For this reason, some authors like Göllner et al. strictly prohibit any provisional prosthesis to bridge the time till the definitive prosthesis installation [26].

Under special circumstances and a close and stringent recall, temporary prosthesis could be planed and inserted (Fig. 16.5a–c). These arrangements should be adapted to the patients' wishes and possibilities and, of course, adapted to the personal MRONJ risk – once more – as discussed above.

### Conclusion

Oral rehabilitation is of major importance for patients receiving bisphosphonates or denosuamb who often face critical illnesses and the respective treatment protocols. Planning, manufacturing, and maintenance of dental prostheses have to take the individual situation of each patient into account. Misfits and sore spots should be avoided whenever possible.

## References


1. Waller A, Groff SL, Hagen N, Bultz BD, Carlson LE. Characterizing distress, the 6th vital sign, in oncology pain clinic. Curr Oncol. 2012;19(2):e53–9.
2. Ringe JD. Therapie chronischer Schmerzen des Bewegungsapparates mit Opioiden. J Mineralsoffw. 2002;9:23–5.
3. Fueki K, Yoshida E, Igarashi Y. A structural equation model relating objective and subjective masticatory function and oral health-related quality of life in patients with removable partial dentures. J Oral Rehabil. 2011;38(11):810–7.
4. Veyrune JL, Tubert-Jeannin S, Dutheil C, Riordan PJ. Impact of new prostheses on the oral health related quality of life of edentulous patients. Gerodontology. 2005;22(1):3–9.
5. Hantsch ROA, Al-Omiri MK, Yunis MA, Dar-Odeh N, Lynch E. Relationship between impacts of complete denture treatment on daily living, satisfaction and personality profiles. J Contemp Dent Pract. 2011;12(3):200–7.
6. Fehm T, Felsenberg D, Krimmel M, Solomayer E, Wallwiener D, Hadjii P. Bisphosphonate-associated osteonecrosis of the jaw in breast cancer patients: recommendations for prevention and treatment. Breast. 2009;18(4):213–7.
7. Özhayat EB, Gotfredsen K. Effect of treatment with fixed and removable dental prostheses. An oral health-related quality of life study. J Oral Rehabil. 2012;39(1):28–36.
8. AWMF-Register Nr. 007/091. Bisphosphonat-assoziierte Kiefernekrosen (BP-ONJ) und andere Medikamenten-assoziierte Kiefernekrosen. 2012. http://www.awmf.org/uploads/tx_szleitlinien/007-091l_S3_Bisphosphonat-assoziierte_Kiefernekrose_2012-04.pdf (Stand 3/2014).
9. Ruggiero SL, Didson TB, Assael LA, Landesberg R, Marx RE, Mehrotra B. American Association of Oral and Maxillofacial Surgeons Position Paper on Bisphosphonate-related osteonecrosis of the jaws-2009 update. J Oral Maxillofac Surg. 2009;67 Suppl 1:2–12.
10. Gallego L, Junquera L, Pelaz A, Diaz-Bobes C. Rubber dam clamp trauma during endodontic treatment: a risk factor of bisphosphonate-related osteonecrosis of the jaw? J Oral Maxillofac Surg. 2011;69:e93–5.
11. Vahtsevanos K, Kyrgidis A, Verrou E, Katodritou E, Triaridis S, Andreadis CG, Boukovinas I, Koloutsos GE, Teleioudis Z, Kitikidou K, Paraskevopoulos P, Zervas K, Antoniades K. Longitudinal cohort study of risk factors in cancer patients of bisphosphonate-related osteonecrosis of the jaw. J Clin Oncol. 2009;27(32):5356–62.
12. Kyrigidis A, Vahtsevanos K, Koloutsos G, Andreadis C, Boukovinas J, Teleioudis Z, Patrikidou A, Triaridis S. Bisphosphonate-related osteonecrosis of the jaws: a case-control study of risk factors in breast cancer patients. J Clin Oncol. 2008;26(6):4634–8.
13. Vescovi P, Campisi G, Fusco V, Mergoni G, Manfredi M, Merigo E, Solazzo L, Gabriele M, Gaeta GM, Favia G, Peluso F, Coltella G. Surgery-triggered and non surgery-triggered bisphosphonate-related osteonecrosis of the jaws (BRONJ): a retrospective analysis of 567 cases in an Italian multicenter study. Oral Oncol. 2011;47(3):191–4.
14. Hoff AO, Toth BB, Altundag K, Johnson MM, Warneke CL, Hu M, Nooka A, Sayegh G, Guarneri V, Desrouleaux K, Cui J, Adamus A, Gagel R, Hortobagyi GH. Frequency and risk factors associated with osteonecrosis of the jaw in cancer patients treated with intravenous bisphosphonates. J Bone Miner Res. 2008;23(6):826–36.
15. Yarom N, Yahalom R, Shoshani Y, Hamed W, Regev E, Elad S. Osteonecrosis of the jaw induced by orally administered bisphosphonates: incidence, clinical features, predisposing factors and treatment outcome. Osteoporos Int. 2007;18(10):1363–70.
16. Levin L, Laviv A, Schwarts-Arad D. Denture-related osteonecrosis of the maxilla associated with oral bisphosphonate treatment. J Am Dent Assoc. 2007;138(8):1218–20.
17. Hoefert S. Prothesendruckstellen als Risiko einer Bisphosphonat-assoziierten Kiefernekrose. ZWR. 2012;121(11):564–71.
18. Hasegawa Y, Kawabe M, Kimura H, Kurita K, Kukuta J, Urade M. Influence of dentures in the initial occurrence site on the prognosis of bisphosphonate-related osteonecrosis of the jaw: a retrospective study. Oral Surg Oral Med Oral Pathol Oral Radiol. 2012;114(3):318–24.
19. Ravosa MJ, Ning J, Liu Y, Stack MS. Bisphosphonates effects on the behaviour of oral epithelial cells and oral fibroblasts. Arch Oral Biol. 2011;56(5):491–8.
20. Pabst AM, Ziebart T, Koch FP, Taylor KY, Al-Nawas B, Walter C. The influence of bisphosphonates on viability, migration, and apoptosis of human oral keratinocytes – in vitro study. Clin Oral Investig. 2012;16(1):87–93.
21. Sedghizadeh PP, Kumar SK, Gorur A, Schaudinn C, Schuler CF, Costerton JW. Identification of microbial biofilms in osteonecrosis of the jaws secondary to bisphosphonates therapy. J Oral Maxillofac Surg. 2008;66(4):767–75.

22. Kivovics P, Jahn M, Borbely J, Marton K. Frequency and location of traumatic ulcerations following placement of complete dentures. Int J Prosthodont. 2007; 20(4):397–401.

23. Ruggiero SL. An office-based approach to the diagnosis and management on osteonecrosis. Atlas Oral Maxillofac Surg Clin North Am. 2013;21(2): 167–73.

24. Tripathi A, Pandey S, Singh SV, Sharma NK, Singh R. Bisphosphonate therapy for skeletal malignancies and metastases: impact on jaw bones and prosthodontic concerns. J Prosthodont. 2011;20(7):601–3.

25. Garret NR, Kapur KK, Perez P. Effects of improvements of poorly fitting dentures and new dentures on patients satisfaction. J Prosthet Dent. 1996;76(10):403–13.

26. Göllner M, Holst S, Fenner M, Schmitt J. Prosthodontic treatment of a patient with bisphosphonate-induced osteonecrosis of the jaw using a removable dental prosthesis with a heat-polymerized resilient liner: a clinical report. J Prosthet Dent. 2010;103(4):196–201.

27. Kawano F, Tada N, Nagao K, Matsumoto N. The influence of soft lining materials on pressure distribution. J Prosthet Dent. 1991;6(4):567–75.

28. Maruta H, Haberham RC, Hamada T, Taguchi N. Settings and stress relaxation behaviour of resilient denture liners. J Prosthet Dent. 1998;80(6):714–22.

29. Taguchi N, Murata H, Hamada T, Hong G. Effect of viscoelastic properties of resilient venture liners on pressures under dentures. J Oral Rehabil. 2001;28(11): 1003–8.

30. Wagner WC, Kawano F, Dootz ER, Koran A. Dynamic viscoelastic properties of processed soft denture liners: part II-effect of aging. J Prosthet Dent. 1995;74(3):299–304.

31. Okita N, Orstavik D, Ostavik J, Ostby K. In vivo and in vitro studies on soft denture materials: microbial adhesion and tests for antibacterial activity. Dent Mater. 1991;7:155–60.

32. Döring K, Linek W, Spieckermann J. Die Bisphosphonat-assoziierte Kiefernekrose. Oralchirurgie J. 2007;1:26–30.

33. Felton D, Cooper L, Duqum I, Minsley G, Guckes A, Haug S, Meredith P, Solie C, Avery D, Chandler ND. Evidence-based guidelines for the care and maintenance of complete dentures: a publication of the American College of Prosthodontics. J Prosthodont. 2011;20 Suppl 1:S1–12.

34. Stark H, Wolowski A, Ehmke B. Nachsorgestrategien für Zahnersatz. ZM. 2011;101(8):60–4.

35. Depprich R, Naujoks C, Lind D, Ommerborn M, Meyer U, Kübler J, Hendschel J. Evaluation of the quality of life of patients with maxillofacial defects after prosthodontic therapy with obturator prostheses. Int J Oral Maxillofac Surg. 2011;40(1):71–9.

# Dental Implants in the Context Antiresorptive Drugs and Medication-Related Osteonecrosis of the Jaw

Yorck Alexander Zebuhr

**Abstract**

Antiresorptive drugs and dental implants both target on bone. So, relationships between bisphosphonates and RANKL-Inhibitor (denosumab) as antiresorptive drugs, the occurrence of MRONJ as an entity of osteonecrosis of jaw, and dental implants are multidimensional: Implants can trigger the occurrence of MRONJ; bisphosphonates and denosumab can alter implant osseointegration and clinical success, but implants are maybe useful in prophylaxis of MRONJ and can even help in rehabilitation after MRONJ. Furthermore, as antiresorptive medication and especially bisphosphonate medication is frequent, and need for implant is frequent, too, there is emerging question on indication of dental implants in these increasing patient groups.

## Introduction

Dental implants, which revolutionized prosthodontic therapy and modern antiresorptive drugs, namely, bisphosphonates, which revolutionized therapy in bone disease, both are about 40 years old. The topic of dental implants in the context of antiresorptive drugs therefore opens a wide field of interests with respect to clinical and scientific impact: Implant surgery and periimplantitis are known risk factors for medication-related osteonecrosis of the jaw (MRONJ). Age is a risk factor for tooth loss and therefore for implant need as well as it is for osteoporosis and solid metastatic tumor. As these two are the most important indications for antiresorptive drugs, there is a big overlap of these two patient groups. On the other hand, implants may be useful in rehabilitation after tooth and jaw bone loss in MRONJ. Implants may also be of prophylactic use for MRONJ, as bad-fitting dentures or denture sores can lead to MRONJ. Last, coating of implants with antiresorptive drugs may be useful in osseointegration and prevention of bone loss around dental implants or even in periimplantitis, as bone resorption is an important process in both conditions.

## Implants, Bisphosphonates, and MRONJ

Undoubtedly, Marx recognized bisphosphonate-induced osteonecrosis of the jaw as an entity and its impact in his famous 2003 publication [1]. But as early as 1995, Stark et al. reported a case of loss of previously osseointegrated implants in a patient after bisphosphonate medication was started [2],

Y.A. Zebuhr, MD, DMD
Klinikum Wels-Grieskirchen GmbH,
Department of Oral and Maxillofacial Surgery,
Head: DDr. W.P. Poeschl, PhD,
Grieskirchnerstr. 42, Wels A-4600, Austria
e-mail: yorck@zebuhr.at

S. Otto (ed.), *Medication-Related Osteonecrosis of the Jaws: Bisphosphonates, Denosumab, and New Agents*,
DOI 10.1007/978-3-662-43733-9_17, © Springer-Verlag Berlin Heidelberg 2015

which could be named the first case of MRONJ in the literature, retrospectively. Later, it was shown in a lot of reports that iatrogenic trauma like implant surgery can trigger MRONJ. So, there is evidence that implant surgery may be a risk factor or a trigger event for MRONJ, and vice versa, bisphosphonate medication may affect implant success, but the impact of both of them is not known.

## Implants as a Trigger for MRONJ

Generally, implant surgery is a highly elective procedure. Therefore, there is an important demand on safety of dental implantology, especially with regard on potential consequences with a relevant morbidity like MRONJ undoubtedly may enfold. Implant surgery has the potential for bacterial contamination which is a known initiator for MRONJ. Nonetheless, MRONJ also occurs as a late effect of implant rehabilitation: In a recent case collection study, only the minority of patients developed BRONJ as a surgical site complication, while in a majority of cases, MRONJ formed after months or even years of implant osseointegration [3]. Similarly, in another case series of 14 patients with BRONJ after implant therapy, mean onset time between implant insertion and MRONJ was 20.9 months [4]. A recent report demonstrated spontaneous onset of MRONJ in a long-term stable previously grafted sinus [5], which emphasizes that long intervals between surgery or implant surgery and MRONJ onset are possible.

First recommendations totally neglected elective jaw surgery like implant surgery in patients with bisphosphonate history [6]. Some authors [7] and also the AAOMS guidelines [8] advise against implants in patients with a history of intravenous bisphosphonate medication, while they do not contraindicate them in oral drug users under special conditions and informed consent, including late failure and morbidity. But implant-related MRONJ does not only occur in intravenous bisphosphonate users but also in oral route therapy [4, 9, 10]. Furthermore, there is emerging impact of MRONJ generally as a consequence of not only intravenous medication both also oral medication due to epidemiological reasons [9]. Though there is lack of data, high risk is attributed to dental implants in cancer patients on intravenous medication, and long drug holidays of up to 6 years are recommended [11], which effec-

tively would exclude many of these patients from implant therapy. Then again, successful implant therapy in intravenous bisphosphonate users was followed in single cases [12], and implants can even heal and keep in function after cured MRONJ [13]. Subsequently, there is neither evidence for nor against dental implants in bisphosphonate medication, but potential late-onset problems should be taken into account. By now, no reports exist on MRONJ as effect of implants in patients on RANKL-inhibitor (denosumab) medication. Probably, these medications are stated as contraindications from implantologists. So there is lack of information on this topic, and one could only speculate if implant therapy could be safely performed in these patients, as shorter half-life of RANKL-inhibitor than of bisphosphonates may allow effective drug-holidays for surgery.

## Bisphosphonates as a Risk Factor in Implantology

From a theoretical point of view, one can distinguish two impacts of bisphosphonate medication on implantology: Firstly, the process of osseointegration of dentals implants could be disturbed by systemic bisphosphonate medication, and secondly, correctly osseointegrated implants could be affected.

Reports on successful osseointegration of dental implants overweigh informations on disturbed integration [14, 15], but late loss seems to be an important problem: Late loss of previously osseo-integrated implants was first described in 1995: A patient lost five implants 6 months after bisphosphonate therapy for osteoporosis was started [2]. Implant failure rate was shown to be slightly increased in women with oral bisphosphonate medication when compared to nonusers [16], but this may not justify an absolute contraindication for these patient groups, as survival of implants in postmenopausal women showed no difference whether they were on bisphosphonate medication or not [17]. Furthermore, there may be an overlap for underlying common risk factors for osteoporosis as a bisphosphonate indication and for implant failure, like smoking and steroid intake.

An overview on the existing literature on the impact of bisphosphonates on implant failure and induction of MRONJ by implant surgery is given in Table 17.1.

**Table 17.1** The Impact of Bisphosphonates on Dentals Implants: Implant Success or Failure in Patients under Bisphosphonate Therapy, BRONJ related to Implants and Implants in Rehabilitation after BRONJ

| Author, year | Study population | Medication (indication) | Implant complication | Time of onset or follow-up | Development of BRONJ |
| --- | --- | --- | --- | --- | --- |
| Starck, 1995 [2] | 1 patient with 5 implants | Not given | Implant loss, bone exposure | 6 months | Yes? |
| Kushner, 2005 [18] | 2 cases | Alendronate | BRONJ and implant loss (both cases) pathological fracture (one case) | 3 and 4 months | Yes |
| Marx, 2005 [6] | 119 patients with BRONJ | 116 IV (oncologic)<br><br>3 p.o. (osteoporotic) | Implant loss, bone exposure | Not given | 4 (3,4 %) of BRONJ cases induced by implants (1 on IV rest not given) |
| Jeffcoat, 2006 [19] | 50 patients with 210 implants | 25 patients p.o.<br>25 controls (no medication) | Success >99 % in both groups | Longer than 3 years | No |
| Brooks, 2007 [9] | 1 patient with 10 implants and grafting | p.o. (osteoporotic) for 2 years | Infection, explantation of 1 implant with sequestrotomy | 2 years | Yes |
| Wang, 2007 [20] | 1 patient with 5 implants | p.o. for >10 years | Infection, implants kept | 1 year | Yes |
| Marx, 2007 [21] | 30 patients with BRONJ, thereof 2 caused by implant placement | p.o. | | | Yes |
| Fugazzotto, 2007 [22] | 61 patients with 169 implants, 22/39 thereof put at time of tooth removal | p.o. (4 patients osteoporotic dose, 57 patients prophylactic dose) for 3.3 years on average | 1 case with bone exposure and spontaneous healing | 12–24 months | No |
| Yarom, 2007 [23] | 11 patients with BRONJ, thereof 2 with implants and 1 with "implant extraction" | Oral | BRONJ, implant loss | 2, 7, and 14 months in these 3 patients | Yes |
| Grant, 2008 [24] | 115 patients with 468 implants | Oral | 2 failed, 1 was successfully replaced, 1 was not replaced | 2–10 years | None |

(continued)

**Table 17.1** (continued)

| Author, year | Study population | Medication (indication) | Implant complication | Time of onset or follow-up | Development of BRONJ |
|---|---|---|---|---|---|
| Bell, 2008 [25] | 42 patients with 100 implants and 68 bone grafts | Oral | 5 implants failed but were successfully replaced | 4–89 months average: 37 months | None |
| Kasai, 2009 [26] | 65 women of more than 36 years of age | 11 on oral BP for osteoporosis with 35 implants | 5 implants without osseointegration in 3 patients (14, 3 %) | | None |
| | | 40 on no medication with 161 implants | 7 implants without osseointegration in 7 patients (4, 3 %) | | |
| Goss, 2010 [27] | 16.000 patients with 28.000 implants | Unselected dental implant clientele | 7 cases of implant failure in patients with oral bisphosphonate medication | 3 cases: no osseointegration 4 cases: late failure | None |
| Bedogni, 2010 [28] | 1 patient with 2 implants and bone augmentation | Oral BP for osteoporosis | Primary osseointegration, late infection | 2 years | Yes |
| Lazarovici, 2010 [29] | 114 BRONJ patients with 27 implant-related BRONJ cases | 11 implant-related BRONJ cases on oral BP | Early infection or primary osseointegration and late infection | 16,2 months mean duration until BRONJ development | Yes |
| | | 16 implant-related BRONJ cases on i.v. BP | | | |
| Martin, 2010 [30] | 8,752 patients, 589 of them with implants | Oral BP | 16 patients with 26 implant complications | Early and late implant failure (4 weeks to 11 years) | None did meet AAOMS criteria |
| Shabestari, 2010 [31] | 21 patients with 46 implants | Oral BP | None | | No |
| Koka, 2010 [17] | 137 postmenopausal women | 55 on oral BP | 1 of 121 implants lost | | No |
| | | 88 without BP therapy | 3 of 166 implants lost | | |
| Bojer, 2011 [12] | 1 patient with 4 mandibular implants | IV (steroid-induced osteoporosis) | Uneventful healing | 35 months | No |
| Famili, 2011 [32] | 23 patients with 75 implants | p. o. | 1 lost but replaced | 1–3 years | No |
| Zahid, 2011 [33] | 26 patients with 51 implants | p. o. | 3 implants lost | | No |
| Ferlito, 2011 [34] | 1 patient with extractions and immediate implants | IV for multiple myeloma | BRONJ in the only extraction site where no implant was put (!) | | Yes |
| Zebuhr, 2012 [13] | 2 patients with cured BRONJ, 9 implants | p.o. (osteoporotic) | None | 9 and 12 months | No |

| Diniz-Freitas, 2012 [35] | 20 consecutive BRONJ cases, 2 thereof after implant surgery | p.o. (osteoporotic) | | | Yes |
|---|---|---|---|---|---|
| Flichy-Fernandez, 2012 [36] | 1 patient (drug holiday and CTX test before implant surgery) | p.o. (osteoporotic) | BRONJ, bone loss, but implants kept | | Yes |
| Subramanian, 2012 [37] | 6 implants in 1 patient | p.o. (osteoporotic) | Primary osseointegration, late implant loss | 8 years after implant surgery, 7 years after BP therapy start | No |
| Gupta, 2012 [38] | 2 implants in 1 patient (CTX test before implant surgery) | p.o. (osteoporotic) | Bone sequestration, implant loosening in 1 implant, 1 implant without problems but no prosthetic use | 6 weeks | No |
| Lopez-Cedrun, 2013 [39] | 9 patients with BRONJ after dental implants | 7 patients: osteoporosis | 7 of 9 recovered | Average BRONJ onset 20,9 months after implant surgery, range 1–34 months | 9 patients with BRONJ after dental implants |
| | | 1 patient: osteoarthritis | | | |
| | | 1 patient: polymyalgia rheumatica | | | |
| Mattheos, 2013 [40] | Implant surgery and augmentation in 1 patient | IV (osteoporotic) | None | 6 months | No |
| Jacobsen, 2013 [4] | 110 BRONJ patients with | Two thirds with oncological indication | Infection, explantation | Average BRONJ onset 20,9 months after implant surgery | 12 cases of BRONJ induced by implants |
| | 12 cases of BRONJ induced by implants | One third with anti-osteoporotic indication | | | |
| | Number of implants=23 | | | | |
| Yip, 2013 [16] | 337 female implant patients, 1,181 implants, aged min. 40 years | Oral BP therapy | In patients with implant failure, odds of oral BP use was 2,69-fold higher (95 %-CI: 1.49-4,86) than in adjusted controls with no implant failure | 6–14 years | No |
| Rugani, 2014 [41] | 1 patient with cured BRONJ | IV (osteoporotic) | None | | No |

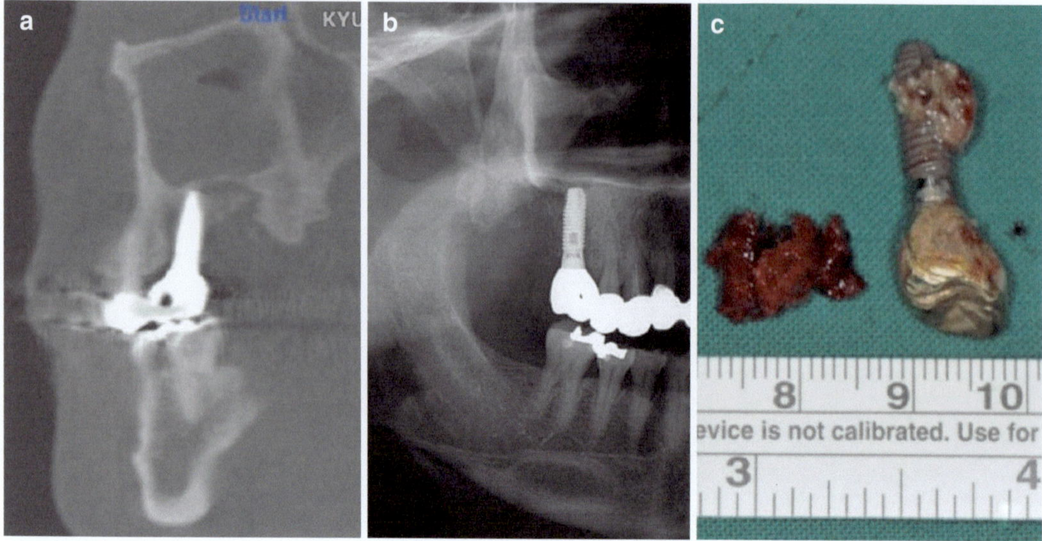

**Fig. 17.1** The patient initiated alendronate 1 year before installation of the two implants at the left maxilla. Four years later after implantation and BP coverage, one posterior implant was removed at a local clinic because of the bone exposure and pain. (**a, b**) Radiographic bone destruction around the remaining implant maintaining the partial bone-implant contact. (**c**) The specimen was sequestrated with surrounding necrotic bone

## Implant-Associated Infections in Bisphosphonate Medication Versus Common Periimplantitis

Periimplantitis in non-bisphosphonate cases usually initiates in the interface between mucosa and implant surface as a mucositis. Then it affects the integrity of the bone-implant junction in a bone resorption process in direction from crestal to apical. If untreated, a gap between implant and bone is generated and osseointegration is lost. Contrarily, it was shown that the jaw bone develops sequestrum which includes the implant itself, but histologically, osseointegration of the implant can persist [3, 42]. One could explain this with regard to the fact that bone resorption is inhibited by the bisphosphonates, especially near to the surface of the bone, while deep in the bone marrow, there is still potential for a process like sequestration (Figs. 17.1 and 17.2).

## Implants in Rehabilitation After MRONJ

MRONJ has a significant impact on quality of life and a big part of this is caused by bad oral conditions like eating discomfort, lack of self-consciousness, and mucosal irritability [43]. MRONJ itself often leads to relevant destruction of the jaw bone (Fig. 17.3), and surgical treatment of the disease regularly sacrifices parts of the jaw bone, additionally (Fig. 17.4). While surgical protocols to treat MRONJ seem to assimilate as they lead to curing in the majority of cases (see treatment chapter), bony reconstruction is problematic, as MRONJ can affect transferred bone [44] like it does in the jaw bone. As well as, there is lack of protocols for rehabilitation after MRONJ: Dentures should be very stable, because denture sores can trigger MRONJ [45]. But often in these patients, teeth and jaw bone loss leads to conditions where dentures cannot be fit in a sufficient manner (Fig. 17.5). Implants can immobilize dentures perfectly, but a history of MRONJ is a risk factor of relevant and highly debated impact, which excludes these patients from implantology, when regarding the AAOMS recommendations [8]. Consequently, leaving patients without dental prosthodontic rehabilitation is a recommendation given [46]. In the last years, the point of view changed from oral surgery as a true risk factor for MRONJ to the idea of oral surgery as a possible trigger of infection and acidic milieu, which then starts the cascade for MRONJ [47]. While still under debate [15, 48],

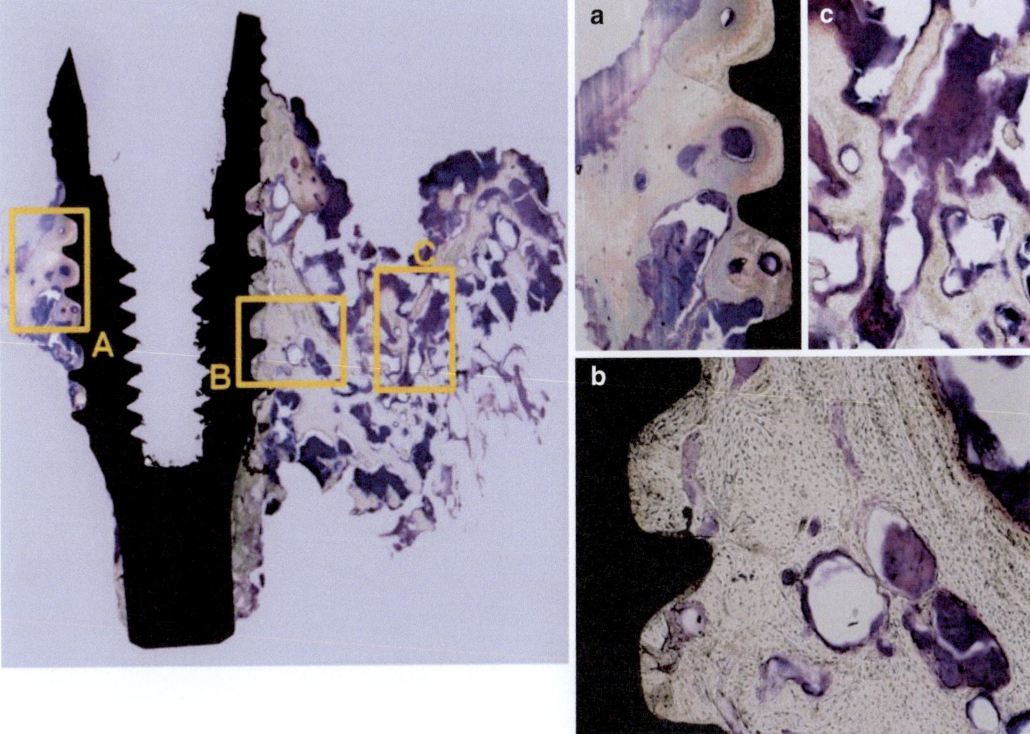

**Fig. 17.2** Histological feature of the specimen from sequestrated bone-implant complex. (**a, b**) Osseointegration was maintained in some part of the implant surface. Microorganisms are dominantly infiltrating to exposed bone surface and not deeply to the implant-bone interface. (**c**) Abundant bacterial colony infiltrating the necrotic osseous structure at the outer side of the specimen. (Villanueva bone stain, × 100) (Figs. 17.1 and 17.2: Courtesy of Tae-Geon Kwon, DDS, PhD, Professor, Department of Oral & Maxillofacial Surgery, School of Dentistry, Kyungpook National University, Samduck 2 Ga, Jung Gu, Daegu, 700-412, Korea, E-mail: kwondk@knu.ac.kr)

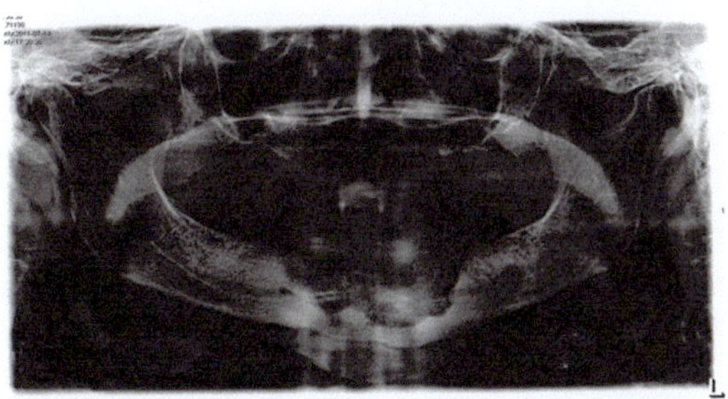

**Fig. 17.3**  Large BRONJ defect in the anterior mandible of a 73-year-old female with a 5-year oral bisphosphonate medication on osteopenia

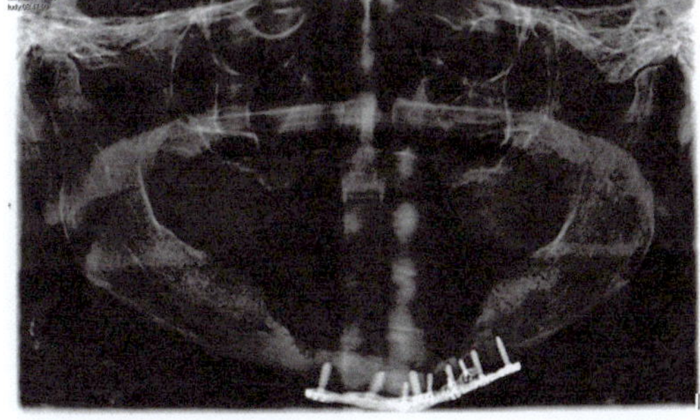

**Fig. 17.4**  Defect after surgical debridement and plating of pathological fracture

some evidence for successful implant therapy in patients on oral bisphosphonate medication also came up in the recent literature.

In the author's opinion, surgeons should use implants as a means of oral rehabilitation in selected cases and under control for other risk factors: In a 73-year-old female, which was on oral bisphosphonates for 5 years, MRONJ and MRONJ-induced pathological fractures were treated (Figs. 17.3, 17.4, and 17.5). After MRONJ was cured, implants were inserted (Fig. 17.6) and a bar-retained removable prosthesis was inserted (Fig. 17.7). The patient is on high-frequency recall and without any clinical or radiographical

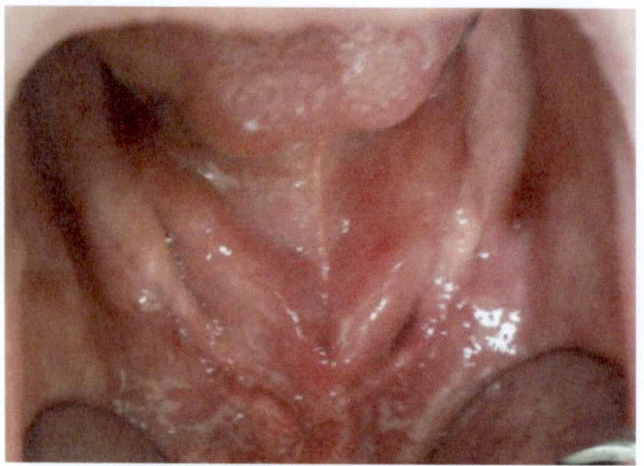

**Fig. 17.5** Closed and sane mucosa in the area of the BRONJ defect in the anterior mandible, but absence of alveolar process and no possibility to wear a total denture (same patient as Figs. 17.1 and 17.2)

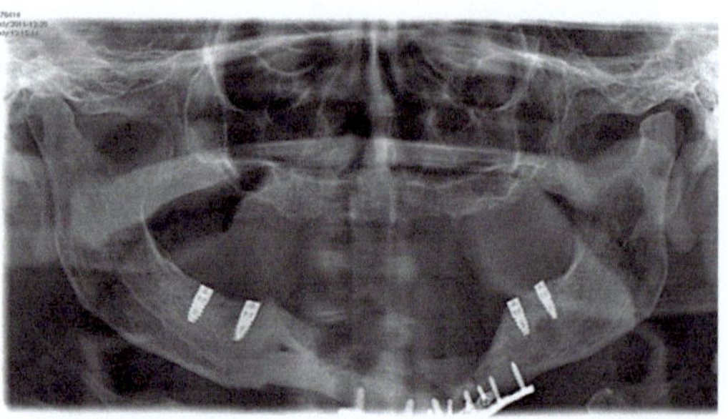

**Fig. 17.6** Insertion of four dental implants, four months after fracture plating

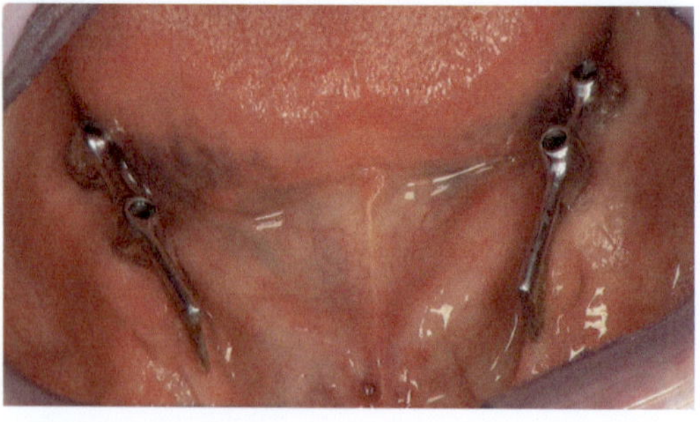

**Fig. 17.7** Bar retainers, nine months after insertion, 13 months after implant insertion

signs of infection (Figs. 17.8 and 17.9). The experience of other authors is consistent with this opinion [41], but of course, there is still lack of data on the topic.

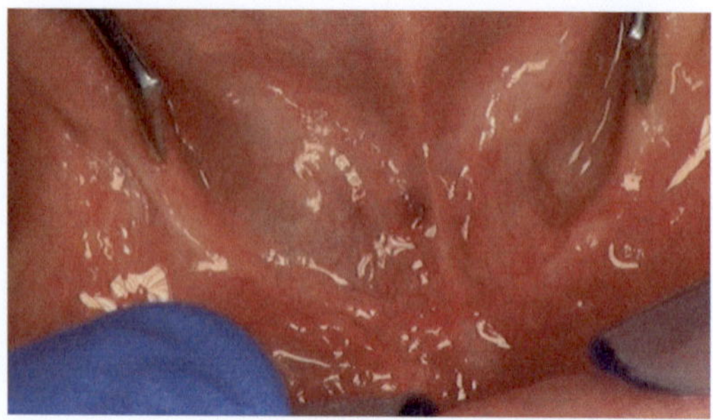

**Fig. 17.8** Healthy conditions at 24-month follow-up exam

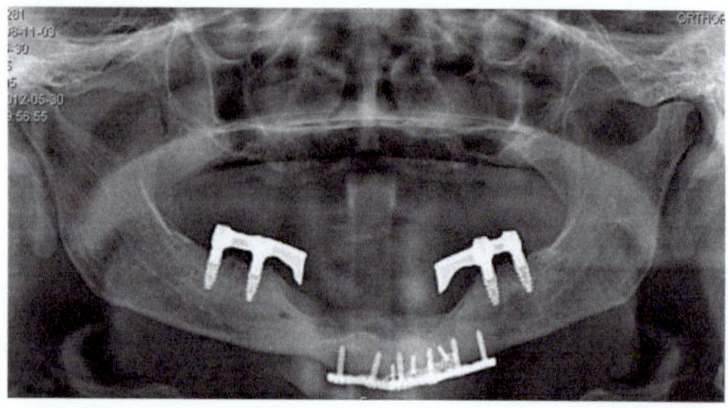

**Fig. 17.9** Panoramic x-ray at 24-month follow-up exam showing no signs of inflammation, sequestration, or bone loss

## Excursus: Antiresorptive Coatings of Dental Implants

Matthias Troeltzsch, Sven Otto, and Yorck Zebuhr

Low doses of bisphosphonates inhibit osteoclasts while stimulating osteoblasts at the same time [49] which may lead to an anabolic effect on bone formation. Therefore, ideas grew to apply these drugs for better osseointegration of dental implants [50]. Animal studies on beagle dogs performed in the late 1990s have provided initial hints that bisphosphonate-coated dental implants might induce peri-implant bone formation and increased bone-implant contact (BIC) [51, 52]. The increased stability is explained by enhanced differentiation, proliferation, and activity of endost and bone marrow-derived osteoprogenitor cells induced by bisphosphonate exposure [49].

These results were confirmed in later studies that examined bone formation and bone density around implants coated with various nitrogen-containing bisphosphonates in dog, rat, and sheep models [53–55]. In a study in rats, tibias improvement of screw pullout forces was shown for both systemically, but even more for alendronate-coated implants [56]. Another animal study found no difference in implant removal torque whether alendronate was systemically administered or not [57]. But enhanced bone formation and a slightly higher level of BIC were observed for bisphosphonate-coated implants in comparison with other chemical surface treatments in micro CT images and histological pictures [49]. A combined coating of calcium phosphate and bisphosphonates has displayed the highest efficacy for the improvement of bone quality around implants [49, 55]. However, there is sparseness of studies that have investigated the influence of bisphosphonate containing surface modification of dental implants in humans [58, 59]. A total of 22 patients who have received 22 bisphosphonate-coated oral implants are reported in the literature [58, 59]. Resonance frequency analysis was used to measure implant stability at various points in time, and peri-implant bone loss was measured on intraoral long cone radiographs. In one study, two implants were removed after 6 months for histological examination [58]. Although increased values in the resonance frequency analysis could be observed for bisphosphonate-coated implants, peri-implant bone loss was detected around bisphosphonate-coated implants as well as for the uncoated controls [58, 59]. The histological analysis showed healthy tissues with no signs of osteonecrosis around those implants [58]. The follow-up period of the human studies was limited to 6 months.

At the present time, bisphosphonate-coated oral implants have to be considered as an experimental treatment, the efficacy of which has yet to be shown in long-term clinical human trials involving more probands as the current evidence on this topic is weak. As discussed elsewhere in this chapter, occurrence of MRONJ in patients receiving systemically administered bisphosphonates may be a late complication even after years.

However, the follow-up period in the available studies was only 6 months. Therefore, the presented data on humans may not be entirely reliable and might not cover the full spectrum of possible adverse side effects of such surface modifications. In a recent animal study in rats, it was shown that bisphosphonate coating on implant surfaces improves osseointegration, while long-term systemic administration of nitrogen-containing bisphosphonates can lead to MRONJ [60]. These findings also indicate that interaction of antiresorptive drugs with osseointegration of dental implants is far from being completely understood.

## Indicating Dental Implants in Patients with Bisphosphonate Therapy

The success story of dental implantology was always influenced by decided contraindications for patients with a wide variety of adverse conditions, like, for example, periodontal disease, diabetes, or osteoporosis. But these hard restrictions softened over the years, as biological and technical knowledge on implantology grew. Bisphosphonate therapy is a relatively new contraindication for elective dental implantology, so it is understandable that restrictive recommendations came up firstly [61–63]. Historically, an intravenous bisphosphonate medication generally was indicated for oncological therapy, and oral medication usually meant an anti-osteoporotic regimen. Nowadays, intravenous formulas also exist for these patients, which must not be overlooked when regarding the risks of dental implant therapy for patients on antiresorptive drugs. This should lead the focus on oncological versus anti-osteoporotic dosage and term of use [40, 64].

In the author's experience, implants can successfully integrate and work in patients on bisphosphonate therapy: In 2004, a 55-year-old female underwent maxillary bone splitting and implant surgery (Fig. 17.10). She received 70 mg oral alendronate for osteoporosis which was diagnosed in 2004 with a 3.8 T-score and a 1.9

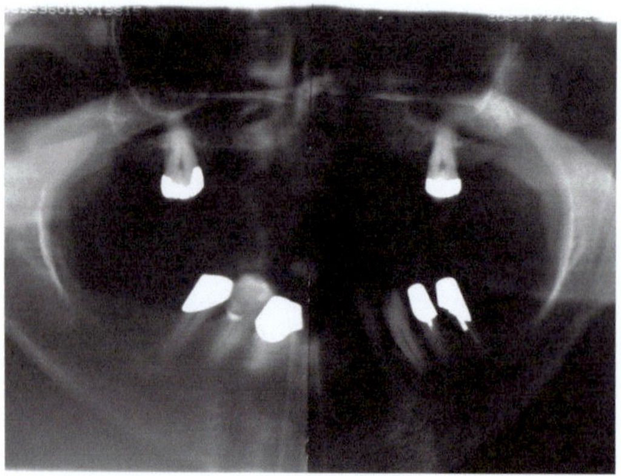

**Fig. 17.10** Panoramic x-ray before maxillary augmentation and implant surgery, 54-year-old female with osteoporosis and oral bisphosphonate therapy (70 mg alendronate/week)

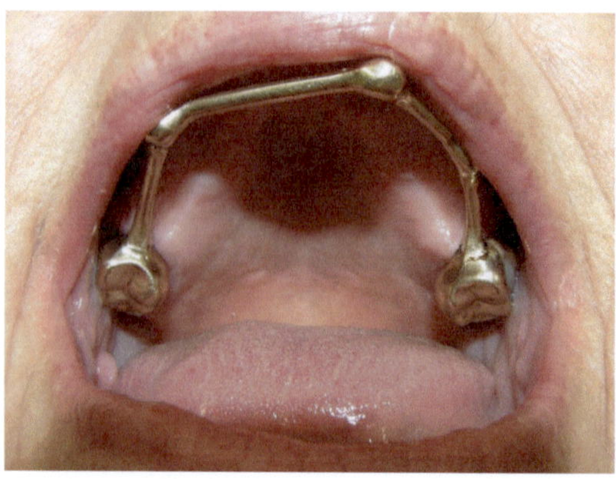

**Fig. 17.12** Gold bar with partial anchor crowns on teeth 17 and 27 and implants 13, 22, and 24 (picture taken at 10-year follow-up examination)

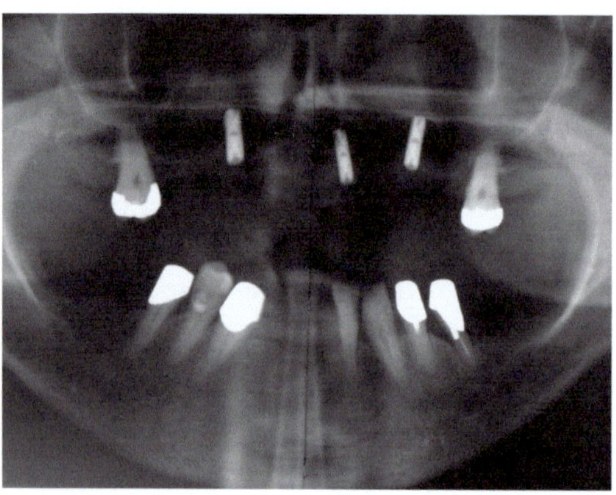

**Fig. 17.11** Panoramic x-ray after augmentation and insertion of three dental implants

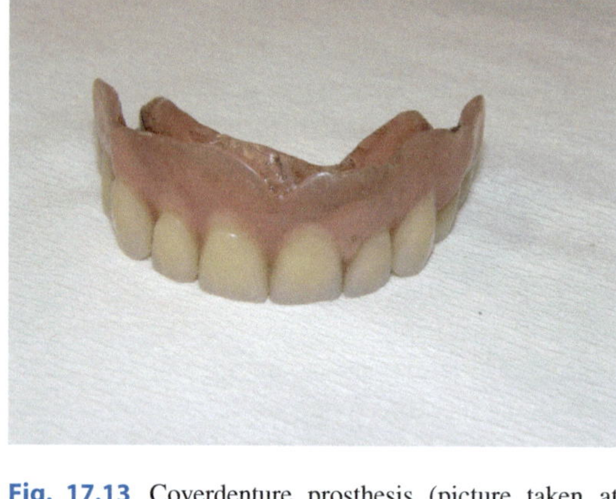

**Fig. 17.13** Coverdenture prosthesis (picture taken at 10-year follow-up examination)

Z-score. Due to lack of bone, only three of the planned four implants were inserted. The implants were placed slightly subcrestal, and primary wound closure was applied surgery (Fig. 17.11). The surgery was performed under IV sedation and under IV antibiotic prophylaxis with 2,000 mg amoxicillin and 200 mg clavulanic acid. Parenteral antibiotic prophylaxis was the standard procedure for implant surgery under IV sedation in the author's office at this time. Moreover, oral antibiotics and chlorhexidine were administered. The second-stage surgery was done 3 months later. Prosthodontic rehabilitation was performed by a gold bar with partial crowns on the remaining teeth 17 and 27 and the three implants (Fig. 17.12) and a partial coverdenture prosthesis (Fig. 17.13). Follow-up examinations were done every 6–12 months. At the 7-year checkup, a purulent mucositis and osseous resorption were detected and treated with a modeling osteotomy and implant surface decontamination (Fig. 17.14). On this occasion, the author inquired the orthopedic surgeon about the lasting alendronate therapy, and cessation of it was decided. Healing after flap surgery was uneventful and the situation remained stable for another 3 years with respect to a recession at the implant 13 (Fig. 17.15). Clinical and radiographical findings at the 10-year checkup were fine (Figs. 17.16 and 17.17).

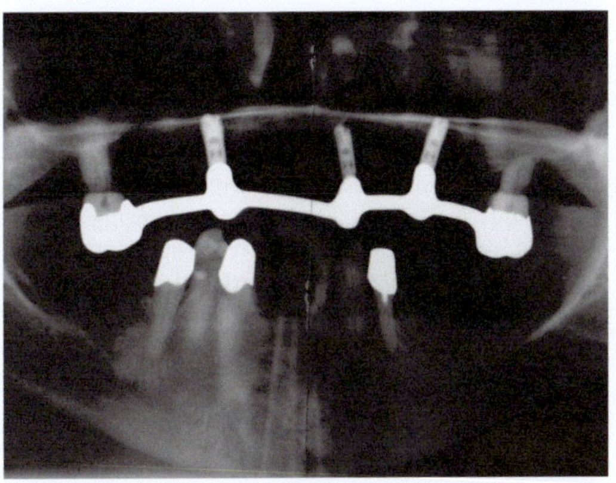

**Fig. 17.14** Osteolytic alteration at the implant 13 at 7-year follow up examination

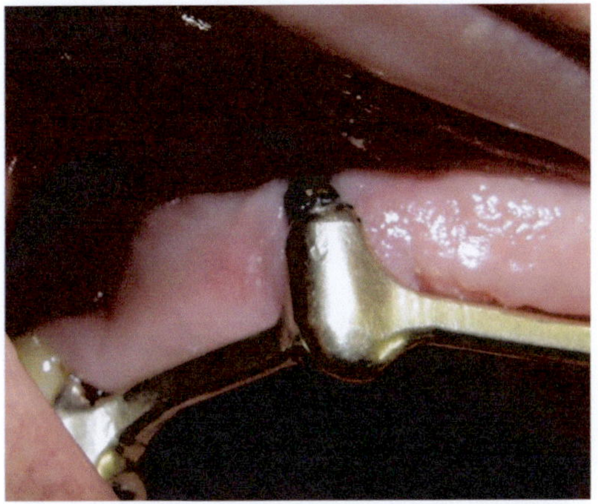

**Fig. 17.15** Stable recession at implant 13, 10 years after insertion, 3 years after flap surgery

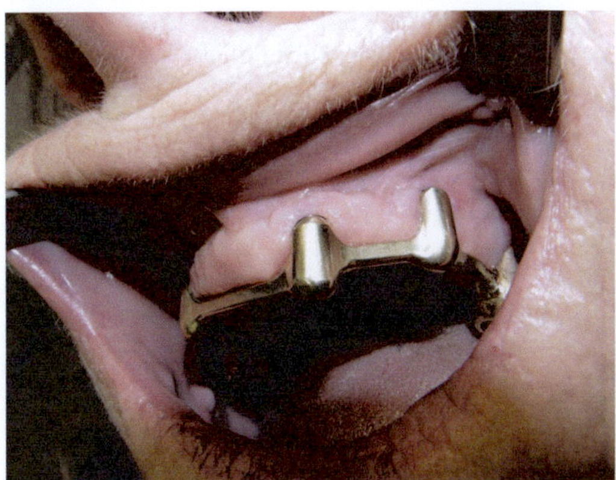

**Fig. 17.16** Implants 22 and 24, without pathological findings, 10 years after insertion

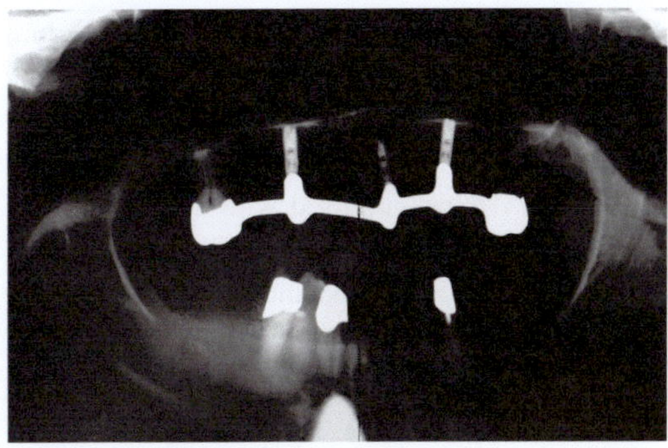

**Fig. 17.17** Follow-up panoramic x-ray, 10 years after implant insertion and augmentation

Indication of dental implants for patients under or after antiresorptive medication should substantially balance risks and benefits: The individual risk for MRONJ, the potential implant rehabilitation has for avoidance of risk factors like denture sores or protection of the remaining teeth, and the need for augmentation are the main topics to be discussed [14]. As the harm of MRONJ is important, and implant surgery is highly elective, special care on informed consent is necessary [64, 65]. Today, augmentation procedures are not recommended, as there is lack of data on the one side [64] and potential for late complications on the other side [5]. As especially anti-osteoporotic bisphosphonate therapy is very common in developed countries [66] as well as implant therapy, there must be a high number of unobserved patients with implants under or after bisphosphonate therapy. This big overlap of patient groups is also indicated in a US single-center study: From 1,319 female implant patients over the age of 40 years, 458 answered a survey, and 115 of these had a history of bisphosphonates [24].

With respect to the mentioned, the author's recommendations for implants on patients on antiresorptive medication are the following: Short operation time, minimal periosteal denudation, and the use of monofilic sutures [67] should apply for minimization of bacterial invasion. Perioperative regimens includes parenteral and oral antibiotics and chlorhexidine mouth rinses. Operation sites are prepared and intraoperatively rinsed with Betadine. Submerged healing and secondary minimally invasive uncovering of the implant with stitch incisions work well in the author's practice. It is a dictum in this kind of surgery always to keep a mucosal coverage, like this indicated from animals studies [68]. Digital planning tools, 3-D images, and positioning devices are used with the intention of avoiding augmentations and saving operating time. Prosthodontic work should anticipate loss of single implants and loss of manual ability for cleaning. With outstanding regard to the special conditions and risks, but also with respect to potential benefits, implant therapy may not be routinely denied for patients with antiresorptive medication, but is an issue of discussion in every single patient. Risk assessment scores [69] could facilitate clinical decision making and be useful for scientific analyses.

## Conclusion

Antiresorptive drugs like bisphosphonates, RANKL-Inhibitors (denosumab), Medication-related osteonecrosis of the jaw (MRONJ), and dental implants offer a wide field for scientific and clinical discussion. Oral surgery like implant surgery can be a trigger for MRONJ but can also safely work for years in patients under bisphosphonate medication and even after MRONJ. On the one hand, as MRONJ also occurs as late and very late complication, we maybe could expect a thunderstorm of complications, when the emerging number of patients with dental implants and augmentations develops indications for antiresorptive therapy regimens. On the other hand, recent insights in the etiology and pathogenesis of MRONJ encourage us as surgeons, not to contraindicate implants in every bisphosphonate user but to consider risks and benefits individually while scientific evidence is missing.

**Acknowledgement** Part of the presented material originates from the thesis of Yorck Alexander Zebuhr (in preparation).

# References

1. Marx RE. Pamidronate (Aredia) and zoledronate (Zometa) induced avascular necrosis of the jaws: a growing epidemic. J Oral Maxillofac Surg. 2003; 61(9):1115–7.

2. Starck WJ, Epker BN. Failure of osseointegrated dental implants after diphosphonate therapy for osteoporosis: a case report. Int J Oral Maxillofac Implants. 1995; 10(1):74–8.

3. Kwon TG, Lee CO, Park JW, Choi SY, Rijal G, Shin HI. Osteonecrosis associated with dental implants in patients undergoing bisphosphonate treatment. Clin Oral Implants Res. 2014;25(5):632–40.

4. Jacobsen C, Metzler P, Rossle M, Obwegeser J, Zemann W, Gratz KW. Osteopathology induced by bisphosphonates and dental implants: clinical observations. Clin Oral Investig. 2013;17(1):167–75.

5. Kim JW, Kwon TG. Bisphosphonate-related osteonecrosis of the jaw at a previously grafted sinus. Implant Dent. 2014;23(1):18–21.

6. Marx RE, Sawatari Y, Fortin M, Broumand V. Bisphosphonate-induced exposed bone (osteonecrosis/osteopetrosis) of the jaws: risk factors, recognition, prevention, and treatment. J Oral Maxillofac Surg. 2005;63(11):1567–75.

7. Favia G, Piattelli A, Sportelli P, Capodiferro S, Iezzi G. Osteonecrosis of the posterior mandible after implant insertion: a clinical and histological case report. Clin Implant Dent Relat Res. 2011;13(1):58–63.

8. Ruggiero SL, Dodson TB, Assael LA, Landesberg R, Marx RE, Mehrotra B, et al. American Association of Oral and Maxillofacial Surgeons position paper on bisphosphonate-related osteonecrosis of the jaws–2009 update. J Oral Maxillofac Surg. 2009;67(5 Suppl): 2–12.

9. Brooks JK, Gilson AJ, Sindler AJ, Ashman SG, Schwartz KG, Nikitakis NG. Osteonecrosis of the jaws associated with use of risedronate: report of 2 new cases. Oral Surg Oral Med Oral Pathol Oral Radiol Endod. 2007;103(6):780–6.

10. Marx RE. Oral and intravenous bisphosphonate-induced osteonecrosis of the jaws. History, etiology, prevention and treatment. Chicago: Quintessence Publishing Co, Inc; 2011.

11. Marx RE. Oral presentation, conference title: Dental Implants vs. Bisphosphonates. 2013; Zurich.

12. Bojer SB, Th., Spitzer W. Erfolgreiche Implantatinsertion trotz parenteraler Bisphosphonattherapie. DGKMG Gemeinschaftstagung; Berlin; 2011.

13. Zebuhr Y. Rehabilitation in patients after BRONJ – are implants possible or forbidden? EACMFS Congress; Dubvrovnik; 2012.

14. Groetz KA. In which bisphosphonate patients am I allowed to place implants? A systematic review. Z Zahnärztl Impl, 2010;26(2), DOI 10.3238/ZZI.2010.0153.

15. Javed F, Almas K. Osseointegration of dental implants in patients undergoing bisphosphonate treatment: a literature review. J Periodontol. 2010; 81(4):479–84.

16. Yip JK, Borrell LN, Cho SC, Francisco H, Tarnow DP. Association between oral bisphosphonate use and dental implant failure among middle-aged women. J Clin Periodontol. 2012;39(4):408–14.

17. Koka S, Babu NM, Norell A. Survival of dental implants in post-menopausal bisphosphonate users. J Prosthodont Res. 2010;54(3):108–11.

18. Kushner GMA, B. Bisphosphonate Induced Osteonecrosis of the Jaws (ONJ). AO Dialogue 2005;02/2005.
19. Jeffcoat MK. Safety of oral bisphosphonates: controlled studies on alveolar bone. Int J Oral Maxillofac Implants. 2006;21(3):349–53.
20. Wang HL, Weber D, McCauley LK. Effect of long-term oral bisphosphonates on implant wound healing: literature review and a case report. J Periodontol. 2007;78(3):584–94.
21. Marx RE, Cillo Jr JE, Ulloa JJ. Oral bisphosphonate-induced osteonecrosis: risk factors, prediction of risk using serum CTX testing, prevention, and treatment. J Oral Maxillofac Surg. 2007;65(12):2397–410.
22. Fugazzotto PA, Lightfoot WS, Jaffin R, Kumar A. Implant placement with or without simultaneous tooth extraction in patients taking oral bisphosphonates: postoperative healing, early follow-up, and the incidence of complications in two private practices. J Periodontol. 2007;78(9):1664–9.
23. Yarom N, Yahalom R, Shoshani Y, Hamed W, Regev E, Elad S. Osteonecrosis of the jaw induced by orally administered bisphosphonates: incidence, clinical features, predisposing factors and treatment outcome. Osteoporos Int. 2007;18(10):1363–70.
24. Grant BT, Amenedo C, Freeman K, Kraut RA. Outcomes of placing dental implants in patients taking oral bisphosphonates: a review of 115 cases. J Oral Maxillofac Surg. 2008;66(2):223–30.
25. Bell BM, Bell RE. Oral bisphosphonates and dental implants: a retrospective study. J Oral Maxillofac Surg. 2008;66(5):1022–4.
26. Kasai T, Pogrel MA, Hossaini M. The prognosis for dental implants placed in patients taking oral bisphosphonates. J Calif Dent Assoc. 2009;37(1):39–42.
27. Goss A, Bartold M, Sambrook P, Hawker P. The nature and frequency of bisphosphonate-associated osteonecrosis of the jaws in dental implant patients: a South Australian case series. J Oral Maxillofac Surg. 2010;68(2):337–43.
28. Bedogni A, Bettini G, Totola A, Saia G, Nocini PF. Oral bisphosphonate-associated osteonecrosis of the jaw after implant surgery: a case report and literature review. J Oral Maxillofac Surg. 2010;68(7):1662–6.
29. Lazarovici TS, Yahalom R, Taicher S, Schwartz-Arad D, Peleg O, Yarom N. Bisphosphonate-related osteonecrosis of the jaw associated with dental implants. J Oral Maxillofac Surg. 2010;68(4):790–6.
30. Martin DC, O'Ryan FS, Indresano AT, Bogdanos P, Wang B, Hui RL, et al. Characteristics of implant failures in patients with a history of oral bisphosphonate therapy. J Oral Maxillofac Surg. 2010;68(3):508–14.
31. Shabestari GO, Shayesteh YS, Khojasteh A, Alikhasi M, Moslemi N, Aminian A, et al. Implant placement in patients with oral bisphosphonate therapy: a case series. Clin Implant Dent Relat Res. 2010;12(3):175–80.
32. Famili P, Quigley S, Mosher T. Survival of dental implants among post-menopausal female dental school patients taking oral bisphosphonates: a retrospective study. Compend Contin Educ Dent. 2011;32(6):E106–9.
33. Zahid TM, Wang BY, Cohen RE. Influence of bisphosphonates on alveolar bone loss around osseointegrated implants. J Oral Implantol. 2011;37(3):335–46.
34. Ferlito S, Liardo C, Puzzo S. Bisphosphonates and dental implants: a case report and a brief review of literature. Minerva Stomatol. 2011;60(1–2):75–81.
35. Diniz-Freitas M, Lopez-Cedrun JL, Fernandez-Sanroman J, Garcia-Garcia A, Fernandez-Feijoo J, Diz-Dios P. Oral bisphosphonate-related osteonecrosis of the jaws: clinical characteristics of a series of 20 cases in Spain. Med Oral Patol Oral Cir Bucal. 2012;17(5):e751–8.
36. Flichy-Fernandez AJ, Gonzalez-Lemonnier S, Balaguer-Martinez J, Penarrocha-Oltra D, Penarrocha-Diago MA, Bagan-Sebastian JV. Bone necrosis around dental implants: a patient treated with oral bisphosphonates, drug holiday and no risk according to serum CTX. J Clin Exp Dent. 2012;4(1):e82–5.
37. Subramanian G, Fritton JC, Iyer S, Quek SY. Atypical dental implant failure with long-term bisphosphonate treatment–akin to atypical fractures? Oral Surg Oral Med Oral Pathol Oral Radiol. 2012;114(6):e30–5.
38. Gupta R. Early dental implant failure in patient associated with oral bisphosphonates. Indian J Dent Res. 2012;23(2):298.
39. Lopez-Cedrun JL, Sanroman JF, Garcia A, Penarrocha M, Feijoo JF, Limeres J, et al. Oral bisphosphonate-related osteonecrosis of the jaws in dental implant patients: a case series. Br J Oral Maxillofac Surg. 2013;51(8):874–9.
40. Mattheos N, Caldwell P, Petcu EB, Ivanovski S, Reher P. Dental implant placement with bone augmentation in a patient who received intravenous bisphosphonate treatment for osteoporosis. J Can Dent Assoc. 2013;79:d2.
41. Rugani P, Kirnbauber B, Acham S, Truschnegg A, Jakse N. Implant placement adjacent to successfully treated Bisphosphonate-related osteonecrosis of the jaw (BRONJ). J Oral implantol. 2014.
42. Shirota T, Nakamura A, Matsui Y, Hatori M, Nakamura M, Shintani S. Bisphosphonate-related osteonecrosis of the jaw around dental implants in the maxilla: report of a case. Clin Oral Implants Res. 2009;20(12):1402–8.
43. Miksad RA, Lai KC, Dodson TB, Woo SB, Treister NS, Akinyemi O, et al. Quality of life implications of bisphosphonate-associated osteonecrosis of the jaw. Oncologist. 2011;16(1):121–32.
44. Pautke C, Otto S, Reu S, Kolk A, Ehrenfeld M, Sturzenbaum S, et al. Bisphosphonate related osteonecrosis of the jaw–manifestation in a microvascular iliac bone flap. Oral Oncol. 2011;47(5):425–9.
45. Hasegawa Y, Kawabe M, Kimura H, Kurita K, Fukuta J, Urade M. Influence of dentures in the initial occurrence site on the prognosis of bisphosphonate-related osteonecrosis of the jaws: a retrospective study. Oral Surg Oral Med Oral Pathol Oral Radiol. 2012;114(3):318–24.
46. Groetz KA, Al-Nawas B. Persisting alveolar sockets-a radiologic symptom of BP-ONJ? J Oral Maxillofac Surg. 2006;64(10):1571–2.

47. Otto S, Hafner S, Mast G, Tischer T, Volkmer E, Schieker M, et al. Bisphosphonate-related osteonecrosis of the jaw: is pH the missing part in the pathogenesis puzzle? J Oral Maxillofac Surg. 2010;68(5):1158–61.
48. Chadha GK, Ahmadieh A, Kumar SK, Sedghizadeh PP. Osseointegration of dental implants and osteonecrosis of the jaw in patients treated with bisphosphonate therapy: a systematic review. J Oral Implantol. 2013; 39(4):510–20.
49. Kajiwara H, Yamaza T, Yoshinari M, Goto T, Iyama S, Atsuta I, et al. The bisphosphonate pamidronate on the surface of titanium stimulates bone formation around tibial implants in rats. Biomaterials. 2005; 26(6):581–7.
50. Berardi D, Carlesi T, Rossi F, Calderini M, Volpi R, Perfetti G. Potential applications of bisphosphonates in dental surgical implants. Int J Immunopathol Pharmacol. 2007;20(3):455–65.
51. Meraw SJ, Reeve CM. Qualitative analysis of peripheral peri-implant bone and influence of alendronate sodium on early bone regeneration. J Periodontol. 1999;70(10): 1228–33.
52. Meraw SJ, Reeve CM, Wollan PC. Use of alendronate in peri-implant defect regeneration. J Periodontol. 1999;70(2):151–8.
53. Gao Y, Zou S, Liu X, Bao C, Hu J. The effect of surface immobilized bisphosphonates on the fixation of hydroxyapatite-coated titanium implants in ovariectomized rats. Biomaterials. 2009;30(9): 1790–6.
54. Ferguson SJ, Langhoff JD, Voelter K, von Rechenberg B, Scharnweber D, Bierbaum S, et al. Biomechanical comparison of different surface modifications for dental implants. Int J Oral Maxillofac Implants. 2008; 23(6):1037–46.
55. Yoshinari M, Oda Y, Inoue T, Matsuzaka K, Shimono M. Bone response to calcium phosphate-coated and bisphosphonate-immobilized titanium implants. Biomaterials. 2002;23(14):2879–85.
56. Linderback P, Areva S, Aspenberg P, Tengvall P. Sol-gel derived titania coating with immobilized bisphosphonate enhances screw fixation in rat tibia. J Biomed Mater Res A. 2010;94(2):389–95.
57. Chacon GE, Stine EA, Larsen PE, Beck FM, McGlumphy EA. Effect of alendronate on endosseous implant integration: an in vivo study in rabbits. J Oral Maxillofac Surg. 2006;64(7):1005–9.
58. Abtahi J, Tengvall P, Aspenberg P. A bisphosphonate-coating improves the fixation of metal implants in human bone. A randomized trial of dental implants. Bone. 2012;50(5):1148–51.
59. Abtahi J, Tengvall P, Aspenberg P. Bisphosphonate coating might improve fixation of dental implants in the maxilla: a pilot study. Int J Oral Maxillofac Surg. 2010;39(7):673–7.
60. Abtahi J, Agholme F, Sandberg O, Aspenberg P. Effect of local vs. systemic bisphosphonate delivery on dental implant fixation in a model of osteonecrosis of the jaw. J Dent Res. 2013;92(3):279–83.
61. Serra MP, Llorca CS, Donat FJ. Oral implants in patients receiving bisphosphonates: a review and update. Med Oral Patol Oral Cir Bucal. 2008;13(12):E755–60.
62. Scully C, Madrid C, Bagan J. Dental endosseous implants in patients on bisphosphonate therapy. Implant Dent. 2006;15(3):212–8.
63. Hwang D, Wang HL. Medical contraindications to implant therapy: part I: absolute contraindications. Implant Dent. 2006;15(4):353–60.
64. Grötz KA, Al-Nawas B, Terheyden H. Implantate und Bisphosphonat-Therapie. Implantologie. 2013;21(1): 53–9.
65. Stoopler ET. The importance of informed consent. J Can Dent Assoc. 2013;79:d81.
66. Marx RE. Bisphosphonat-induzierte Osteonekrose der Kiefer. Berlin: Qiuntessenz; 2013.
67. Banche G, Roana J, Mandras N, Amasio M, Gallesio C, Allizond V, et al. Microbial adherence on various intraoral suture materials in patients undergoing dental surgery. J Oral Maxillofac Surg. 2007;65(8):1503–7.
68. Abtahi J, Agholme F, Aspenberg P. Prevention of osteonecrosis of the jaw by mucoperiosteal coverage in a rat model. Int J Oral Maxillofac Surg. 2013;42(5):632–6.
69. Zebuhr A. Epidemiologie der bisphosphonatinduzierten Osteonekrose der Kiefer unter besonderer Berücksichtigung ihrer Risikofaktoren [Master Thesis]. Linz: JKU Linz; 2013.

# Osteonecrosis of the Jaw in Association with Targeted Therapy

**18**

Matthias Troeltzsch, Markus Troeltzsch, Christoph Pache, and Timothy Woodlock

**Abstract**

Various non-bisphosphonate drugs seem to be associated with the etiology of osteonecrosis of the jaw (ONJ). The human monoclonal antibodies denosumab and bevacizumab and the tyrosine kinase inhibitor sunitinib have been suspected to increase the risk for ONJ development. Very recent reports have identified the mTOR (mammalian target of rapamycin) inhibitor everolimus to be implicated in the evolution of ONJ. Current evidence supports the theory that denosumab treatment in isolation may trigger ONJ. Bevacizumab and sunitinib as part of oncologic treatment protocols which include bisphosphonates may increase the likelihood for ONJ and reduce the latency period until ONJ occurrence. Dentoalveolar surgeries in patients on these drugs should be performed with the same precautions as for bisphosphonate patients.

M. Troeltzsch, MD, DMD (⊠) • C. Pache, MD, DMD
Department of Oral and Maxillofacial Surgery,
Ludwig – Maximilians Universität München,
München, Germany
e-mail: matthias_troeltzsch@hotmail.com

M. Troeltzsch, MD, DMD
Department of Maxillofacial Surgery,
Universitätsmedizin Göttingen, Göttingen, Germany
e-mail: troeltzsch@gmx.net

T. Woodlock, MD
Department of Hematology and Oncology,
School of Medicine and Dentistry,
University of Rochester, Rochester, NY, USA

Unity Health System, Rochester, NY, USA

## Introduction

The association between bisphosphonate treatment and the emergence of osteonecrosis of the jaw (ONJ) is well documented [1, 2], and plausible theories for its pathogenesis have been established [3–5]. The management of bisphosphonate-related osteonecrosis of the jaw (BRONJ) and its sequelae has become a challenge for dentists, oral and maxillofacial surgeons, as well as oncologists all over the world [2, 6]. However, the risk of ONJ development is not limited to patients receiving bisphosphonate treatment [7]. Topical research has recently identified other drugs that seem to be capable of triggering ONJ or at least increasing the risk of its development [7, 8]. Namely, these are the

S. Otto (ed.), *Medication-Related Osteonecrosis of the Jaws: Bisphosphonates, Denosumab, and New Agents*,   193
DOI 10.1007/978-3-662-43733-9_18, © Springer-Verlag Berlin Heidelberg 2015

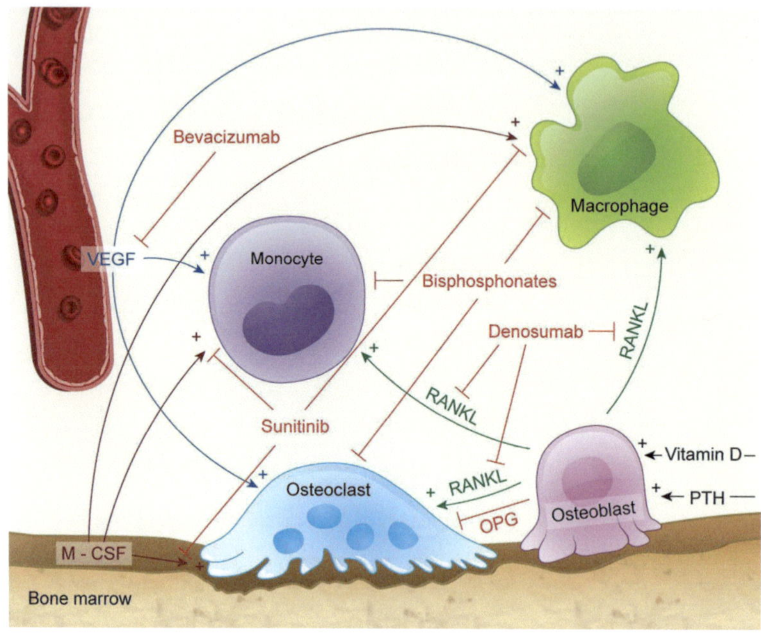



**Fig. 18.1** Molecular mechanisms of action of denosumab, bevacizumab and sunitinib in bone physiology and angiogenesis in comparison to bisphosphonates (Reprinted from Troeltzsch et al [7] with kind permission of The Canadian Dental Association)

monoclonal antibodies denosumab (XGEVA®, Prolia®) and bevacizumab (Avastin®) and the tyrosine kinase inhibitor sunitinib (Sutent®). They belong to the group of targeted therapy drugs which specifically aim at certain molecules instead of inhibiting all cells in a similar manner [8]. As mentioned in previous chapters, denosumab acts as a decoy receptor on RANKL (receptor activator of nuclear factor kB ligand) and prevents the interaction between RANK and RANK-L (RANK ligand) which is an important stimulus for osteoclast differentiation and maturation [9, 10]. Biologically, denosumab behaves similarly as osteoprotegerin (OPG), mainly secreted by osteoblasts and stromal cells [9, 10]. Bevacizumab is an antagonist on the vascular endothelial growth factor A (VEGF-A) and inhibits blood vessel formation [11, 12]. Sunitinib is an inhibitor of various tyrosine kinase receptors implicated in VEGF-, PDGF (platelet-derived growth factor)-, c-KIT- or RET-mediated signaling pathways and decreases neoangiogenesis, bone remodelling, and immunological processes [13]. The specific mechanisms of action of the mentioned drugs are displayed in Fig. 18.1 (from Troeltzsch et al. [7]).

## Denosumab

The indications for denosumab use are similar to those of bisphosphonates [10, 14], and their clinical use has been advocated and increased in recent years [15]. Although denosumab in general displays a low-toxicity profile [16], various well-designed randomized studies have proven the significance of denosumab in the etiology of ONJ [15, 17–23] (Table 18.1). Denosumab-related osteonecrosis of the jaw (DRONJ) is reported at a similar rate as BRONJ [15, 17–21]. This is remarkable, as denosumab and bisphosphonates have significantly different mechanisms of action [16]. The risk of ONJ development after denosumab exposure seems to rise with increased denosumab doses and reduced application intervals [16]. Unlike bisphosphonates, denosumab is not incorporated into the bone matrix and has a shorter tissue half-life [14, 16]. In contrast to bisphosphonates which take effect in all cell lines, denosumab is targeted against the RANKL-RANK system controlling osteoclast differentiation [10]. Osteoclasts originate from the monocyte-macrophage cell lineage and exert immunologic

**Table 18.1** Relevant randomized controlled trials investigating the risk of DRONJ development compared to the risk of BRONJ development

| | BRONJ rate/examined patients receiving bisphosphonates | DRONJ rate/examined patients receiving denosumab | Reason for drug use |
|---|---|---|---|
| Stopeck et al. [15] | 2.0 %/1,020 | 1.6 %/1,026 | Metastatic breast cancer |
| Henry et al. [17] | 1.3 %/878 | 1.1 %/878 | Various malignancies with lytic bone disease |
| Fizazi et al. [19] | 1 %/951 | 2 %/950 | Disseminated prostate cancer |
| Kyrgidis et al. [23] | 1.5 %/1,914 | 1.3 %/1,908 | Bone metastases of various cancers |
| Bone et al. [21] | N/A | 0.13 %/4,550 | Osteoporosis in postmenopausal women |
| Henry et al. [18] | 0.8 %/792 | 1.1 %/786 | Bone metastases of solid tumors |
| Saad et al. [22] | 1.3 %/2,860 | 1.8 %/2,862 | Bone metastases of solid tumors and patients with multiple myeloma |
| Scagliotti et al. [20] | 0.8 %/395 | 0.7 %/406 | Bone metastases in lung cancer patients |

functions [7, 9, 24, 25]. It is unclear whether the reduction of bone turnover or the inhibition of immunological processes, which can be induced by denosumab, is the decisive step in the development of DRONJ [25]. More research will be necessary to elucidate this matter.

## Bevacizumab

Bevacizumab is a human monoclonal antibody inhibiting blood vessel formation with applications in the treatment of breast, ovarian, lung, renal, central nervous, and colon cancer as well as in the treatment of macular degeneration which received approval of the American Food and Drug administration (FDA) in 2004 [7, 12, 26, 27]. The antineoplastic effect of bevacizumab is enhanced when administered in combination with conventional chemotherapy drugs when compared to isolated bevacizumab therapy [12]. Common side effects of bevacizumab employment are hypertension, thromboembolic events, gastrointestinal perforations, and wound healing complications [12]. Bevacizumab as an addition to chemotherapy regimens may increase the frequency and severity of these side effects [28].

A possible association between ONJ etiology and bevacizumab was reported recently [7, 24]. The implications of bevacizumab in the etiology of ONJ are unclear. The limited number of reported bevacizumab-associated ONJ cases raises considerable doubt whether bevacizumab alone can cause ONJ [7, 29]. Until 2012, 55 cases of bevacizumab-associated ONJ had been reported to the British and French drug regulatory agencies in a cohort of 800,000 patients in therapy [30]. There is clinical suspicion that the simultaneous application of bevacizumab and bisphosphonates increases the risk of ONJ development and leads to spontaneous, sometimes multilocular, ONJ lesions [8, 28, 31, 32]. A considerable amount of cases have been reported in the literature [26, 27, 29, 33–39] (Table 18.2). In most of those cases, bevacizumab was administered as part of a complex chemotherapeutic regimen, and dentoalveolar surgical procedures had not been performed [27, 29, 33, 35, 37, 38]. Although bisphosphonates and bevacizumab decrease the bone blood supply, ONJ lesions usually exhibit an intact vascular architecture [7, 14, 29, 40, 41]. On the other hand, there are reports of the importance of VEGF for osteoclast activity [42]. VEGF increases osteoclastic bone resorption and is therefore essential in the control of bone turnover [42]. Furthermore, the presence of VEGF triggers immunologic processes [42]. Limited bone turnover and debilitated immunologic response in combination with soft tissue toxicity by small vessel breakdown [43] may

**Table 18.2** Compilation of reported cases of bevacizumab-related ONJ until December 2013; only cases of ONJ development in patients who never received bisphosphonates are listed

| | Number of reported cases | Reason for bevacizumab administration | Circumstances of ONJ development |
| --- | --- | --- | --- |
| Estilo et al. [27] | 2 | Breast cancer | Unclear, no dentoalveolar surgeries performed |
| Greuter et al. [35] | 1 | Breast cancer | ONJ development after tooth extraction |
| Serra et al. [36] | 1 | Lung cancer | ONJ development after tooth extraction |
| Guarneri et al. [37] | 2 | Disseminated colon, breast, and renal cancer | N/A |
| Disel et al. [33] | 1 | Colon cancer | Unclear, no dentoalveolar surgeries performed |
| Hopp et al. [26] | 1 | Intravitreal injection for the treatment of retinal vein thrombosis | Unclear, no dentoalveolar surgeries performed |
| Santos-Silva et al. [29] | 1 | Renal cancer | Unclear, no dentoalveolar surgeries performed |
| Sato et al. [38] | 1 | Colon cancer | Unclear, no dentoalveolar surgeries performed |
| Pakosch et al. [34] | 1 | Pancreatic carcinoma | Mandibular abscess surgical drainage |
| Brunamonti et al. [39] | 1 | Adenocarcinoma of the parotid gland | Pericoronitis of mandibular wisdom tooth |

create a scenario in which ONJ can develop. It is therefore conceivable that bevacizumab is associated with ONJ, and precautions should be undertaken before the performance of dentoalveolar surgeries in these patients [7].

## Sunitinib

Sunitinib belongs to the group of small-molecule multikinase inhibitors [44]. The main effect of sunitinib is the inhibition of receptor tyrosine kinases with implications in neoangiogenesis [44]. The exact molecular mechanism of action of sunitinib is very complex as it blocks multiple intracellular signaling pathways at the same time [44, 45]. Macrophage maturation, mobility, and maturation may be impeded by sunitinib effects such as antagonism on M-CSF (macrophage-colony stimulating factor, Fig. 18.1) [7, 24]. Therefore, an inhibition of macrophage function by sunitinib is conceivable [24]. Sunitinib was approved by the FDA in 2007 and is administered orally [45]. The range of application for sunitinib comprises gastrointestinal stromal tumors (GIST), neuroendocrine tumors, and advanced renal cell cancer [44–47]. The main side effects of sunitinib application are mucositis, thrombocytopenia, neutropenia, gastrointestinal symptoms, and fatigue [44].

Several case reports of ONJ development in patients treated with sunitinib alone or in combination with other chemotherapy regimens have surfaced since 2009 (Table 18.3) [8, 13, 32, 46–54]. At the present time, there is very little evidence that sunitinib therapy alone may be associated with an increased risk for ONJ development [7, 50, 51]. The British and French drug regulatory agencies registered 27 cases of sunitinib-associated ONJ in a cohort of 100,000 patients receiving sustained sunitinib treatment until the end of 2012 [30]. However, there is considerable evidence that patients receiving chemotherapy, bisphosphonates, and sunitinib at the same time are at a higher risk to develop ONJ [7, 8, 13, 32, 46, 48, 49, 52, 53]. The underlying reasons have yet to be elucidated [24]. Impaired macrophage function, depletion of blood supply, and decay of the epithelial barrier as side effects of sunitinib treatment may contribute to the evolution of ONJ [24, 46].

**Table 18.3** Compilation of reported cases of sunitinib-related ONJ until December 2013; cases of ONJ development after sunitinib treatment alone and in combination with BP are listed

| Author | Number of reported cases | Reason for treatment | Bisphosphonate (BP) therapy | Outcome |
|---|---|---|---|---|
| Brunello et al. [13] | 1 | Renal cancer | Intravenous BP therapy prior to sunitinib treatment | Healing after surgical intervention and antibiotic treatment |
| Christodoulou et al. [32] | 1 | Renal cancer | Intravenous BP therapy prior to sunitinib treatment | Improvement of symptoms after conservative therapy |
| Bozas et al. [48] | 1 | Renal cancer | Concurrent treatment with intravenous BP and sunitinib | Healing after BP drug holiday and hyperbaric oxygen treatment |
| Hoefert et al. [49] | 3 | Patients 1–3: renal cancer | Patients 1 and 2: concurrent intravenous BP therapy | Patients 1 and 2: healing after discontinuation of sunitinib and surgical/antibiotic therapy |
| | | | Patient 3: previous intravenous BP therapy | Patient 3: healing after two surgical interventions, antibiotic treatment, and discontinuation of sunitinib |
| Koch et al. [47] | 1 | Renal cancer | Sunitinib treatment alone | Healing after surgical intervention and antibiotic treatment |
| Bonacina et al. [50] | 3 | N/A | Concurrent intravenous BP therapy and sunitinib | N/A |
| Fleissig et al. [46] | 1 | Renal cancer | Sunitinib treatment alone | Healing after surgical intervention and antibiotic treatment |
| Nicolatou-Galitis et al. [51] | 1 | Metastatic renal cancer | Sunitinib treatment alone | Healing after conservative treatment and antibiotic administration |
| Agrillo et al. [52] | 2 | Patient 1 and 2: renal cancer | Patients 1 and 2: concurrent intravenous BP therapy and sunitinib | Patient 1 and 2: relapse of ONJ lesion after surgical and antibiotic therapy and death of both patients due to oncologic complications |
| Beuselink et al. [53] | 5 | All patients: metastatic renal cancer | Concurrent intravenous BP therapy and sunitinib | N/A |
| Yildiz et al. [54] | 3 | All patients: metastatic renal cancer | Sunitinib treatment alone | N/A |
| Smidt-Hansen et al. [8] | 6 | All patients: metastatic renal cancer | Concurrent intravenous BP therapy | Healing in 1 patient reported after surgical and antibiotic therapy |

## Everolimus

Reports about everolimus-associated ONJ have been published recently (Table 18.4) [55, 56]. Everolimus is an orally available inhibitor of mTOR (mammalian target of rapamycin), a serine/threonine kinase with controlling functions for various cell-signaling pathways which are critical in the pathogenesis of many malignant tumors and the control of immunologic reactions [57]. The main effects of everolimus

**Table 18.4** Compilation of case reports of everolimus-related ONJ

| Author | Number of cases reported | Reason for administration of everolimus | Treatment with bisphosphonates | Clinical course |
|---|---|---|---|---|
| Giancola et al. [55] | 1 | Metastatic renal cancer | Simultaneous treatment with intravenous bisphosphonates | Surgical treatment, no complete healing reported |
| Kim et al. [56] | 1 | Metastatic thyroid cancer | 11 years prior to everolimus administration | Conservative treatment, no complete healing reported |

are decreased angiogenesis, deceleration of cell maturation, and inhibition of osteoclasts [56]. Everolimus was approved by the FDA in 2003 for the treatment of organ transplant rejection, advanced renal cell carcinoma, neuroendocrine tumors, breast cancer, and some other cancers [57]. Unwanted side effects of everolimus treatment comprise mucositis, nausea, immunosuppression, gastrointestinal symptoms, and cough [57]. The limited evidence of everolimus-related ONJ does not allow any conclusions about cause and effect relationships at this time.

> **Conclusion**
>
> The array of new drugs with implications in the etiology of ONJ has constantly increased in the past years. Denosumab has already been proven to increase the risk for ONJ [15]. The combination of bisphosphonates with antiangiogenetic drugs (bevacizumab and sunitinib) in various oncologic treatment regimens may enhance the risk for ONJ and decrease the latency period until ONJ occurrence [28]. The pathomechanisms of denosumab-, bevacizumab-, and sunitinib-related ONJ have yet to be explored. The latest drug that has been associated with ONJ is everolimus [55–57]. All the mentioned drugs have some inhibitory effect on osteoclast maturation and activity and curb the immunologic host response. This may eventually explain their role in the pathogenesis of ONJ. Meticulous dental examination and special precautions in the performance of dentoalveolar surgeries have to be provided for patients prior to treatment or in active treatment with the mentioned drugs to reduce the risk of ONJ development.

## References


1. Marx RE. Pamidronate (Aredia) and zoledronate (Zometa) induced avascular necrosis of the jaws: a growing epidemic. J Oral Maxillofac Surg. 2003;61(9):1115–7.
2. Colella G, Campisi G, Fusco V. American Association of Oral and Maxillofacial Surgeons position paper: bisphosphonate-related osteonecrosis of the jaws-2009 update: the need to refine the BRONJ definition. J Oral Maxillofac Surg. 2009;67(12):2698–9.
3. Otto S, Hafner S, Mast G, Tischer T, Volkmer E, Schieker M, et al. Bisphosphonate-related osteonecrosis of the jaw: is pH the missing part in the pathogenesis puzzle? J Oral Maxillofac Surg. 2010;68(5):1158–61.
4. Otto S, Pautke C, Opelz C, Westphal I, Drosse I, Schwager J, et al. Osteonecrosis of the jaw: effect of bisphosphonate type, local concentration, and acidic milieu on the pathomechanism. J Oral Maxillofac Surg. 2010;68(11):2837–45.
5. Otto S, Schreyer C, Hafner S, Mast G, Ehrenfeld M, Sturzenbaum S, et al. Bisphosphonate-related osteonecrosis of the jaws – characteristics, risk factors, clinical features, localization and impact on oncological treatment. J Craniomaxillofac Surg. 2012;40(4):303–9.
6. Pautke C, Bauer F, Otto S, Tischer T, Steiner T, Weitz J, et al. Fluorescence-guided bone resection in bisphosphonate-related osteonecrosis of the jaws: first clinical results of a prospective pilot study. J Oral Maxillofac Surg. 2011;69(1):84–91.
7. Troeltzsch M, Woodlock T, Kriegelstein S, Steiner T, Messlinger K. Physiology and pharmacology of non-bisphosphonate drugs implicated in osteonecrosis of the jaw. J Can Dent Assoc. 2012;78:c85.
8. Smidt-Hansen T, Folkmar TB, Fode K, Agerbaek M, Donskov F. Combination of zoledronic acid and targeted therapy is active but may induce osteonecrosis of the jaw in patients with metastatic renal cell carcinoma. J Oral Maxillofac Surg. 2013;71(9):1532–40.
9. Boyle WJ, Simonet WS, Lacey DL. Osteoclast differentiation and activation. Nature. 2003;423(6937):337–42.
10. Baron R, Ferrari S, Russell RG. Denosumab and bisphosphonates: different mechanisms of action and effects. Bone. 2011;48(4):677–92.
11. Van Poznak C. Osteonecrosis of the jaw and bevacizumab therapy. Breast Cancer Res Treat. 2010;122(1):189–91.

12. Ortega J, Vigil CE, Chodkiewicz C. Current progress in targeted therapy for colorectal cancer. Cancer Control. 2010;17(1):7–15.

13. Brunello A, Saia G, Bedogni A, Scaglione D, Basso U. Worsening of osteonecrosis of the jaw during treatment with sunitinib in a patient with metastatic renal cell carcinoma. Bone. 2009;44(1):173–5.

14. Compston J. Pathophysiology of atypical femoral fractures and osteonecrosis of the jaw. Osteoporos Int. 2011;22(12):2951–61.

15. Stopeck AT, Lipton A, Body JJ, Steger GG, Tonkin K, de Boer RH, et al. Denosumab compared with zoledronic acid for the treatment of bone metastases in patients with advanced breast cancer: a randomized, double-blind study. J Clin Oncol. 2010;28(35):5132–9.

16. Malan J, Ettinger K, Naumann E, Beirne OR. The relationship of denosumab pharmacology and osteonecrosis of the jaws. Oral Surg Oral Med Oral Pathol Oral Radiol. 2012;114(6):671–6.

17. Henry D, Vadhan-Raj S, Hirsh V, von Moos R, Hungria V, Costa L, et al. Delaying skeletal-related events in a randomized phase 3 study of denosumab versus zoledronic acid in patients with advanced cancer: an analysis of data from patients with solid tumors. Support Care Cancer. 2013;22(3):679–87.

18. Henry DH, Costa L, Goldwasser F, Hirsh V, Hungria V, Prausova J, et al. Randomized, double-blind study of denosumab versus zoledronic acid in the treatment of bone metastases in patients with advanced cancer (excluding breast and prostate cancer) or multiple myeloma. J Clin Oncol. 2011;29(9):1125–32.

19. Fizazi K, Carducci M, Smith M, Damiao R, Brown J, Karsh L, et al. Denosumab versus zoledronic acid for treatment of bone metastases in men with castration-resistant prostate cancer: a randomised, double-blind study. Lancet. 2011;377(9768):813–22.

20. Scagliotti GV, Hirsh V, Siena S, Henry DH, Woll PJ, Manegold C, et al. Overall survival improvement in patients with lung cancer and bone metastases treated with denosumab versus zoledronic acid: subgroup analysis from a randomized phase 3 study. J Thorac Oncol. 2012;7(12):1823–9.

21. Bone HG, Chapurlat R, Brandi ML, Brown JP, Czerwinski E, Krieg MA, et al. The effect of three or six years of denosumab exposure in women with postmenopausal osteoporosis: results from the FREEDOM extension. J Clin Endocrinol Metab. 2013;98(11):4483–92.

22. Saad F, Brown JE, Van Poznak C, Ibrahim T, Stemmer SM, Stopeck AT, et al. Incidence, risk factors, and outcomes of osteonecrosis of the jaw: integrated analysis from three blinded active-controlled phase III trials in cancer patients with bone metastases. Ann Oncol. 2012;23(5):1341–7.

23. Kyrgidis A, Toulis KA. Denosumab-related osteonecrosis of the jaws. Osteoporos Int. 2011;22(1):369–70.

24. Pazianas M. Osteonecrosis of the jaw and the role of macrophages. J Natl Cancer Inst. 2011;103(3):232–40.

25. Sivolella S, Lumachi F, Stellini E, Favero L. Denosumab and anti-angiogenetic drug-related osteonecrosis of the jaw: an uncommon but potentially severe disease. Anticancer Res. 2013;33(5):1793–7.

26. Hopp RN, Pucci J, Santos-Silva AR, Jorge J. Osteonecrosis after administration of intravitreous bevacizumab. J Oral Maxillofac Surg. 2011;70(3):632–5.

27. Estilo CL, Fornier M, Farooki A, Carlson D, Bohle 3rd G, Huryn JM. Osteonecrosis of the jaw related to bevacizumab. J Clin Oncol. 2008;26(24):4037–8.

28. Lescaille G, Coudert AE, Baaroun V, Ostertag A, Charpentier E, Javelot MJ, et al. Clinical study evaluating the effect of bevacizumab on the severity of zoledronic acid-related osteonecrosis of the jaw in cancer patients. Bone. 2014;58:103–7.

29. Santos-Silva AR, Belizario Rosa GA, Castro Junior G, Dias RB, Prado Ribeiro AC, Brandao TB. Osteonecrosis of the mandible associated with bevacizumab therapy. Oral Surg Oral Med Oral Pathol Oral Radiol. 2013;115(6):e32–6.

30. Bevacizumab, sunitinib: osteonecrosis of the jaw. Prescrire Int. 2011;20(117):155.

31. Aragon-Ching JB, Ning YM, Chen CC, Latham L, Guadagnini JP, Gulley JL, et al. Higher incidence of Osteonecrosis of the Jaw (ONJ) in patients with metastatic castration resistant prostate cancer treated with anti-angiogenic agents. Cancer Invest. 2009;27(2):221–6.

32. Christodoulou C, Pervena A, Klouvas G, Galani E, Falagas ME, Tsakalos G, et al. Combination of bisphosphonates and antiangiogenic factors induces osteonecrosis of the jaw more frequently than bisphosphonates alone. Oncology. 2009;76(3):209–11.

33. Disel U, Besen AA, Ozyilkan O, Er E, Canpolat T. A case report of bevacizumab-related osteonecrosis of the jaw: old problem, new culprit. Oral Oncol. 2011; 48(2):e2–3.

34. Pakosch D, Papadimas D, Munding J, Kawa D, Kriwalsky MS. Osteonecrosis of the mandible due to anti-angiogenic agent, bevacizumab. Oral Maxillofac Surg. 2013;17(4):303–6.

35. Greuter S, Schmid F, Ruhstaller T, Thuerlimann B. Bevacizumab-associated osteonecrosis of the jaw. Ann Oncol. 2008;19(12):2091–2.

36. Serra E, Paolantonio M, Spoto G, Mastrangelo F, Tete S, Dolci M. Bevacizumab-related osteonecrosis of the jaw. Int J Immunopathol Pharmacol. 2009;22(4):1121–3.

37. Guarneri V, Miles D, Robert N, Dieras V, Glaspy J, Smith I, et al. Bevacizumab and osteonecrosis of the jaw: incidence and association with bisphosphonate therapy in three large prospective trials in advanced breast cancer. Breast Cancer Res Treat. 2010;122(1):181–8.

38. Sato M, Ono F, Yamamura A, Onochi S. A case of osteonecrosis of the jaw during treatment by bevacizumab for sigmoid colon cancer. Nihon Shokakibyo Gakkai Zasshi. 2013;110(4):655–9.

39. Brunamonti Binello P, Bandelloni R, Labanca M, Buffoli B, Rezzani R, Rodella LF. Osteonecrosis of the jaws and bevacizumab therapy: a case report. Int J Immunopathol Pharmacol. 2012;25(3):789–91.

40. Hansen T, Kunkel M, Springer E, Walter C, Weber A, Siegel E, et al. Actinomycosis of the jaws – histopathological study of 45 patients shows significant involvement in bisphosphonate-associated osteonecrosis and infected osteoradionecrosis. Virchows Arch. 2007;451(6):1009–17.

41. Hansen T, Kunkel M, Weber A, James Kirkpatrick C. Osteonecrosis of the jaws in patients treated with bisphosphonates – histomorphologic analysis in comparison with infected osteoradionecrosis. J Oral Pathol Med. 2006;35(3):155–60.

42. Aldridge SE, Lennard TW, Williams JR, Birch MA. Vascular endothelial growth factor receptors in osteoclast differentiation and function. Biochem Biophys Res Commun. 2005;335(3):793–8.

43. Magremanne M, Lahon M, De Ceulaer J, Reychler H. Unusual bevacizumab-related complication of an oral infection. J Oral Maxillofac Surg. 2013; 71(1):53–5.

44. Mena AC, Pulido EG, Guillen-Ponce C. Understanding the molecular-based mechanism of action of the tyrosine kinase inhibitor: sunitinib. Anticancer Drugs. 2010;21 Suppl 1:S3–11.

45. Goodman VL, Rock EP, Dagher R, Ramchandani RP, Abraham S, Gobburu JV, et al. Approval summary: sunitinib for the treatment of imatinib refractory or intolerant gastrointestinal stromal tumors and advanced renal cell carcinoma. Clin Cancer Res. 2007;13(5):1367–73.

46. Fleissig Y, Regev E, Lehman H. Sunitinib related osteonecrosis of jaw: a case report. Oral Surg Oral Med Oral Pathol Oral Radiol Endod. 2012;113(3):e1–3.

47. Koch FP, Walter C, Hansen T, Jager E, Wagner W. Osteonecrosis of the jaw related to sunitinib. Oral Maxillofac Surg. 2011;15(1):63–6.

48. Bozas G, Roy A, Ramasamy V, Maraveyas A. Osteonecrosis of the jaw after a single bisphosphonate infusion in a patient with metastatic renal cancer treated with sunitinib. Onkologie. 2010;33(6):321–3.

49. Hoefert S, Eufinger H. Sunitinib may raise the risk of bisphosphonate-related osteonecrosis of the jaw: presentation of three cases. Oral Surg Oral Med Oral Pathol Oral Radiol Endod. 2010;110(4):463–9.

50. Bonacina R, Mariani U, Villa F, Villa A. Preventive strategies and clinical implications for bisphosphonate-related osteonecrosis of the jaw: a review of 282 patients. J Can Dent Assoc. 2011;77:b147.

51. Nicolatou-Galitis O, Migkou M, Psyrri A, Bamias A, Pectasides D, Economopoulos T, et al. Gingival bleeding and jaw bone necrosis in patients with metastatic renal cell carcinoma receiving sunitinib: report of 2 cases with clinical implications. Oral Surg Oral Med Oral Pathol Oral Radiol. 2012;113(2):234–8.

52. Agrillo A, Nastro Siniscalchi E, Facchini A, Filiaci F, Ungari C. Osteonecrosis of the jaws in patients assuming bisphosphonates and sunitinib: two case reports. Eur Rev Med Pharmacol Sci. 2012;16(7):952–7.

53. Beuselinck B, Wolter P, Karadimou A, Elaidi R, Dumez H, Rogiers A, et al. Concomitant oral tyrosine kinase inhibitors and bisphosphonates in advanced renal cell carcinoma with bone metastases. Br J Cancer. 2012;107(10):1665–71.

54. Yildiz I, Sen F, Basaran M, Ekenel M, Agaoglu F, Darendeliler E, et al. Response rates and adverse effects of continuous once-daily sunitinib in patients with advanced renal cell carcinoma: a single-center study in Turkey. Jpn J Clin Oncol. 2011;41(12):1380–7.

55. Giancola F, Campisi G, Russo LL, Muzio LL, Di Fede O. Osteonecrosis of the jaw related to everolimus and bisphosphonate: a unique case report? Ann Stomatol (Roma). 2013;4 Suppl 2:20–1.

56. Kim DW, Jung YS, Park HS, Jung HD. Osteonecrosis of the jaw related to everolimus: a case report. Br J Oral Maxillofac Surg. 2013;51(8):e302–4.

57. Lebwohl D, Anak O, Sahmoud T, Klimovsky J, Elmroth I, Haas T, et al. Development of everolimus, a novel oral mTOR inhibitor, across a spectrum of diseases. Ann N Y Acad Sci. 2013;1291:14–32.

# History of Osteonecrosis of the Jaw

**19**


Sebastian Hoefert, Claudia Sade Hoefert,
and Martin Widmann



## Abstract

Medication-related osteonecrosis of the jaw and phosphorous necrosis are strikingly similar. Phosphorous necrosis (phossy jaw) was caused by close contact with yellow phosphorous. In the nineteenth century, the knowledge concerning cause and prevention of osteonecrosis was astonishingly accurate. Rules concerning prevention and treatment were similar to those of our days. The Bern convention banned the use of yellow phosphorous. In the following decades, the disease gradually disappeared from common knowledge, until Robert Marx described the first modern bisphosphonate-related osteonecrosis of the jaw in 2003.


## Introduction

Osteonecrosis of the jaw is – quite contrary to common view – not a recently discovered side effect and complication of antiresorptive medication.

This might come as a surprise, taking into consideration that literature concerning the disease (PubMed.gov; US National Library of Medicine National Institute of Health) was virtually nonexistent before 2003, rising steadily to more or less 200 articles per year since 2007.

This is hardly surprising since bisphosphonates (originally called diphosphonates) were not introduced until 1969, when etidronate entered the market, and highly effective formulas were not available until the introduction of pamidronate and zoledronate [1]. Side effects of this new medication were not observed until 2003, when Robert Marx described the first cases of osteonecrosis of the jaw, which he attributed to the use of bisphosphonates [2].


S. Hoefert, MD, DDS (✉)
Department of Oral- and Maxillofacial Surgery,
University Hospital Tuebingen,
Osianderstrasse 2-8, 72076 Tuebingen, Germany
e-mail: sebastian.hoefert@med.uni-tuebingen.de,
sebastian.hoefert@uni-tuebingen.de

C.S. Hoefert, DDS
Dental Practice Reutlingen Dr. Ruoff,
Albstrasse 2, 72764 Reutlingen, Germany

M. Widmann, MD
Department of Anaesthesiology,
Intensive Care Medicine and Pain Therapy,
Berufsgenossenschaftliche Unfallklinik Tuebingen,
University Hospital Tuebingen,
Schnarrenbergstrasse 95, 72076 Tuebingen, Germany



S. Otto (ed.), *Medication-Related Osteonecrosis of the Jaws: Bisphosphonates, Denosumab, and New Agents*,
DOI 10.1007/978-3-662-43733-9_19, © Springer-Verlag Berlin Heidelberg 2015

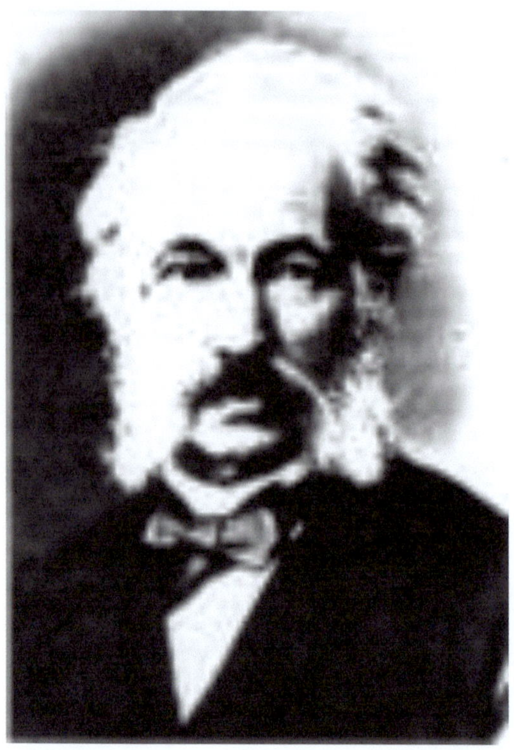



**Fig. 19.1** Friedrich Wilhelm Lorinser (1817–1895) (Reprinted from Lecky [10])

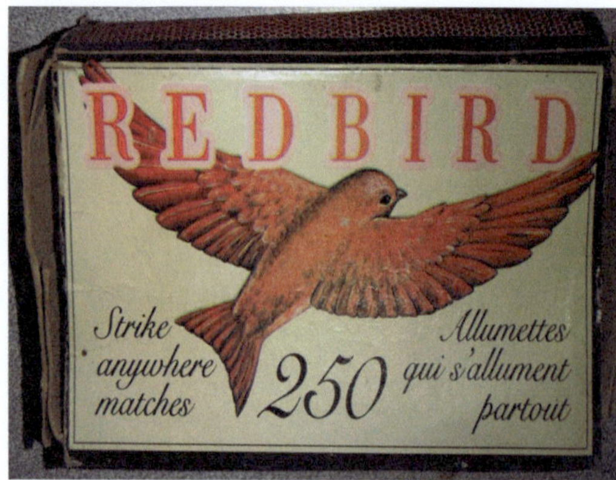

**Fig. 19.2** Strike anywhere matches incorporating yellow phosphorus in the match head (Reprinted from R.E. Marx Introduction in "Bisphosphonates and Osteonecrosis of the Jaw" by Francesco Saverio de Ponte with kind permission of Springer Science+Business Media)

## Phosphorous Necrosis and Match Making

The history of phosphorous-associated osteonecrosis of the jaw, also called phosphorous necrosis, however goes back in time considerably. As early as in 1845, Friedrich Wilhelm Lorinser described nine cases of serious necrosis of the jaw that came to his attention in the year 1839 (Fig. 19.1). He published his report in "Österreichische medicinische Jahrbücher" with the original title "Necrose der Kieferknochen in folge der Einwirkung von Phosphordämpfen/ Necrosis of the jaw following exposure to phosphorous fumes." Friedrich Wilhelm Lorinser (1817–1895) was a physician from Vienna, who practiced at the local hospital in Vienna. All in all, Lorinser observed 126 patients suffering from osteonecrosis, who had come in close contact with yellow phosphorous, while working in matchmaking factories [3].

Yellow phosphorous was used in manufacturing "strike anywhere" matches (Fig. 19.2). The yellow phosphorus-tipped match was developed around 1830 [4] and named Lucifer matches by Samuel Jones in 1829 [5]. Primarily, factory workers called "dippers," "mixers," and "boxers" came to close contact with yellow phosphorous. "Mixers" had to heat phosphorous for the dippers, who dipped the wooden pins of the matches into it. After drying, the "boxers" sorted and packed the finished matches into matchboxes [4–6]. Match production did not require strength or special skills and was ideal for low-income families working from home. A nursery rhyme dating back to those times describes the practice of child labor in that context: "The match box, the match box was hard to make at three, but now I am four or rather more, it is easier for me" [5].

## Phosphorous Necrosis and Clinical Observation

As in contemporary medication-related osteonecrosis of the jaw, the workers of the nineteenth century developed severe jaw infections, mostly after tooth extractions. Mortality in those pre-antibiotic days was as high as 20 % [4, 7]. Besides palatal spreading (a stage 3 equivalent) to the

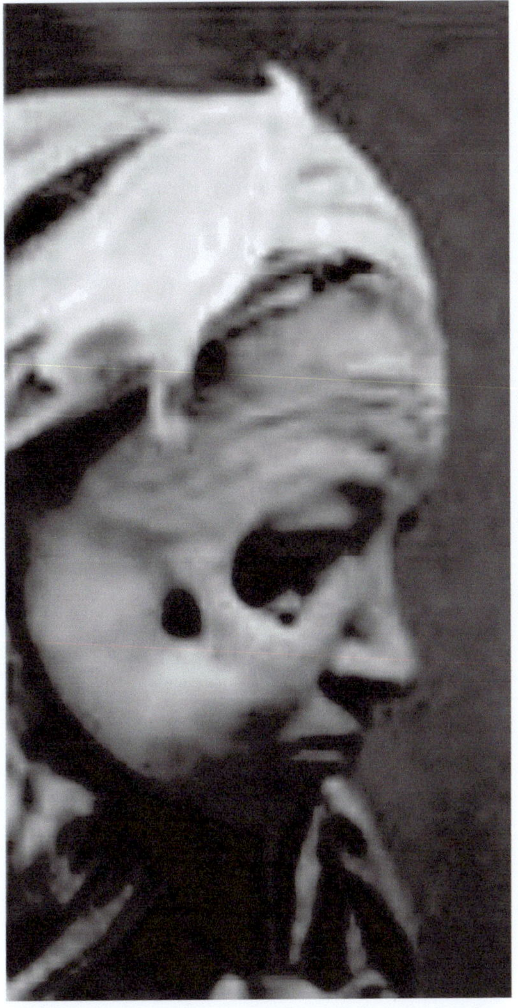

**Fig. 19.3** Necrosis of the upper jaw with destruction of the eyeball. Case presented by Teleky (Reprinted with kind permission of Springer Science+Business Media from Ludwig Teleky L 1955 "Gewerbliche Vergiftungen" Springer)

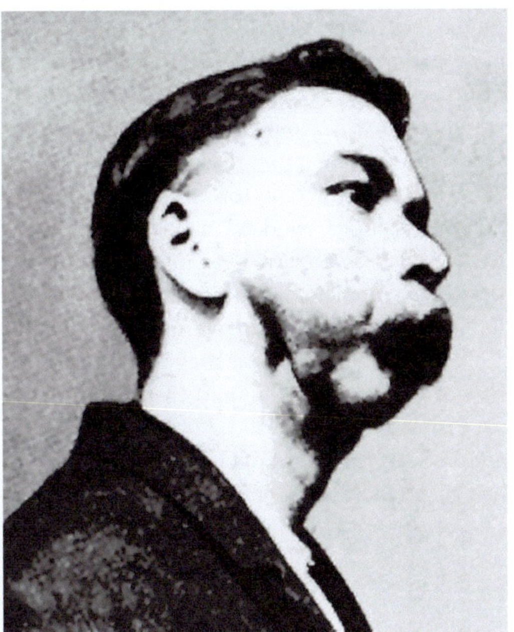

**Fig. 19.4** Match factory worker at the end of 19th century suffering from phossy jaw with pathological fracture of the mandible and fistula formation (Reprinted from R.E. Marx "Introduction" in "Bisphosphonates and Osteonecrosis of the Jaw" by Francesco Saverio de Ponte with kind permission of Springer Science+Business Media)

orbital bones, the infection could also affect the eyes with subsequent atrophy of the eyeball (Fig. 19.3). Besides that pathological fractures of the mandible and fistula formations have also been described (Fig. 19.4). Meningeal inflammation and cerebral abscesses were feared complications [8, 9]. The connection between osteonecrosis and extraction of infected teeth was obvious [4, 6, 9–11]. According to Miles, the typical course was described by Simon as follows: "Typically a dull red area developed on the gum, usually in relation to an infected tooth. An indolent ulcer formed or, following the extraction of the tooth, the socket refused to heal and the soft tissue inflammation persisted. There was relatively slow progressive extension with eventual separation of a sequestrum which is classically described as porous and light in weight and presenting a worm-eaten appearance likened to pumice-stone" [12].

## History of Prevention and Precaution of Phosphorous Necrosis

It soon became obvious that prevention and precaution was the key to reduce the number of necrosis cases. Due to the severity of these cases and the frequently fatal outcome of phosphorous necrosis in those days, politicians were forced to act. Rules for match makers and special medical and dental examinations were introduced.

Employees, who worked in the dipping room for more than 28 days straight, had to be examined by an appointed dentist. Regular medical examinations every 3 months were mandatory. All cases of toothache or swelling of the jaw had to be examined and reported immediately. After tooth extractions, workers had to be excluded from match making till a final examination showed a complete restoration to health. Owing to these measures, Goadby was able to report in 1909 during an annual meeting in England that between 1900 and 1907, only 13 cases of osteonecrosis out of a total of 1,378 workers (0.9 %) had been observed, as opposed to 73 cases that had been reported out of a total of 1,908 workers (3.8 %) before [13]. In contrast, Austria assessments addressed 350–400 non-registered cases between the years 1896 and 1905 [9].

An American patent from 1863 provided a novel technique for dipping splints in phosphorous compositions, putting an end to close contact to the phosphorous fumes [8], but was not able to stop the phosphorous necrosis.

## The Berne Convention

The plight of match makers suffering from phosphorous necrosis drew wide public attention that in 1906, the International Association for Labour Legislation called an international conference at Berne. The Berne convention put a ban on the use of yellow phosphorous for match making. The agreement was signed by a number of nations. Russia and Japan had not sent delegates due to hostilities between both nations. England joined the law later in 1908, after considerable public pressure. Early in 1931, yellow phosphorous disappeared in the United States, when a high tax on these matches made them cost prohibitive [4, 7, 8]. Yellow phosphorus was subsequently replaced by red phosphorus. Matches made with red phosphorus or with phosphorus sesquisulfide (trisulfurated phosphorus) had additional benefits. They were safer regarding fire hazards (spontaneous ignitions) and poisoning after ingestion was less severe [4].

Even before the Berne convention, the salvation army of England had introduced matches made from red phosphorous advertising them as "Lights in darkest England" [5]. They even advertised them with the remark of "health-preserving principles" in production.

## After the Berne Ban

After solving the problem of phosphorous necrosis, the disease gradually faded from common knowledge. Interestingly, the awareness of phosphorus necrosis was very much alive in 1924 that a new disease was described as: "Somewhat similar to phosphorus necrosis, which, however, was caused by some radio-active substance" referring to osteoradionecrosis [14]. In 1951, phosphorous necrosis was described as follows: "Phosphorus causes osteomyelitis of the jaws in workers in the manufacture of matches who pay little or no attention to hygiene of the mouth. The phosphorus in its solid form or by its fumes probably gains entrance to the jaw bone through devitalized pulps of carious teeth or through an inflamed periodontal membrane" [15]. Interestingly, all previous knowledge about osteonecrosis seems to have disappeared by then, being replaced by relatively simple mechanical thinking.

In 2003, Marx described the first cases of BRONJ after bisphosphonate medication [2]. In September 2004, Novartis, the manufacturer of the intravenous bisphosphonates pamidronate (Aredia) and zoledronate (Zometa), notified healthcare professionals of the risk of osteonecrosis of the jaw in connection with bisphosphonate medication.

This was followed in 2005 by a drug class warning concerning the above described complication for all bisphosphonates including oral preparations [16].

## Phosphorous Necrosis and Bisphosphonate-Related Osteonecrosis of the Jaw

Critics will emphasize the differences between bisphosphonate-related osteonecrosis of the jaw and phosphorous necrosis. Marx offered the following solution to this puzzle [7]. He assumed that yellow phosphorous is transformed into some kind of bisphosphonate in the human body by biological processes. Yellow phosphorus with its simple formula $P_4O_{10}$ might be combined with $H_2O$, $CO_2$ and amino acids like lysine. The chemical product could be identical to a (medical) bisphosphonate. The human body would act as a bioreactor producing so-called "auto" bisphosphonates. Technically speaking, the pyrophosphate molecule ($P_2H_4O_7$) is derived from the basic molecular structure of yellow phosphorous with the addition of $2H_2O$ molecules. This diphosphonate is transformed into a bisphosphonate, when a carbon atom is substituted for an oxygen atom. This carbon backbone could be derived from $CO_2$ or carbonic acid, a reaction possibly aided by $N^5$ methyl tetrahydrofolate and dihydrofolate reductase. The result would be a so-called first-generation bisphosphonate – originally derived from simple yellow phosphorous. To create a bisphosphonate of higher potency, the nitrogen could either come from ammonia ($NH_3$) or, more likely, from amino acids, such as lysine. Interestingly, such a molecule has similarities with alendronate or pamidronate [7]. In all honesty, it must be admitted, however, that no additional reports have so far confirmed Marx's ingenious theory.

In conclusion, there are striking similarities between phosphorous necrosis (phossy jaw) and bisphosphonate-related osteonecrosis of the jaw. Even though it is not proven that it is the same entity or that there is a common etiology, the clinical presentation and preventive measurements were obviously similar to nowadays medication-related osteonecrosis of the jaw.

## References

1. Russel RGG. Bisphosphonates: the first 40 years. Bone. 2011;49:2–19.
2. Marx RE. Pamidronate (Aredia) and Zoledronate (Zometa) induced avascular necrosis of the jaws: a growing epidemic. J Oral Maxillofac Surg. 2003;61:1115–7.
3. Müller M, Böcher A, Buchter A. Phosphor-induzierte Kieferknochennekrose, eine "alte" "aktuelle" Berufserkrankung. [Homepage of Universitätsklinikum des Saarlandes], [Online]. 2012. http://scidok.sulb.uni-saarland.de/volltexte/2007/992/pdf/phosphor_poster.pdf. [07.06.2012].
4. Vance MA. Osteonecrosis of the jaw and bisphosphonates: a comparison with white phosphorus, radium, and osteopetrosis. Clin Toxicol. 2007;45:753–62.
5. Felton JS. Phosphorus necrosis – a classical occupational disease. Am J Indust Med. 1982;3:77–120.
6. Traves F. Phosphorus necrosis. Lancet. 1882;119:206.
7. Marx RE. Uncovering the cause of "phossy jaw" circa 1858 to 1906: oral and maxillofacial surgery closed case files – case closed. J Oral Maxillofac Surg. 2008;66:2356–63.
8. Crass MF. A history of the match industry. J Chem Educ. 1941;18:428–31.
9. Teleky L. Phosphor. In: Tekely L, editor. Gewerbliche Vergiftungen. Heidelberg: Springer; 1955. p. 146–50.
10. Lecky E. Die Phosphornekrose, klassisches Beispiel einer Berufskrankheit. Wien Klin Woch. 1966;78:601–4.
11. Thompson WG. The occupational diseases. New York: D. Appleton and Company; 1914. p. 334–56.
12. Simon J. "Fifth report of the medical officer of the Privy council". London: HMSO. Cited by Miles AEW. Phosphorus necrosis of the jaw: "Phossy jaw." Br Dent J. 1972;133:203–6.
13. Goadby KW. General results of the special rules in force in match factories. Proc R Soc Med (Odontolo Sect). 1909;2:53–70.
14. Hoffman FL. Malignancy in radio-active persons. Lancet. 1933;221:441–2.
15. Blair VP, Ivy RH, Brown JB. Essential in oral surgery. In: Blair VP, Ivy RH, Brown JB, editors. Essentials of oral surgery. St. Louis: The C.V. Mosby Company; 1951. p. 232.
16. Ruggiero SL, Dodson TB, Assael LA, Landesberg R, Marx RE, Mehrotra B. American Association of Oral and Maxillofacial Surgeons position paper 72 on bisphosphonate-related osteonecrosis of the jaws-2009 update. J Oral Maxillofac Surg. 2009;67:2–12.

Ralf Smeets, Henning Hanken, Ole Jung,
and Max Heiland

**Abstract**

Today, bisphosphonates are already used in a variety of indications, which by far exceed the commonly known applications. Closely related to their anorganic compound pyrophosphate, organic bisphosphonates are already used in everyday products like toothpastes and reagents for anticalculus and anti-calcification purposes. Besides that, bisphosphonates were successfully applied within experimental, animal, and clinical trial studies for dental socket preservations, periodontitis, and periimplantitis. Thereby, among other positive aspects like distinctive antibacterial profiles, more bone formation and fewer bone resorption were detected. Several other conditions commonly seen in oral and maxillofacial surgery might also benefit from administrations of antiresorptive drugs. In addition, bisphosphonates can also be successfully administered in uranyl intoxications as well as for hard and soft tissue calcifications. The primary aim of the ongoing research in this field can be defined in the detection of the ideal dose-effect relationship of different bisphosphonates when applied intravenously, orally, or topically.

## Introduction

Bisphosphonates represent the organic analogue (P-C-P) for inorganic pyrophosphate (P-O-P), which, as the simplest of the condensed phosphates, denoted the starting point for the development of today's commonly used bisphosphonates (Fig. 20.1) [24, 26, 55, 87]. This fact is also reflected in the currently pervasive use of both bisphosphonates and pyrophosphates in various everyday products besides the broad use in the treatment regimen for osteoporosis and bone tumors (Table 20.1) [22, 24, 25]. While bisphosphonates were earlier used to prevent calcium carbonate precipitation (e.g., boiler stones), they have been implemented in various everyday products like toothpastes and therapy patterns in order to avoid dental calculus, caries, and general soft

R. Smeets, MD, DMD, PhD (✉)
H. Hanken, MD, DMD • O. Jung, MD
M. Heiland, MD, DMD, PhD
Department of Oral and Maxillofacial Surgery,
University Medical Center Hamburg-Eppendorf,
Martinistraße 52, Hamburg D-20246, Germany
e-mail: r.smeets@uke.de

S. Otto (ed.), *Medication-Related Osteonecrosis of the Jaws: Bisphosphonates, Denosumab, and New Agents*, 207
DOI 10.1007/978-3-662-43733-9_20, © Springer-Verlag Berlin Heidelberg 2015

**Fig. 20.1** Chemical structure of pyrophosphate and bisphosphonates

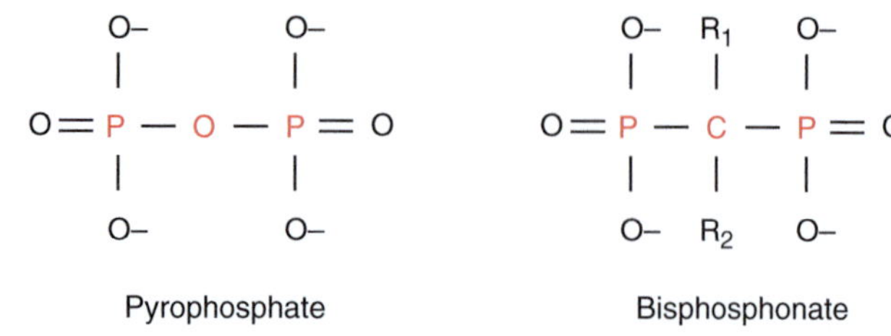



**Table 20.1** Daily commodities containing bisphosphonates and pyrophosphates

| Application | Examples |
| --- | --- |
| Crystal, metal, and other surfaces | Prevention of stone formation, corrosion, and pollution |
| Solutions | Softener of water |
| | Textile dyes |
| | Plasticizer in wool |
| | Synthetic detergents |
| Plastics and polymer industry | Stabilization, adhesion |
| Daily commodities | Cosmetics, photograph, toothpaste, hair shampoos, soap, disinfectant, dispersant |

and hard tissue calcifications [39, 50, 63, 67, 77, 103–105]. Due to their high bone affinity, pyrophosphates are also used in bone scintigraphy with $^{99m}$technetium [48, 59, 85, 95, 101].

With regard to their pharmacokinetic and pharmacodynamic profile, pyrophosphates can only be administered intravenously and exhibit a poor pharmacological impact, which antagonizes their broad use. On the other hand, bisphosphonates feature superior modes of action and can also be applied locally or orally [22, 24, 25].

Besides the already known indications for bisphosphonates like osteoporosis and bone tumors, especially maxillofacial and dental application purposes have become a developing field with new indications for broader implementations of bisphosphonates [55, 87].

## Perspectives of Bisphosphonates in Dentistry

### Anticalculus and Anticaries Effects

Like pyrophosphates, various studies revealed that bisphosphonates are also capable of preventing dental calculus and caries [100]. This also applies to TRK-530, a new bisphosphonate, which Sikder and Shinoda et al. administered topically for anticalculus purposes in rats [83, 86].

Considering clinical usage, Koch et al. were able to reveal a significant anticaries profile by the use of bisphosphonates in a 3-year controlled clinical trial with more than 1,000 patients [45]. Thereby, toothpastes with 250 or 1,000 ppm fluoride were either applied with 1-hydroxyethylidene-1.1-bisphosphonate (HEBP), azacycloheptylidene-2.2-bisphosphonate (AHBP) or as control group in more than 1,100 children at 11 and 12 years of age. After 3 years of unsupervised brushing, AHBP exhibited significant better results compared to single fluoride treatments.

## Dental Implant Coating

Based on pharmacological perceptions, bisphosphonates can increase bone mineralization.

In a study with beagle dogs, Yoshinari et al. showed that the coating of titanium implants with calcium phosphate followed by pamidronate immobilization for 24 h at 37 °C results in higher osseointegration and bone formation rates than in the uncoated control groups [111]. Moon et al. interpreted this fact to generally enhanced alkaline phosphatase (*ALP*) and osteoclast inhibition rates [60]. In several more studies, Stadelmann et al. could reveal higher bone densities, bone thickness, and bone mineralization by the application of zoledronate in orthopedic applications [89–91, 94]. In dentistry, subsequent patient studies showed generally higher stability quotient rates for bisphosphonate-coated dental titanium implants [2, 3].

## Socket Preservation

Teeth loosening, loss of teeth, and teeth extraction often result in elevated bone resorption processes, which makes bone augmentation prior to implant treatment mandatory.

In animal experiments, intravenous or subcutaneous application of zoledronate or alendronate results in diminished bone resorption after teeth extraction [6, 31, 42]. Jee et al. detected significant differences in vertical and horizontal alveolar crests after subcutaneous application of alendronate (1 mg/kg/day), whereas Abtahi and Kuroshima et al. only accomplished satisfactory results by using soft tissue coverage therapies characterized by a mucoperiosteal flap or parathyroid hormone usage [1, 40, 46]. Vertical and horizontal higher alveolar crests were also detected by Graziani et al. in a randomized clinical trial [35].

Other animal studies showed that prolonged systemic applications of zoledronate can induce BRONJ, inhibit angiogenesis, and lead to bacterial colonization, whereas these effects could not be proven for alendronate and etidronate [5, 44, 109]. However, pharmacological actions and side effects of bisphosphonates have to be interpreted with special regard to the dose and frequency of application (cumulative dose) [8, 64].

When reimplanting teeth after accidents or surgical procedures demanding teeth extraction, topical application of alendronate, zoledronate, and etidronate can be used to prevent inflammatory resorptive processes [17, 61, 81].

## Periodontitis

Periodontitis must be seen as one of the major risk factors for the development of teeth loosening, loss of teeth, and periimplantitis after implant treatment. Besides systematically planned mechanical interventions and control appointments, medications for plaque prevention and removal are necessary and highly questioned.

Various animal studies showed positive effects of alendronate, clodronate, etidronate, risedronate, tiludronate, TRK-530, and zoledronate on the inhibition of bone resorption, bone mineralization, and bone formation after experimentally induced periodontitis [4, 12, 20, 30, 33, 58, 65, 71, 72, 75, 83, 84, 102, 107]. In an ovariectomized rat model that simulated postmenopausal estrogen deficiency, Said, Xiong, and Duarte et al. were not able to completely restore bone balance by the application of bisphosphonates [20, 75, 107]. For the overall suppression of osteoclasts, Goes and Price et al. were able, among others, to show additive suppressive effects for alendronate and statins [30, 34, 70, 102]. In two studies, Buduneli et al. revealed additive antiresorptive effects by using alendronate and doxycycline [13, 14]. Furthermore, Buduneli, as well as Menezes et al., demonstrated anti-inflammatory and antibacterial effects of alendronate [13, 33, 56]. Alendronate was also capable to lower bone specific alkaline phosphatase and alveolar bone loss significantly [33]. Topical application of 1 % alendronate gel improved the overall gingival index as well as probing depth and clinical attachment level [71].

Shoji and Aguirre et al. detected dose-dependent actions of risedronate and zoledronate on osteoclastogenesis and therefore bone resorption [4, 84]. Thereby, higher doses of subcutaneous risedronate enhance bone-protecting effects, whereas 80 µg/kg zoledronate results in further periodontal bone defects. Within all mentioned animal studies, the route of drug administration (oral, intravenous, subcutaneous, subperiosteal) does not seem to determine positive or negative effects as well as side effects of bisphosphonate application. However, some bisphosphonates, as shown by Cetinkaya and Kim et al., seem to have negative effects on bone microcirculation [15, 42]. Thus, disturbances in bone circulation were connected to the occurrence of BRONJ [22, 23, 64].

In several clinical controlled study trials with at least 52 periodontal defects and a follow-up between 6 and 12 months, Pradeep and Sharma et al. revealed positive effects of 1 % alendronate gel on probing depth, bleeding index, clinical attachment level, and overall bone deposition [68, 69, 79, 80]. These results were also detected by Lane et al. in a study with 27 patients [47]. In two other studies, radiologic evidence of the positive effects of alendronate was shown by

El-Shinnawi and Veena et al. [21, 99]. Besides alendronate, also etidronate has positive effects on bone resorption over 5 years as shown by Takaishi et al. in a study with four women [92]. While Rocha et al. revealed positive effects of alendronate on periodontal bone resorption and cementoenamel junction, Jeffcoat et al. only detected an overall positive impact of alendronate in the prevention and development of manifesting periodontitis [41, 74].

With regard to drug administration developments, Samdancioglu et al. developed microspheres with alendronate on chitosan and poly(lactide-co-glycolide) acid (PLGA) basis that showed slower and faster drug release kinetics [76].

## Bisphosphonates and Periimplantitis

Overall, positive effects of bisphosphonates on bone resorption, bone formation, and periodontal processes were shown in the enumerated studies above.

Meraw and Shibutani et al. detected macroscopic and radiologic bone formation and less bone resorption by topical and intramuscular application of alendronate and pamidronate in a dog model [57, 82]. Thereby, Shibutani et al. did not detect significant differences of the serum markers osteocalcin and deoxypyridinoline [82].

As a prognostic marker in peri-implant inflammatory processes, detection of matrix metalloproteinases (MMPs) in the peri-implant sulcus fluid and periodontal ligament cells plays a crucial role [43]. In vitro and in vivo studies of Ozdemir, Nakaya, and Teronen et al. showed the inhibition of MMP-1, MMP-3, MMP-8 and MMP-9 by clodronate and tiludronate [62, 66, 93]. Despite these significant results, RNA levels were not affected [62].

## Potential Applications in Other Diseases of the Maxillofacial Region

Bisphosphonates can also be applied for other diseases and indications of the maxillofacial area. Numerous studies revealed beneficial effects of bisphosphonates in the treatment of Paget's disease, osteogenesis imperfecta, osteoradionecrosis, giant cell granuloma, and fibrous dysplasia [10, 16, 18, 19, 38, 48, 51, 73, 78, 112]. In diffuse sclerosing osteomyelitis and SAPHO syndrome, bisphosphonates successfully reduced pain, bone resorption, and bone turnover [7, 36, 49, 52, 88, 106, 110].

Against all presumptions, the vast majority of studies did not reveal any hard or soft tissue necrosis after systemic or topical application of various bisphosphonates. Besides even more application possibilities in the future, the great advantages of bisphosphonates influencing bone resorption should not be forgotten in oral and maxillofacial surgery and other medical specialties.

## Additional Applications for Bisphosphonates

Intoxications with uranyl nitrate are another major field of experimental bisphosphonate application. Uranyl nitrate is, among other applications, important for the nuclear processing of enriched uranium. In a study with rats, Ubios and Bozal et al. systematically applied ethane-1-hydroxy-1,1-bisphosphonate after uranyl intoxication [11, 97]. Thereby, bone growth, bone and cartilage thickness, and metaphyseal activity were not different to control groups. In this case, bisphosphonates act as uranyl chelating agents [27–29, 37, 53, 54, 96, 108].

Additional applications were described by van Dyck, Göcmen, and Bereket et al. [9, 32, 98]. In these studies, bisphosphonates were applied in order to treat infantile arterial calcification, pulmonary alveolar microlithiasis, and vitamin D intoxication.

### Conclusion

Overall, bisphosphonates as well as pyrophosphates can be used in a broad and still expanding range of indications in maxillofacial surgery, dentistry, and other medical specialties.

Besides the prevalent application in osteoporosis and bone metastasis, the substances are already regularly used in daily products like toothpastes and chemical reagents for anticalculus, anti-calcification, and cleaning purposes. In various studies, bisphosphonates were applied for periodontitis, periimplantitis, socket preservations, and uranyl intoxications and in coated implants. In these studies, bisphosphonates successfully antagonize bone resorption and even stimulated bone growth. In radiology, bisphosphonates and pyrophosphates can be used with radioactive nuclides as bone markers.

However, additional research has to be done regarding advantages and disadvantages, side effects, pharmacokinetics, and application profiles of bisphosphonates, before evidence-based recommendations for new indications can be given.

# References


1. Abtahi J, Agholme F, Aspenberg P. Prevention of osteonecrosis of the jaw by mucoperiosteal coverage in a rat model. Int J Oral Maxillofac Surg. 2013;42(5):632–6. PubMed PMID: 23499148.

2. Abtahi J, Tengvall P, Aspenberg P. Bisphosphonate coating might improve fixation of dental implants in the maxilla: a pilot study. Int J Oral Maxillofac Surg. 2010;39(7):673–7. PubMed PMID: 20452185.

3. Abtahi J, Tengvall P, Aspenberg P. A bisphosphonate-coating improves the fixation of metal implants in human bone. A randomized trial of dental implants. Bone. 2012;50(5):1148–51. PubMed PMID: 22348981.

4. Aguirre JI, Akhter MP, Kimmel DB, Pingel JE, Williams A, Jorgensen M, et al. Oncologic doses of zoledronic acid induce osteonecrosis of the jaw-like lesions in rice rats (Oryzomys palustris) with periodontitis. J Bone Miner Res. 2012;27(10):2130–43. PubMed PMID: 22623376.

5. Aguirre JI, Altman MK, Vanegas SM, Franz SE, Bassit ACF, Wronski TJ. Effects of alendronate on bone healing after tooth extraction in rats. Oral Dis. 2010;16(7):674–85. PubMed PMID: 20846154.

6. Allen MR, Kubek DJ, Burr DB, Ruggiero SL, Chu TG. Compromised osseous healing of dental extraction sites in zoledronic acid-treated dogs. Osteoporos Int. 2011;22(2):693–702. PubMed PMID: 20458574.

7. Armstrong DJ, Wright SA, Coward SM, Finch MB. Bone marker response in chronic diffuse sclerosing osteomyelitis treated with intravenous ibandronate. Ann Rheum Dis. 2006;65(7):976–7. PubMed PMID: 16769790.

8. Assaf AT, Smeets R, Riecke B, Weise E, Gröbe A, Blessmann M, et al. Incidence of bisphosphonate-related osteonecrosis of the jaw in consideration of primary diseases and concomitant therapies. Anticancer Res. 2013;33(9):3917–24. PubMed PMID: 24023329.

9. Bereket A, Erdogan T. Oral bisphosphonate therapy for vitamin D intoxication of the infant. Pediatrics. 2003;111(4 Pt 1):899–901. PubMed PMID: 12671131.

10. Bolland MJ, Cundy T. Paget's disease of bone: clinical review and update. J Clin Pathol. 2013;66(11):924–7. PubMed PMID: 24043712.

11. Bozal CB, Martinez AB, Cabrini RL, Ubios AM. Effect of ethane-1-hydroxy-1,1-bisphosphonate (EHBP) on endochondral ossification lesions induced by a lethal oral dose of uranyl nitrate. Arch Toxicol. 2005;79(8):475–81. PubMed PMID: 15798912.

12. Brunsvold MA, Chaves ES, Kornman KS, Aufdemorte TB, Wood R. Effects of a bisphosphonate on experimental periodontitis in monkeys. J Periodontol. 1992;63(10):825–30. PubMed PMID: 1328593.

13. Buduneli E, Buduneli N, Vardar-Sengül S, Kardeşler L, Atilla G, Lappin D, et al. Systemic low-dose doxycycline and alendronate administration and serum interleukin-1beta, osteocalcin, and C-reactive protein levels in rats. J Periodontol. 2005;76(11):1927–33. PubMed PMID: 16274312.

14. Buduneli E, Vardar S, Buduneli N, Berdeli AH, Türkoğlu O, Başkesen A, et al. Effects of combined systemic administration of low-dose doxycycline and alendronate on endotoxin-induced periodontitis in rats. J Periodontol. 2004;75(11):1516–23. PubMed PMID: 15633329.

15. Cetinkaya BO, Keles GC, Ayas B, Gurgor P. Effects of risedronate on alveolar bone loss and angiogenesis: a stereologic study in rats. J Periodontol. 2008;79(10):1950–61. PubMed PMID: 18834251.

16. Chapurlat RD, Gensburger D, Jimenez-Andrade JM, Ghilardi JR, Kelly M, Mantyh P. Pathophysiology and medical treatment of pain in fibrous dysplasia of bone. Orphanet J Rare Dis. 2012;7 Suppl 1:S3. PubMed PMID: 22640953.

17. Choi SC, Kwon Y, Kim KC, Kim G. The effects of topical application of bisphosphonates on replanted rat molars. Dent Traumatol. 2010;26(6):476–80. PubMed PMID: 21078072.

18. Cundy T. Recent advances in osteogenesis imperfecta. Calcif Tissue Int. 2012;90(6):439–49. PubMed PMID: 22451222.

19. D'Eufemia P, Finocchiaro R, Villani C, Zambrano A, Lodato V, Palombaro M, et al. Serum brain-type creatine kinase increases in children with osteogenesis imperfecta during neridronate treatment. Pediatr Res. 2014;75(5):626–30.

20. Duarte PM, de Assis DR, Casati MZ, Sallum AW, Sallum EA, Nociti FH. Alendronate may protect against increased periodontitis-related bone loss in estrogen-deficient rats. J Periodontol. 2004;75(9):1196–202. PubMed PMID: 15515333.

21. El-Shinnawi UM, El-Tantawy SI. The effect of alendronate sodium on alveolar bone loss in periodontitis (clinical trial). J Int Acad Periodontol. 2003;5(1):5–10. PubMed PMID: 12666950.

22. Fleisch H. Bisphosphonates. Pharmacology and use in the treatment of tumour-induced hypercalcaemic

and metastatic bone disease. Drugs. 1991;42(6):919–44. PubMed PMID: 1724640.

23. Fleisch H. Bisphosphonates: pharmacology. Semin Arthritis Rheum. 1994;23(4):261–2. PubMed PMID: 8009246.

24. Fleisch H. Development of bisphosphonates. Breast Cancer Res. 2002;4(1):30–4. PubMed PMID: 11879557.

25. Fleisch H. Bisphosphonates in osteoporosis. Eur Spine J. 2003;12 Suppl 2:S142–6. PubMed PMID: 13680318.

26. Fleisch H. Einführung in die Bisphosphonate. Geschichte und Wirkungsmechanismen. Orthopade. 2007;36(2):103–4, 106–9. PubMed PMID: 17277961.

27. Fukuda S. Chelating agents used for plutonium and uranium removal in radiation emergency medicine. Curr Med Chem. 2005;12(23):2765–70. PubMed PMID: 16305471.

28. Fukuda S, Ikeda M, Nakamura M, Katoh A, Yan X, Xie Y, et al. The effects of bicarbonate and its combination with chelating agents used for the removal of depleted uranium in rats. Hemoglobin. 2008;32(1–2):191–8. PubMed PMID: 18274996.

29. Fukuda S, Ikeda M, Nakamura M, Yan X, Xie Y. Effects of pH on du intake and removal by CBMIDA and EHBP. Health Phys. 2007;92(1):10–4. PubMed PMID: 17164594.

30. Furlaneto FAC, Nunes NLT, Oliveira Filho IL, Frota NPR, Yamamoto KO, Lisboa MRP, et al. Effects of locally-administered tiludronic acid on experimental periodontitis in rats. J Periodontol. 2014;85(9):1291–301.

31. Gerard DA, Carlson ER, Gotcher JE, Pickett DO. Early inhibitory effects of zoledronic acid in tooth extraction sockets in dogs are negated by recombinant human bone morphogenetic protein. J Oral Maxillofac Surg. 2014;72(1):61–6. PubMed PMID: 23891015.

32. Göcmen A, Toppare MF, Kiper N, Büyükpamukcu N. Treatment of pulmonary alveolar microlithiasis with a diphosphonate–preliminary results of a case. Respiration. 1992;59(4):250–2. PubMed PMID: 1485012.

33. Goes P, Melo IM, Dutra CS, Lima APS, Lima V. Effect of alendronate on bone-specific alkaline phosphatase on periodontal bone loss in rats. Arch Oral Biol. 2012;57(11):1537–44. PubMed PMID: 23062673.

34. Goes P, Melo IM, Silva LMCM, Benevides NMB, Alencar NMN, Ribeiro RA, et al. Low-dose combination of alendronate and atorvastatin reduces ligature-induced alveolar bone loss in rats. J Periodontal Res. 2014;49(1):45–54. PubMed PMID: 23742139.

35. Graziani F, Rosini S, Cei S, La Ferla F, Gabriele M. The effects of systemic alendronate with or without intraalveolar collagen sponges on postextractive bone resorption: a single masked randomized clinical trial. J Craniofac Surg. 2008;19(4):1061–6. PubMed PMID: 18650733.

36. Hatano H, Shigeishi H, Higashikawa K, Shimasue H, Nishi H, Oiwa H, et al. A case of SAPHO syndrome with diffuse sclerosing osteomyelitis of the mandible treated successfully with prednisolone and bisphosphonate. J Oral Maxillofac Surg. 2012;70(3):626–31. PubMed PMID: 21816533.

37. Henge-Napoli MH, Ansoborlo E, Chazel V, Houpert P, Paquet F, Gourmelon P. Efficacy of ethane-1-hydroxy-1,1-bisphosphonate (EHBP) for the decorporation of uranium after intramuscular contamination in rats. Int J Radiat Biol. 1999;75(11):1473–7. PubMed PMID: 10597920.

38. Hennedige AA, Jayasinghe J, Khajeh J, Macfarlane TV. Systematic review on the incidence of bisphosphonate related osteonecrosis of the jaw in children diagnosed with osteogenesis imperfecta. J Oral Maxillofac Res. 2013;4(4):e1. PubMed PMID: 24478911.

39. Huang MS, Sage AP, Lu J, Demer LL, Tintut Y. Phosphate and pyrophosphate mediate PKA-induced vascular cell calcification. Biochem Biophys Res Commun. 2008;374(3):553–8. PubMed PMID: 18655772.

40. Jee J, Lee W, Lee BD. The influence of alendronate on the healing of extraction sockets of ovariectomized rats assessed by in vivo micro-computed tomography. Oral Surg Oral Med Oral Pathol Oral Radiol Endod. 2010;110(2):e47–53. PubMed PMID: 20591699.

41. Jeffcoat MK, Cizza G, Shih WJ, Genco R, Lombardi A. Efficacy of bisphosphonates for the control of alveolar bone loss in periodontitis. J Int Acad Periodontol. 2007;9(3):70–6. PubMed PMID: 17715838.

42. Kim J, Park Y, Li Z, Shim J, Moon H, Jung H, et al. Effect of alendronate on healing of extraction sockets and healing around implants. Oral Dis. 2011;17(7):705–11. PubMed PMID: 21771209.

43. Kivelä-Rajamäki M, Maisi P, Srinivas R, Tervahartiala T, Teronen O, Husa V, et al. Levels and molecular forms of MMP-7 (matrilysin-1) and MMP-8 (collagenase-2) in diseased human peri-implant sulcular fluid. J Periodontal Res. 2003;38(6):583–90. PubMed PMID: 14632921.

44. Kobayashi Y, Hiraga T, Ueda A, Wang L, Matsumoto-Nakano M, Hata K, et al. Zoledronic acid delays wound healing of the tooth extraction socket, inhibits oral epithelial cell migration, and promotes proliferation and adhesion to hydroxyapatite of oral bacteria, without causing osteonecrosis of the jaw, in mice. J Bone Miner Metab. 2010;28(2):165–75. PubMed PMID: 19882100.

45. Koch G, Bergmann-Arnadottir I, Bjarnason S, Finnbogason S, Höskuldsson O, Karlsson R. Caries-preventive effect of fluoride dentifrices with and without anticalculus agents: a 3-year controlled clinical trial. Caries Res. 1990;24(1):72–9. PubMed PMID: 2403486.

46. Kuroshima S, Mecano RB, Tanoue R, Koi K, Yamashita J. Distinctive tooth-extraction socket healing: bisphosphonate versus parathyroid hormone therapy. J Periodontol. 2014;85(1):24–33. PubMed PMID: 23688101.

47. Lane N, Armitage GC, Loomer P, Hsieh S, Majumdar S, Wang H, et al. Bisphosphonate therapy improves the outcome of conventional periodontal treatment: results of a 12-month, randomized, placebo-controlled study. J Periodontol. 2005;76(7):1113–22. PubMed PMID: 16018754.

48. de Lange J, Rosenberg AJ, van den Akker HP, Koole R, Wirds JJ, van den Berg H. Treatment of central giant cell granuloma of the jaw with calcitonin. Int J Oral Maxillofac Surg. 1999;28(5):372–6. PubMed PMID: 10535540.

49. Le Goff B, Berthelot J, Maugars Y, Romas E. Alternative use of bisphosphonate therapy for rheumatic disease. Curr Pharm Des. 2010;16(27): 3045–52. PubMed PMID: 20722620.

50. Lomashvili KA, Garg P, Narisawa S, Millan JL, O'Neill WC. Upregulation of alkaline phosphatase and pyrophosphate hydrolysis: potential mechanism for uremic vascular calcification. Kidney Int. 2008;73(9):1024–30. PubMed PMID: 18288101.

51. Mäkitie AA, Törnwall J, Mäkitie O. Bisphosphonate treatment in craniofacial fibrous dysplasia–a case report and review of the literature. Clin Rheumatol. 2008;27(6):809–12. PubMed PMID: 18247080.

52. Marshall H, Bromilow J, Thomas AL, Arden NK. Pamidronate: a novel treatment for the SAPHO syndrome? Rheumatology (Oxford). 2002;41(2): 231–3. PubMed PMID: 11886977.

53. Martínez AB, Cabrini RL, Ubios AM. Orally administered ethane-1-hydroxy-1,1-biphosphonate reduces the lethal effect of oral uranium poisoning. Health Phys. 2000;78(6):668–71. PubMed PMID: 10832926.

54. Martinez AB, Mandalunis PM, Bozal CB, Cabrini RL, Ubios AM. Renal function in mice poisoned with oral uranium and treated with ethane-1-hydroxy-1,1-bisphosphonate (EHBP). Health Phys. 2003;85(3):343–7. PubMed PMID: 12938724.

55. Maruotti N, Corrado A, Neve A, Cantatore FP. Bisphosphonates: effects on osteoblast. Eur J Clin Pharmacol. 2012;68(7):1013–8. PubMed PMID: 22318756.

56. Menezes AMA, Rocha FAC, Chaves HV, Carvalho CBM, Ribeiro RA, Brito GAC. Effect of sodium alendronate on alveolar bone resorption in experimental periodontitis in rats. J Periodontol. 2005;76(11):1901–9. PubMed PMID: 16274309.

57. Meraw SJ, Reeve CM, Wollan PC. Use of alendronate in peri-implant defect regeneration. J Periodontol. 1999;70(2):151–8. PubMed PMID: 10102552.

58. Mitsuta T, Horiuchi H, Shinoda H. Effects of topical administration of clodronate on alveolar bone resorption in rats with experimental periodontitis. J Periodontol. 2002;73(5):479–86. PubMed PMID: 12027248.

59. Monte GU, Drager LF, Souza FS, Avila LF, Parga Filho JR, César LAM, et al. Magnetic resonance vs technetium-99m pyrophosphate scintigraphy in the detection of perioperative myocardial necrosis. Arq Bras Cardiol. 2008;91(2):113–8. PubMed PMID: 18709263.

60. Moon H, Yun Y, Han C, Kim MS, Kim SE, Bae MS, et al. Effect of heparin and alendronate coating on titanium surfaces on inhibition of osteoclast and enhancement of osteoblast function. Biochem Biophys Res Commun. 2011;413(2):194–200. PubMed PMID: 21888898.

61. Mori GG, Janjacomo DM, Nunes DC, Castilho LR. Effect of zoledronic acid used in the root surface treatment of late replanted teeth: a study in rats. Braz Dent J. 2010;21(5):452–7. PubMed PMID: 21180803.

62. Nakaya H, Osawa G, Iwasaki N, Cochran DL, Kamoi K, Oates TW. Effects of bisphosphonate on matrix metalloproteinase enzymes in human periodontal ligament cells. J Periodontol. 2000;71(7):1158–66. PubMed PMID: 10960024.

63. O'Neill WC, Lomashvili KA, Malluche HH, Faugere M, Riser BL. Treatment with pyrophosphate inhibits uremic vascular calcification. Kidney Int. 2011;79(5):512–7. PubMed PMID: 21124302.

64. Otto S, Pautke C, Hafner S, Hesse R, Reichardt LF, Mast G, et al. Pathologic fractures in bisphosphonate-related osteonecrosis of the jaw-review of the literature and review of our own cases. Craniomaxillofac Trauma Reconstr. 2013;6(3):147–54. PubMed PMID: 24436752.

65. O'uchi N, Nishikawa H, Yoshino T, Kanoh H, Motoie H, Nishimori E, et al. Inhibitory effects of YM175, a bisphosphonate, on the progression of experimental periodontitis in beagle dogs. J Periodontal Res. 1998;33(4):196–204. PubMed PMID: 9689615.

66. Ozdemir SP, Kurtiş B, Tüter G, Bozkurt Ş, Gültekin SE, Sengüven B, et al. Effects of low-dose doxycycline and bisphosphonate clodronate on alveolar bone loss and gingival levels of matrix metalloproteinase-9 and interleukin-1β in rats with diabetes: a histomorphometric and immunohistochemical study. J Periodontol. 2012;83(9):1172–82. PubMed PMID: 22220769.

67. Pfarrer AM, White DJ, Featherstone JD. Anticaries profile qualification of an improved whitening dentifrice. J Clin Dent. 2001;12(2):30–3. PubMed PMID: 11476010.

68. Pradeep AR, Kumari M, Rao NS, Naik SB. 1% alendronate gel as local drug delivery in the treatment of Class II furcation defects: a randomized controlled clinical trial. J Periodontol. 2013;84(3):307–15. PubMed PMID: 22554293.

69. Pradeep AR, Sharma A, Rao NS, Bajaj P, Naik SB, Kumari M. Local drug delivery of alendronate gel for the treatment of patients with chronic periodontitis with diabetes mellitus: a double-masked controlled clinical trial. J Periodontol. 2012;83(10):1322–8. PubMed PMID: 22264208.

70. Price U, Le HT, Powell SE, Schmid MJ, Marx DB, Zhang Y, et al. Effects of local simvastatin-alendronate conjugate in preventing periodontitis bone loss. J Periodontal Res. 2013;48(5):541–8. PubMed PMID: 23278592.

71. Reddy GT, Kumar TMP, Veena. Formulation and evaluation of Alendronate Sodium gel for the treatment of bone resorptive lesions in Periodontitis. Drug Deliv. 2005;12(4):217–22. PubMed PMID: 16044536.

72. Reddy MS, Weatherford TW, Smith CA, West BD, Jeffcoat MK, Jacks TM. Alendronate treatment of naturally-occurring periodontitis in beagle dogs. J Periodontol. 1995;66(3):211–7. PubMed PMID: 7776166.

73. Reid IR. Pharmacotherapy of Paget's disease of bone. Expert Opin Pharmacother. 2012;13(5): 637–46. PubMed PMID: 22339140.

74. Rocha M, Nava LE, La Vázquez de Torre C, Sánchez-Márin F, Garay-Sevilla ME, Malacara JM. Clinical and radiological improvement of periodontal disease in patients with type 2 diabetes mellitus treated with alendronate: a randomized, placebo-controlled trial. J Periodontol. 2001;72(2):204–9. PubMed PMID: 11288794.

75. Said F, Ghoul-Mazgar S, Khemiss F, El Ayeb H, Saidane D, Berdal A, et al. The effect of etidronate on the periodontium of ovariectomized rats. J Periodontol. 2012;83(8):1063–8. PubMed PMID: 22166164.

76. Samdancioglu S, Calis S, Sumnu M, Atilla Hincal A. Formulation and in vitro evaluation of bisphosphonate loaded microspheres for implantation in osteolysis. Drug Dev Ind Pharm. 2006;32(4):473–81. PubMed PMID: 16638686.

77. Schneider VS, LeBlanc A, Huntoon CL. Prevention of space flight induced soft tissue calcification and disuse osteoporosis. Acta Astronaut. 1993;29(2):139–40. PubMed PMID: 11543594.

78. Seton M. Paget disease of bone: diagnosis and drug therapy. Cleve Clin J Med. 2013;80(7):452–62. PubMed PMID: 23821690.

79. Sharma A, Pradeep AR. Clinical efficacy of 1% alendronate gel as a local drug delivery system in the treatment of chronic periodontitis: a randomized, controlled clinical trial. J Periodontol. 2012;83(1):11–8. PubMed PMID: 21542734.

80. Sharma A, Pradeep AR. Clinical efficacy of 1% alendronate gel in adjunct to mechanotherapy in the treatment of aggressive periodontitis: a randomized controlled clinical trial. J Periodontol. 2012;83(1): 19–26. PubMed PMID: 21609254.

81. Shibata T, Komatsu K, Shimada A, Shimoda S, Oida S, Kawasaki K, et al. Effects of alendronate on restoration of biomechanical properties of periodontium in replanted rat molars. J Periodontal Res. 2004;39(6):405–14. PubMed PMID: 15491345.

82. Shibutani T, Inuduka A, Horiki I, Luan Q, Iwayama Y. Bisphosphonate inhibits alveolar bone resorption in experimentally-induced peri-implantitis in dogs. Clin Oral Implants Res. 2001;12(2):109–14. PubMed PMID: 11251659.

83. Shinoda H, Takeyama S, Suzuki K, Murakami S, Yamada S. Pharmacological topics of bone metabolism: a novel bisphosphonate for the treatment of periodontitis. J Pharmacol Sci. 2008;106(4):555–8. PubMed PMID: 18431039.

84. Shoji K, Horiuchi H, Shinoda H. Inhibitory effects of a bisphosphonate (risedronate) on experimental periodontitis in rats. J Periodontal Res. 1995;30(4): 277–84. PubMed PMID: 7562325.

85. Shukla G, Tiwari AK, Sinha D, Srivastava R, Cahndra H, Mishra AK. Synthesis and assessment of 99mTc chelate-conjugated alendronate for development of specific radiopharmaceuticals. Cancer Biother Radiopharm. 2009;24(2):209–14. PubMed PMID: 19409043.

86. Sikder MNH, Itoh M, Iwatsuki N, Shinoda H. Inhibitory effect of a novel bisphosphonate, TRK-530, on dental calculus formation in rats. J Periodontol. 2004;75(4):537–45. PubMed PMID: 15152817.

87. Silverman SL. Bisphosphonate use in conditions other than osteoporosis. Ann N Y Acad Sci. 2011;1218:33–7. PubMed PMID: 20946575.

88. Soubrier M, Dubost JJ, Ristori JM, Sauvezie B, Bussière JL. Pamidronate in the treatment of diffuse sclerosing osteomyelitis of the mandible. Oral Surg Oral Med Oral Pathol Oral Radiol Endod. 2001;92(6):637–40. PubMed PMID: 11740481.

89. Stadelmann VA, Bonnet N, Pioletti DP. Combined effects of zoledronate and mechanical stimulation on bone adaptation in an axially loaded mouse tibia. Clin Biomech (Bristol, Avon). 2011;26(1):101–5. PubMed PMID: 20869796.

90. Stadelmann VA, Gauthier O, Terrier A, Bouler JM, Pioletti DP. Implants delivering bisphosphonate locally increase periprosthetic bone density in an osteoporotic sheep model. A pilot study. Eur Cell Mater. 2008;16:10–6. PubMed PMID: 18671203.

91. Stadelmann VA, Terrier A, Gauthier O, Bouler J, Pioletti DP. Prediction of bone density around orthopedic implants delivering bisphosphonate. J Biomech. 2009;42(9):1206–11. PubMed PMID: 19380139.

92. Takaishi Y, Ikeo T, Miki T, Nishizawa Y, Morii H. Suppression of alveolar bone resorption by etidronate treatment for periodontal disease: 4- to 5-year follow-up of four patients. J Int Med Res. 2003;31(6):575–84. PubMed PMID: 14708423.

93. Teronen O, Konttinen YT, Lindqvist C, Salo T, Ingman T, Lauhio A, et al. Human neutrophil collagenase MMP-8 in peri-implant sulcus fluid and its inhibition by clodronate. J Dent Res. 1997;76(9):1529–37. PubMed PMID: 9294486.

94. Toksvig-Larsen S, Aspenberg P. Bisphosphonate-coated external fixation pins appear similar to hydroxyapatite-coated pins in the tibial metaphysis and to uncoated pins in the shaft. Acta Orthop. 2013;84(3):314–8. PubMed PMID: 23621808.

95. Tsuchimochi M, Higashino N, Okano A, Kato J. Study of combined technetium 99m methylene diphosphonate and gallium 67 citrate scintigraphy in diffuse sclerosing osteomyelitis of the mandible:

case reports. J Oral Maxillofac Surg. 1991;49(8): 887–97. PubMed PMID: 2072205.

96. Ubios AM, Braun EM, Cabrini RL. Lethality due to uranium poisoning is prevented by ethane-1-hydroxy-1,1-biphosphonate (EHBP). Health Phys. 1994;66(5):540–4. PubMed PMID: 8175360.

97. Ubios AM, Braun EM, Cabrini RL. Effect of biphosphonates on abnormal mandibular growth of rats intoxicated with uranium. Health Phys. 1998;75(6):610–3. PubMed PMID: 9827507.

98. van Dyck M, Proesmans W, van Hollebeke E, Marchal G, Moerman P. Idiopathic infantile arterial calcification with cardiac, renal and central nervous system involvement. Eur J Pediatr. 1989;148(4):374–7. PubMed PMID: 2707283.

99. Veena HR, Prasad D. Evaluation of an aminobisphosphonate (alendronate) in the management of periodontal osseous defects. J Indian Soc Periodontol. 2010;14(1):40–5. PubMed PMID: 20922078.

100. Volpe AR, Petrone ME, Davies RM. A review of calculus clinical efficacy studies. J Clin Dent. 1993;4(3):71–81. PubMed PMID: 8003237.

101. Wang K, Allen L, Fung E, Chan CC, Chan JCS, Griffith JF. Bone scintigraphy in common tumors with osteolytic components. Clin Nucl Med. 2005;30(10):655–71. PubMed PMID: 16166837.

102. Weinreb M, Quartuccio H, Seedor JG, Aufdemorte TB, Brunsvold M, Chaves E, et al. Histomorphometrical analysis of the effects of the bisphosphonate alendronate on bone loss caused by experimental periodontitis in monkeys. J Periodontal Res. 1994;29(1):35–40. PubMed PMID: 8113951.

103. White DJ, Cox ER. In vitro studies of the anticalculus efficacy of an improved whitening dentifrice. J Clin Dent. 2001;12(2):38–41. PubMed PMID: 11476012.

104. White DJ, Cox ER, Suszcynskymeister EM, Baig AA. In vitro studies of the anticalculus efficacy of a sodium hexametaphosphate whitening dentifrice. J Clin Dent. 2002;13(1):33–7. PubMed PMID: 11507930.

105. White DJ, Gerlach RW. Anticalculus effects of a novel, dual-phase polypyrophosphate dentifrice: chemical basis, mechanism, and clinical response. J Contemp Dent Pract. 2000;1(4):1–19. PubMed PMID: 12167947.

106. Wright SA, Millar AM, Coward SM, Finch MB. Chronic diffuse sclerosing osteomyelitis treated with risedronate. J Rheumatol. 2005;32(7):1376–8. PubMed PMID: 15996085.

107. Xiong H, Peng B, Wei L, Zhang X, Wang L. Effect of an estrogen-deficient state and alendronate therapy on bone loss resulting from experimental periapical lesions in rats. J Endod. 2007;33(11):1304–8. PubMed PMID: 17963952.

108. Xu K, Ge W, Liang G, Wang L, Yang Z, Wang Q, et al. Bisphosphonate-containing supramolecular hydrogels for topical decorporation of uranium-contaminated wounds in mice. Int J Radiat Biol. 2008;84(5):353–62. PubMed PMID: 18464065.

109. Yamamoto-Silva FP, Bradaschia-Correa V, Lima LAPA, Arana-Chavez VE. Ultrastructural and immunohistochemical study of early repair of alveolar sockets after the extraction of molars from alendronate-treated rats. Microsc Res Tech. 2013;76(6):633–40. PubMed PMID: 23564359.

110. Yamazaki Y, Satoh C, Ishikawa M, Notani K, Nomura K, Kitagawa Y. Remarkable response of juvenile diffuse sclerosing osteomyelitis of mandible to pamidronate. Oral Surg Oral Med Oral Pathol Oral Radiol Endod. 2007;104(1):67–71. PubMed PMID: 17197211.

111. Yoshinari M, Oda Y, Inoue T, Matsuzaka K, Shimono M. Bone response to calcium phosphate-coated and bisphosphonate-immobilized titanium implants. Biomaterials. 2002;23(14):2879–85. PubMed PMID: 12069328.

112. Zhao X, Yan S. Recent progress in osteogenesis imperfecta. Orthop Surg. 2011;3(2):127–30. PubMed PMID: 22009598.

# Index

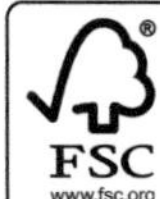